New Insights on Cardiomyopathy

Edited by Sameh M. Said

Published in London, United Kingdom

New Insights on Cardiomyopathy
http://dx.doi.org/10.5772/intechopen.100931
Edited by Sameh M. Said

Contributors
Claudio Stefano Centorbi, Enrica Garau, Leonardo Borsi, Valerio Brambilla, Davide Lazzeroni, Lorenzo Brambilla, Neelima Katukuri, Shivangi Patel, Mario Madruga, Saima Sharif, Saira Rafaqat, Shagufta Naz, Jessica Bugbee, Diana Cimiotti, Kornelia Jaquet, Seyyed-Reza Sadat-Ebrahimi, Andreas Mügge, Valeri Kapelko, Sameh M. Said, Eduard Quintana, Khaled F. Salhab, Sonia Vicenty-Rivera, Ingrid Bonilla-Mercado, Margaret A. Schwarz, Gowthami Mahendran, Jaipaul Singh, Manal Smail, Sunil Rupee, Khemraj Rupee, Abla Mohammed Ahmed Ismail, Sara Sultan, Frank Christopher Howarth, Ernest A. Adeghate

First published in London, United Kingdom, 2024 by IntechOpen
IntechOpen is the global imprint of INTECHOPEN LIMITED, registered in England and Wales, registration number: 11086078, 5 Princes Gate Court, London, SW7 2QJ, United Kingdom

British Library Cataloguing-in-Publication Data
A catalogue record for this book is available from the British Library

Additional hard and PDF copies can be obtained from orders@intechopen.com

New Insights on Cardiomyopathy
Edited by Sameh M. Said
p. cm.
Print ISBN 978-1-83969-857-6
Online ISBN 978-1-83969-858-3
eBook (PDF) ISBN 978-1-83969-859-0

For EU product safety concerns:
IN TECH d.o.o., Prolaz Marije Krucifikse Kozulić 3, 51000 Rijeka, Croatia,
info@intechopen.com or visit our website at intechopen.com.

Meet the editor

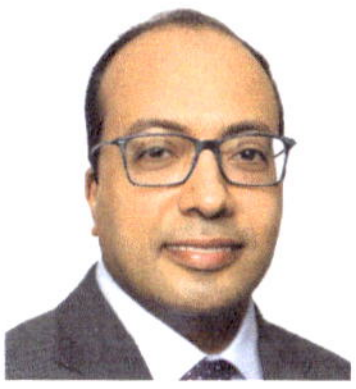

Dr. Sameh M. Said is a pediatric and adult congenital cardiac surgeon and the current chief of the Division of Pediatric and Adult Congenital Cardiac Surgery, Maria Fareri Children's Hospital, Westchester Medical Center Health Network, USA. He is also a Professor of Surgery and Pediatrics at New York Medical College. He previously worked as a pediatric and adult cardiac surgeon at Mayo Clinic, USA, and the University of Minnesota, USA. Dr. Said graduated from Alexandria University, Egypt, in 1998, where he also completed his cardiothoracic surgical residency. This was followed by an advanced cardiovascular surgery fellowship at Mayo Clinic, where he also completed an integrated general and thoracic surgery residency. He also completed an accredited pediatric congenital cardiac surgery fellowship at Lucile Packard's Children's Hospital, USA. Dr. Said is board-certified in general, thoracic, and pediatric cardiac surgery and has special expertise and interest in neonatal surgery, complex cardiac reoperation, unifocalization and pulmonary artery branch rehabilitation, Ebstein's anomaly, hypertrophic cardiomyopathy, and the Ross procedure. He has co-authored more than 200 peer-reviewed publications and 24 book chapters and edited two books. He is an active member of many cardiothoracic surgical societies and associations.

Contents

Preface

The World Health Organization, in defining cardiomyopathy, recognizes that ventricular dysfunction can result from volume and/or pressure overload in valve disease or to control hypertension. Severe ventricular dysfunction can also be the result of coronary artery disease with subsequent loss of viable myocardium. These conditions are what define specific cardiomyopathies, however, there are several intrinsic disorders of the myocardium itself that can lead to different types of cardiomyopathies.

This book highlights some of the unique types of cardiomyopathies. It starts with a brief introduction in Chapter 1 highlighting the peculiar features of the pump function of the heart, followed by a review of metabolic syndromes and cardiomyopathy that is included in two chapters. Chapter 2 discusses the biomarkers of metabolic syndrome and Chapter 3 is a review of the effects of diabetes mellitus on the conduction system of the heart.

Chapter 4 highlights the surgical perspectives of left ventricular septal myectomy along with the various tips and pitfalls of the technique. Chapter 5 is a review of cardiac amyloidosis as an example of infiltrative cardiomyopathies. Chapter 6 discusses pediatric cardiomyopathies. The final section includes four additional chapters that highlight some miscellaneous topics related to cardiomyopathies. Chapter 2 examines imaging modalities for Takotsubo cardiomyopathy, while Chapter 8 reviews the effects of stimulants on the heart and the countereffect that beta-blockers may have. Chapters 8 and 9 discuss left ventricular non-compaction. Finally, Chapter 10 presents a discussion about the long-term effects of COVID-19 on the cardiovascular system.

I am very grateful to all the contributing authors for their excellent chapters, as well as the editorial staff at IntechOpen.

Sameh M. Said, MBBCh, MD, FACC, FACS
Professor of Surgery and Pediatrics,
New York Medical College,
Valhalla, New York, USA

Chief,
Division of Pediatric and Adult Congenital Cardiac Surgery,
Maria Fareri Children's Hospital,
Valhalla, New York, USA

Westchester Medical Center,
Valhalla, New York, USA

Section 1

Introduction

Chapter 1

Peculiar Features of the Pumping Function of the Heart in Three Types of Cardiomyopathy of Various Genesis

Valeri Kapelko

Abstract

The review considers changes in the pumping and contractile function of the heart in three types of cardiomyopathies. Isoproterenol cardiomyopathy is closest to ischemic cardiomyopathy, which is most commonly observed in the clinic. Cardiomyopathy caused by chronic administration of doxorubicin represents the closest to the clinic variant of toxic cardiomyopathy. Diabetic cardiomyopathy is increasingly common in our time; the review will consider information about type 1 diabetes. The greatest attention in the review is paid to diastolic dysfunction of the heart, the main causes of its occurrence and compensatory mechanisms are analyzed. The earliest changes in diastolic dysfunction in these types of cardiomyopathies are a slowdown in myocardial relaxation and endothelial dysfunction. Information is given showing that the basis of delayed relaxation is two reasons—impaired transport of Ca^{++} in cardiomyocytes and altered properties of connectin (titin). The ability of mitochondrial oriented antioxidants to prevent cardiac dysfunction caused by doxorubicin has been demonstrated.

Keywords: heart, myocardium, diastolic dysfunction, contractility, relaxability, distensibility, contractile function, Ca^{++} transport, connectin (titin), isoproterenol, doxorubicin, diabetes, vascular tone

1. Introduction

Chronic heart failure (CHF) is the end result of many diseases of the circulatory system. Cardiomyopathy, defined as primary myocardial weakness, is one of the common causes of CHF. Its etiology is very diverse—it can occur due to ischemia, impaired energy formation due to the action of toxic factors, hypertension, diabetes, genetic defects associated with impaired synthesis of myofibrillar proteins, and other factors. Despite the commonality of the final effect, each type of cardiomyopathy has its own special features due to specifics of damaging factors. Consideration of this specificity is the subject of this review, which will mainly present the works of the author's team on the study of the myocardial contractile function and arterial tone in three types of cardiomyopathy. Adrenomimetic isoproterenol in high doses causes ischemic micronecroses of the myocardium, the antibiotic doxorubicin, effective in oncology, selectively damages the function of myocardial mitochondria, and another antibiotic streptozotocin, which damages insulin production and deprives cardiomyocytes of the ability to use glucose to the desired extent.

All experiments have been carried out in male Wistar rats aged 4–6 months accordingly to the principles of the 2000 declaration of Helsinki and the 1985 International Guiding Principles for Biomedical Research Involving Animals (1985). Results are represented as M±SE.

2. Isoproterenol cardiomyopathy

Cardiomyopathy caused by chronic myocardial ischemia occurs most often in the clinic. Studying the pathogenesis of this cardiomyopathy requires an adequate model, which has not yet been created. The model of cardiac ischemia caused by isoproterenol, a nonselective agonist of myocardial beta-adrenergic receptors, is considered a classic model for studying the cardioprotective effect of various compounds [1]. This model was proposed by Rona more than half a century ago, and its main consequence was multiple micronecroses of the myocardium. Subsequent studies have shown the multifactorial genesis of these changes – a violation of microcirculation with the development of local zones of ischemia, the effect of catecholamine oxidation products [2], and the overload of cardiomyocytes with Ca^{++} ions with the development of local cardiomyocyte contractures [3]. Within 2–4 weeks, cardiomyopathy occurs with lower ejection fraction [4, 5].

However, insufficient attention was paid to the study of the pumping and contractile function of the heart in this pathology. In this regard, we conducted a comprehensive study of the action of isoproterenol in various doses, from 85 to 180 mg/kg [6]. The contractile function of the heart was investigated using echocardiography (iE33, Philips Ultrasound, Bothell WA, USA) using the S12–4 sensor (12–4 MHz) and catheterization of the left ventricle (LV) using the Millar precision micromanometer inserted through the carotid artery (SciSense Instruments, Canada) and the strain gauge amplifier Hugo Sachs Elektronik (Germany). Traditional contractility indicators were measured – LV maximal pressure development rate (+dP/dtmax) and the contractility index (+dP/dtmax/P – pressure at the time of reaching the maximum +dP/dt). To characterize the relaxation process, the maximum rate of pressure fall (– dP/dtmin) was used, as well as the time constant of isovolumic relaxation [7]. In total, 4 series of experiments were performed, in which isoproterenol in various doses was administered twice at a daily interval. Mortality in these series ranged from 15 to 40%. The use of isoproterenol, even in a minimal dose (85 mg/kg twice), caused mosaic changes in cardiomyocytes, characterizing diffuse micronecroses of the myocardium. Extensive infiltration by cellular elements and fibroblasts, the organizers of fibrosis was noted [6].

Surviving animals and controls were examined after 2 weeks using echocardiography. In a series of experiments using a cumulative dose of 240 mg/kg, both the cardiac output and LV ejection fraction differed slightly from the control values, but the use of a cumulative dose of 300 mg/kg was accompanied by decreased ejection fraction from 84 ± 1% to 72 ± 3% ($p < 0.01$). This was combined with increased LV end-diastolic volume from 0.84 ± 0.05 to 1.1 ± 0.1 ($p < 0.05$). The heart rate and the thickness of posterior LV wall in diastole and systole did not change, but the structure of the cardiocycle was changed – the duration of isometric phases increased from

21 ± 1.0% to 26 ± 1.4% (+26%, $p < 0.01$), and the duration of the period of LV filling decreased from 36 ± 1.1% to 31 ± 1.1% (– 14%, $p < 0.05$).

Isoproterenol in a dose of 240 mg/kg did not violate the cardiac hemodynamics and LV contractility but was accompanied by a significant, almost twice, slowdown in myocardial relaxation – the time constant of isovolumic relaxation increased from 6.3 ± 0.8 to 12.3 ± 1.8 s^{-1} ($p < 0.05$). But at a dose of 360 mg/kg, delayed myocardial relaxation was combined with decreased myocardial contractility index by 20%. As a result of the deterioration of myocardial contractility and relaxation, the LV end-diastolic pressure was clearly increased from 3 ± 1 to 9 ± 2 mm Hg ($p < 0.05$).

These results, characterizing the dose-dependent occurrence of diastolic and systolic dysfunction after the isoproterenol administration, have been obtained earlier [8] and confirmed recently [9]. Echocardiography of the heart of mice revealed the development of diastolic dysfunction after administration of isoproterenol at a dose of 150 mg/kg and systolic dysfunction after administration of higher doses.

The reasons for CHF development at high doses of isoproterenol are obviously due to the development of oxidative stress that occurs in the myocardium with prolonged action of isoproterenol [10]. A slowdown in myocardial relaxation occurred within 3–7 days after the administration of isoproterenol, but cardiac work [5] or the pressure developed by isolated heart remained unchanged [11]. In this case, the authors found a significant decrease in the expression of proteins involved in calcium transport—Ca^{++} -ATPase of the sarcoplasmic reticulum (SR) and phospholamban, as well as Na^+-K^+-ATPase. These data suggested that calcium transport in cardiomyocytes at higher doses of isoproterenol should be disturbed. This assumption was confirmed in our experiments in cardiomyocytes isolated from rat hearts [6].

The intracellular free Ca^{++} level was measured using fluorescent Ca^{++} indicator Fluo-4 (Invitrogen F-14201), and the signal was recorded using a high-speed digital camera AxioCam HS (Zeiss). To excite the cells, electrical stimulation was used with a rate of 1 Hz and a voltage of 38 V for 10 seconds. In cardiomyocytes from hearts of rats that received isoproterenol, various forms of Ca^{++} signal distortion have been observed – either with an unchanged rhythm of contractions but elevation of Ca^{++} diastolic level with steadily decreased magnitude of subsequent peaks or with a decreased number of signals and the appearance of additional peaks, reflecting a slowdown in Ca^{++} excretion from mycoplasma. At the same time, the ascending arm of the signal (an increase in myoplasmic Ca^{++}, reflecting the work of calcium channels) was less altered, but the peak amplitude decreased by about 1.4 times. Thus, judging by the nature of altered calcium peaks, the process of Ca^{++} removal from the mycoplasma suffered predominantly, while the process of Ca^{++} entry into the mycoplasma was less disturbed.

These results can briefly be summarized in the form of three main points: 1) when using smaller isoproterenol dosages, the diastolic dysfunction arose, manifested by a relaxation slowdown and increased LV end-diastolic pressure; 2) at using higher isoproterenol dosages, the systolic dysfunction arose, manifested by decreased LV ejection fraction and LV cavity dilatation; and 3) in all series, regardless of isoproterenol dosage, the myocardial relaxation suffered to a greater extent than contractility, and it has been based on weakened ability of cardiomyocytes to remove Ca^{++} from myofibrils.

3. Doxorubicin cardiomyopathy

Anthracycline cardiomyopathy is a frequent complication of the treatment of cancer patients. The most effective representative of this group is doxorubicin. This type of cardiomyopathy is characterized by the same symptom complex in humans and animals [12, 13], manifested in the form of LV systolic dysfunction and CHF with decreased LV ejection fraction and animal survival [14].

According to most researchers, the damaging effect of doxorubicin is realized by activating free radical oxidation [15, 16]. Mitochondria, characterized by a high intensity of oxidative processes, are the main cellular target of doxorubicin [16–18]. The abundance of unsaturated fatty acids in the inner membrane of mitochondria favors peroxidation with disruption of the electronic transport chain [19]. Using laser-scanning confocal microscopy with oxidation-sensitive fluorescent tag, it has been shown that the addition of doxorubicin (40–160 μM) to the cardiomyocyte incubation medium enhances oxidative reactions near mitochondria [17]. An increased vulnerability of myocardial mitochondria compared to liver mitochondria is due to the fact that cardiac mitochondria contain a large amount of cardiolipin, which has an increased affinity for doxorubicin [20]. Mitochondrial dysfunction is observed even at nanomolar concentrations of doxorubicin [21] – the formation of superoxide increases rapidly with the subsequent release of cytochrome "c", especially in the presence of aglycone derivatives of doxorubicin [18], later the synthesis of ATP and Ca^{++} transport are disturbed [22]. The biochemical study of mitochondria in skinned fibers after 2 weeks of doxorubicin injection revealed unchanged maximal level of oxygen consumption, but lower respiratory index by 30% and apparent affinity constant for ADP by 35% suggesting an increased permeability of mitochondrial membranes [23].

3.1 Studies in vivo

In recent years, we have tried to trace changes in the cardiodynamics and LV contractile function at various times after doxorubicin administration (2 mg/kg). Invasive study of the cardiac contractile function was performed using a standard PV catheter FTH-1912B-8018 and an ADV500 amplifier (Transonic, Canada), as well as the PowerLab 4/35 ADC with the LabChart 8.1 program (ADInstruments, Australia), which automatically calculated more than 20 parameters of the contractile function. Initially, experiments were performed, in which the cardiac function was studied after 8 weekly injections of doxorubicin (cumulative dose of 16 mg/kg). After 10 weeks, the mortality rate was 27% [24].

According to the results of echocardiography (n = 59), a clear decrease in LV ejection fraction was found in 54%, boundary values in 26%, and no changes in 20%. Experiments with catheterization of LV and aorta, performed after 9–13 weeks, showed a progressive diminution in LV contractility index, LV + dP/dt, and an extension of time to its peak by 1.5 times. A slowdown in LV relaxation was altered to even greater extent, the time constant of isovolumic relaxation was more than doubled. There was a progressive decrease in the heart rate and blood pressure, and respectively, LV systolic pressure decreased and LV diastolic pressure increased. Thus, the progressive deterioration of myocardial contractility and systolic dysfunction development was partially compensated by lower peripheral resistance and prolongation of the diastolic pause.

In the next series of experiments (n = 20), only 4 injections of doxorubicin were used to reduce the degree of damage [25]. In echocardiographic study performed 4 weeks after the start of administration, 73% of rats had diastolic dysfunction, and 27% had systolic dysfunction, but after another 4 weeks, during which doxorubicin was not administered, the ratio of rats with diastolic and systolic dysfunction changed in the opposite direction of 43: 57%. In 7 experiments of the last series, after 8 weeks, it was possible to trace changes in LV ejection fraction – after 4 weeks it was 76 ± 2%, and after 8 weeks it decreased to 57 ± 4% ($p < 0.01$). Rats with systolic dysfunction had the same signs of CHF—reduced myocardial contractility and relaxation, lower heart rate, LV systolic pressure, and heart function. Nevertheless, the cardiac output per unit of body weight was within the normal range. An important factor facilitating the LV ejection was a diminution of average aortic pressure to 94 ± 8 mmHg from the control level of 116 ± 4 mmHg, as well as a decrease in arterial elasticity index by 35%. The group of rats with normal ejection fraction was characterized by the same signs, including delayed relaxation, but they had LV contractility index and the maximum rate of pressure development at a normal level, while the relaxation time constant was significantly increased by 15%, as well as LV end-diastolic pressure from 2.4 ± 1.3 to 6.6 ± 1.0 mmHg ($p < 0.05$).

The measurement of energy metabolism in the myocardium of rats with systolic dysfunction in situ [26] showed a constant content of ATP and the number of adenine nucleotides, but a significant decrease in phosphocreatine content from 27.4 ± 0.3 to 16.4 ± 4.7 μmol/g. Accordingly, the phosphocreatine/ATP ratio was reduced from 2.01 ± 0.12 to 1.26 ± 0.21 (−37%, $p < 0.05$). It is thought that a low FCr/ATP ratio may be a predictor of cardiovascular disease mortality [27]. It should also be noted that a large increase in the myocardial lactate content from 1.7 ± 0.4 to 12.0 ± 1.8 μmol/g ($p < 0.01$) indicates a significant activation of anaerobic glycolysis. In rats with diastolic dysfunction, the contents of ATP and phosphocreatine were close to the control values. However, there was a significant increase in lactate compared to controls (20.0 ± 4.6 and 3.6 ± 0.8 μmol/L, respectively, $p < 0.05$), indicating significant activation of anaerobic glycolysis.

The results of this series showed that the formation of systolic dysfunction with decreased LV ejection fraction passes through the phase of diastolic dysfunction. Delayed myocardial relaxation is an indispensable sign of both diastolic and systolic dysfunction. Two reasons may underlie the delayed relaxation – a weakened absorption of Ca^{++} ions, which activated the act of myofibrillar contraction, in the structures of the sarcoplasmic reticulum (SR) and a change in the elastic properties of connectin (titin).

Experiments with the registration of calcium signals in isolated cardiomyocytes showed changes similar to those observed under the action of isoproterenol – the cleavage of signals with the formation of a delayed Ca^{++} recession. These data are consistent with the results of the study of the myocardium of patients with dilated cardiomyopathy, they showed a significantly reduced expression of SERCA2a not only in relation to the total protein but also in relation to the ryanodine receptor [28]. This means that in systolic dysfunction, the process of Ca^{++} absorption into sarcoplasmic reticulum suffers to a greater extent than Ca^{++} release from the reticulum.

A delayed relaxation may also be associated with a change in the properties of connectin (titin), the largest protein not only in cardiomyocytes but also in the body [29, 30]. It is known that within the sarcomere, one end of connectin is associated with myosin in A-disc region and the other end with the Z-line. Thus, it "anchors" the myosin filaments in the center of the sarcomere, contributing to the maintenance of a highly ordered sarcomere structure. With the development of contraction, myosin filaments, forming bonds with actin ones, shift to the Z line, compressing the connectin spring, and when Ca^{++} is eliminated from myofibrils, the connectin spring straightens, returning the ends of the myosin filaments to their previous position. It is thanks to this that contracting isolated cardiomyocytes that do not experience external stress always return to their original length. Connectin stiffness is the main regulator of contractile activity of striated muscles [31–33]. It can change under the influence of phosphorylation of its isoforms – a more extensible N2BA (having a longer tensile part in the I-disc of the sarcomere) and a more rigid N2B. The ratio of N2BA/N2B varies in the mammalian heart: from the smallest in the myocardium of small animals to the largest in the myocardium of large animals and humans [32].

In our experiments, the properties of connectin were investigated in rats treated with doxorubicin (2 mg/kg) once a week for 4 weeks [34]. The ratio of the content of more extensible connectin N2BA isoform to elastic N2B isoform in control experiments was 14/86%. In the myocardium of doxorubicin rats, it was changed in the direction of predominance of more extensible N2BA isoform; its content was 26 ± 2%. The overall level of connectin phosphorylation was increased by 60 ± 18% compared to controls. The degree of phosphorylation of connectin was inversely correlated ($r = -0.94$) with the content of rigid isoform N2B, and as is known, phosphorylation of this isoform reduces its stiffness, therefore, the myocardial extensibility should increase, contributing to better filling of the ventricular chamber [35].

Results showing increased content of more extensible N2BA isoform and increased connectin phosphorylation, suggesting raised myocardial extensibility, have been obtained for the first time. They allow us to think that in diastolic dysfunction, a delayed relaxation, combined with increased LV diastolic pressure, may be due not only to a violation of Ca^{++} transport but also to increased extensibility of connectin, which slows down the relaxation process.

The analysis of these data shows that the main changes occur in energy-dependent systems that require either ATP production or phosphorylation. These are calcium ATPase of sarcoplasmic reticulum – SERCA2a, phosphorylation of phospholamban, and connectin. This suggests the primacy of disorders of the energy formation system in cardiomyocytes as the basis for the subsequent development of diastolic and systolic dysfunction. This is supported by the activation of anaerobic glycolysis in this pathology.

3.2 Studies in the isolated heart

To understand the pathogenesis of diastolic dysfunction, it is important to determine the initial links to myocardial dysfunction. For this purpose, the technique of retrograde perfusion of the isolated heart was used with the registration of pressure in a latex balloon introduced into LV cavity.

In connection with the widespread opinion about the primary role of oxidative stress in alteration of the contractile function of the heart, we aimed to investigate the resistance of the isolated heart to oxidative stress induced by hydrogen peroxide after administration of doxorubicin in vivo [36]. Since a peak of reactive oxygen species formation under the influence of doxorubicin was observed after 2 hours [37], in the first series of experiments, the heart was isolated 2 hours after the administration of doxorubicin in vivo (2.2 mg/kg). A rise in the perfusion rate from 10 to 20 ml/min/g made it possible to reach the maximal LV systolic pressure up to 200 mmHg. The hearts of rats that received doxorubicin showed a normal level of LV systolic pressure and the maximal rate of its development, but a rise in perfusion pressure by 26% was noted, which indicated an increased tone of coronary vessels. This corresponds to previously obtained results [38, 39]. Our data showed that this phenomenon persisted steadily for 2 hours and even 2 weeks after the administration of doxorubicin in vivo. This is probably due to an increased affinity of endothelial

NO synthase for doxorubicin, which is the basis of its dose-dependent inhibition [40] with a subsequent decrease in NO formation. Myocardial relaxation indices 2 hours after doxorubicin administration remained at the same level, but after 2 weeks were significantly reduced by 11–14%, and LV minimal diastolic pressure increased from 2 ± 1 to 7 ± 1 mmHg, i.e. signs characteristic of diastolic dysfunction were observed.

The introduction of hydrogen peroxide (100 μM) into the perfusate as an inducer of reactive oxygen species (ROS) in the control group was accompanied by a steadily fall in LV developed pressure, as well as + dP/dt, after 40 minutes these values decreased to 60 ± 3% of the initial level. Rat hearts isolated 2 hours after doxorubicin administration showed a greater fall—to 40 ± 2% ($p < 0.001$), and this was combined with a significant rise in LV minimal diastolic pressure to 34 mmHg. However, after 2 weeks LV developed pressure response at H_2O_2 introduction in hearts of rats received doxorubicin practically did not differ from the control values, and LV minimal diastolic pressure did not rise [39].

Thus, the elevated negative inotropic effect in response to oxidative stress was observed only in the early stage after the doxorubicin administration, at the peak of ROS formation in the myocardium. It could be assumed that it is associated with a decrease in the activity of antioxidant enzymes, but this activity, measured in myocardial samples taken after the completion of the experiment, did not change either after 2 hours or after 2 weeks, although the concentration of MDA in both series after doxorubicin use was significantly increased by 23–34%. This coincides with the results of the work [41], in which unchanged activity of GSH-Px, catalase, and MnSOD was also found in the interval from 1 to 24 hours after doxorubicin administration (2.5 mg/kg). The activity of antioxidant enzymes increased 4 weeks after the start of doxorubicin [42].

Another series of experiments was aimed to clarify the state of the calcium transport system in the myocardium under the action of doxorubicin [43]. The amplified signals of the pressure sensors were transmitted to the computer via the NI USB-6210 analog-to-digital converter (ADC) from National Instruments (USA), using a digitization frequency of 1000 Hz. A sudden increase in the rate of excitations from a base rate of 5 Hz to 10 Hz was used with a return to 5 Hz after 10 s. The addition of doxorubicin (3 μM) to the perfusate after 30 minutes was accompanied by a decrease in LV developing pressure by 15–20%. The high-frequency load immediately increased LV developed pressure and the maximal rate of its development, as well as the constant of the relaxation rate (the value inversed to the relaxation time constant) and diastolic pressure (Figure 1 in [43]). After doxorubicin addition to the perfusate, similar phenomena were observed, and the magnitude of studied indices coincided. Maintaining an adequate response to the high-frequency load allows us to suggest that the calcium transport system in these conditions was not disturbed, despite a decrease in the initially developed pressure. It is known that the function of ion pumps is supplied by ATP from glycolysis, while the function of myofibrils is from oxidative phosphorylation. The results of these experiments showed that after a single injection of doxorubicin, the earliest changes are an increased tone of the coronary vessels and a gradual slowdown in myocardial relaxation.

3.3 Prevention of heart dysfunction at doxorubicin cardiomyopathy

The increased vulnerability of the cardiac contractile function to H_2O_2 precisely in the initial period of doxorubicin action suggested that reducing the intensity of oxidative stress in the myocardium during this period may delay or prevent the CHF development at prolonged action of doxorubicin. This assumption is based on the information according to which isolated cardiomyocytes with reduced superoxide dismutase (SOD) activity induced by diethyldithiocarbamate were less resistant to the action of doxorubicin [44], and the preliminary use of SOD, like glutathione peroxidase (GSH-Px), prevented the development of apoptosis in embryonic cardiomyocytes under the influence of doxorubicin [45].

To reduce the degree of myocardial damage, the mitochondrial-oriented antioxidant SkQ1 synthesized at Moscow State University was used [46]. Its active ingredient is plastoquinone, a powerful plant antioxidant that performs the same function in plant mitochondria as coenzyme Q in the myocardium. It penetrates into the cells and then into the mitochondria due to a weak positive charge of triphenylphosphonium.

Two series of in vivo experiments were performed. In the first series, doxorubicin was administered for 5 weeks when systolic dysfunction was observed in most experiments [47]. Echocardiographic examination of rats followed by LV catheterization after another 3 weeks, during which the rats received neither doxorubicin nor plastomitin, showed the presence of LV systolic dysfunction with lower LV ejection fraction and contractility index by 32–34% and a rise in the relaxation time constant by 74%. At the same time, LV maximal developed pressure was reduced by 18%, which closely coincided with lower blood pressure by 23% and diminished arterial stiffness by 35%. A significantly decreased peripheral resistance and prolongation of diastolic pause due to 23% lower heart rate can contribute to maintaining LV maximal ejection rate and cardiac output at normal level. The hearts of rats that were administered plastomitin simultaneously with doxorubicin were characterized by normalization of the ejection fraction, all indices of contractility, heart rate, blood pressure, and arterial stiffness.

In another series of experiments [48], doxorubicin (2 mg/kg) was administered twice in 2 weeks, and half of the rats received plastomitin daily along with it. The use of doxorubicin did not cause significant hemodynamic disturbances, but LV maximal rate of pressure development was reduced by 36% and the contractility index by 23%. Even deeper, by 39–43%, the indices of myocardial relaxation were reduced. In the group of rats that received doxorubicin together with plastomitin, all indices of myocardial contractility and relaxation were significantly higher than in the doxorubicin group, and they did not differ from control values. These changes were combined with reduced LV diastolic pressure.

Thus, the use of plastomitin together with doxorubicin completely eliminated the signs of both systolic and diastolic dysfunction caused by doxorubicin. The positive effect of plastomitin is consistent with the idea of the important role of oxidative stress in the initial period of chronic use of doxorubicin. This can serve as the basis for a preclinical trial of plastomitin in doxorubicin therapy for cancer patients.

The results of our study of the pathogenesis of doxorubicin cardiomyopathy showed: a) the earliest changes in the cardiac contractile function are caused by the action of oxidative stress, which impairs the function of mitochondria; at the same time, the calcium transport system in cardiomyocytes does not seem to suffer; b) the initial changes in LV contractile function are manifested in the form of delayed relaxation, as well as increased myocardial extensibility, which is based on connectin phosphorylation, as well as an increase in the content of its more extensible isoform N2BA; c) with smaller doses of doxorubicin, diastolic dysfunction occurs, the obligatory manifestation of which is delayed relaxation, the pumping function of the heart remains at a normal level; d) with higher doses of doxorubicin or increased duration of the drug, systolic dysfunction develops with a violation of the cardiac pump function; and e) both forms of CHF can be successfully prevented if the effective mitochondrial oriented antioxidant plastomitin (SkQ1) is administered to rats concomitantly with the administration of doxorubicin.

4. Diabetic cardiomyopathy

Diabetes is a special disease in which the consumption of glucose by cells is disturbed. There are two types of diabetes. The first type occurs after a significant decrease or complete cessation of insulin production in the pancreas, the second is characterized by normal insulin production, but with a difficulty in glucose transport into cells. The first type is reproduced through the use of streptozotocin or alloxan, which damages the pancreas. Reproduction of the second type is much more difficult. In our experiments, a type 1 model was used.

It is known that in type 1 diabetes the energy metabolism of cardiomyocytes switches almost exclusively to fatty acids as an energy source due to a deterioration of glucose transport into cells [49]. This is combined with the development of diastolic or systolic dysfunction in both animals and humans [50–52]. Reduced strength and rate of contraction were manifested both in the isolated mouse heart and in isolated papillary muscles [53, 54]. But the causes of the deterioration of myocardial contractility have not been identified.

In our experiments performed 2 weeks after the administration of streptozotocin (60 mg/kg), the level of glucose in the blood increased from 5.4 ± 0.1 mmol/l to 31.0 ± 1.4 mmol/l [55]. Echocardiographic and invasive LV studies showed a decrease in LV ejection fraction by 26% with unchanged LV end-diastolic volume and heart rate. However, all indicators of LV systole – LV systolic pressure, the maximal rate of its development, and the contractility index remained within the normal range, and a decrease in LV ejection fraction was apparently associated with a reduced LV maximal ejection rate by 28%. It is known that cardiac output is determined not only by the force of LV contraction but also by vascular resistance, the components of which are blood pressure and arterial rigidity. The latter is manifested through the elastic expansion of the ascending aorta at the time of LV ejection. In our experiments, blood pressure was normal, but arterial rigidity was significantly increased by almost 1.5 times (from 0.27 ± 0.01 to 0.42 ± 0.07 mmHg/μl, $p < 0.01$). An inverse correlation was established between LV maximal rate of ejection and arterial rigidity ($r = -0.69$). Also specific for cardiomyopathy features, namely delayed relaxation and increased LV minimal diastolic pressure, have been observed.

The results of this work, which showed a deterioration in hemodynamics while maintaining normal myocardial contractility, are in contradiction with the data on reduced contractility in experiments in the isolated heart and papillary muscles [53, 54]. However, it should be kept in mind that these experiments were performed with standard Krebs solution in which glucose was the only energetic source while it is well known that at I-type diabetes the cardiomyocytes almost exclusively used fatty acids as an energetic source [49].

The change in the spectrum of energy substrates in type 1 diabetes raises the question of the state of energy metabolism in the myocardium of diabetic rats. In our experiments, the relationship between LV end-diastolic volume and the area covered by the volume-pressure curve for the cardiac cycle (PVA) reflecting the amount of oxygen consumption was studied with a restriction of the flow to the heart created by short-term clamping of the inferior vena cava [56]. In all experiments, the relationship between these parameters was close to linear, but in experiments in diabetic rat hearts, a reduction in LV end-diastolic volume was accompanied by a steeper PVA drop. This suggests that the myocardium of diabetic rats is more sensitive to the restriction of oxygen flow.

In the study of myocardial energy metabolism in diabetic rats, a reduction in the amount of adenine nucleotides by 21% and ATP content by 29% was found [56]. The formation of phosphocreatine was also impaired, as evidenced by the more than halved ratio of phosphocreatine to free creatine – in diabetes, it was 9 ± 3% and in the control 22 ± 4% ($p < 0.05$). The lactate content in the diabetic myocardium was increased (5.9 ± 0.8 versus 2.1 ± 1.0 μmol/g dry weight, $p < 0.001$) showing that some glycolytic processes are taking place. A negative correlation was found between the content of lactate and phosphocreatine ($r = -0.70$). A reduction in phosphocreatine/ATP ratio was noted by 31P magnetic resonance spectroscopy in the hearts of patients with diabetes [57].

Thus, despite the sufficient supply of oxygen and energy substrates in the form of free fatty acids to the myocardium, the energetic metabolism of cardiomyocytes is altered and not always sufficient. The reason is undoubtedly related to the state of mitochondria in cardiomyocytes, this aspect is discussed in detail in the review [58]. Mitochondria are less efficient and produce less ATP with sufficient oxygen supply [59, 60] and are characterized by higher production of ROS and MDA [61]. This is especially pronounced in the interfibrillary mitochondria in which lower number of Krebs cycle proteins [62] and decreased cardiolipin content in their membranes [63] result in violation of ATP synthesis.

Relaxation slowing and increased LV diastolic pressure are indispensable companions of cardiomyopathy. Recently, it has been shown that myocardial relaxation can be accelerated and LV diastolic pressure is reduced with a restriction of inflow to the heart through a short-term (2–3 s) clamping of the inferior vena cava [64]. The use of this technique was accompanied by a reduction in blood pressure and LV diastolic volume. With the same values of LV volume (0.3 ml) and blood pressure (60 mm Hg), LV ejection fraction, maximal rate of LV ejection, and the index of arterial stiffness in diabetic hearts were already slightly different from control values [56]. But the relaxation time constant was still increased by 36%, and LV minimal diastolic pressure still remained elevated. These data once again confirm that in type 1 diabetes, myocardial contractility is not the main cause of the resulting systolic dysfunction.

In addition to contractility and relaxation, in these experiments, we also investigated myocardial extensibility. It is known that LV wall stretching during diastole occurs unevenly—at first, quickly then more slowly. Since the assessment of myocardial extensibility at each moment of diastole is still a very difficult task, we used an integrative indicator – the ratio of an increase in LV pressure during diastole, i.e. the difference between the final and minimal LV diastolic pressure, to the value of LV filling equally to the stroke volume. This is an indicator of LV diastolic stiffness; its value is inversely proportional to extensibility. The measurement of this index in the hearts of control animals showed its dependence on the heart rate and LV diastolic volume. It turned out that there is a high negative correlation between them ($r = -0.89$ and -0.91, respectively). This means that increased LV diastolic volume or the increased heart rate are combined with a reduced value of the diastolic stiffness index, and, therefore, with increased myocardial distensibility. In this regard, a comparison of this indicator between control and diabetic hearts was carried out in a limited and equal range of LV diastolic volume and heart rate. The diastolic stiffness index in the diabetes group was 9.3 ± 1.0 mmHg/ml, and in the control group 13.8 ± 1.0 ($p < 0.01$). A lower index in the diabetes group means increased myocardial extensibility.

In this regard, in separate experiments of this series, a study of connectin (titin) was performed. Its content in the control and diabetic groups was the same and amounted to 15–16% of the content of heavy chains of myosin. However, the ratio of isoforms changed in the direction of increasing more distensible N2BA isoform: its content increased from 21 ± 1.1% in the control to 27 ± 1.0% in the diabetes group ($p < 0.001$). The results of real-time PCR showed a significant increase in the level of mRNA N2BA isoform by 38%, while for the N2B isoform it changed little. The degree of phosphorylation of connectin increased by 30 ± 7.5% ($p < 0.05$) mainly due to isoforms N2B (+ 15%) and NT (+ 12%). The predominance of the more distensible N2BA isoform, as well as an increase in its transcription, creates a lesser resistance during LV filling, but at the same time its contribution to relaxation decreases – after removing Ca^{++} from myofibrils, less stiff connectin, due to its spring-like structure, may exert a lesser force for myosin filaments to return them to initial position.

To detect diastolic dysfunction in this model of diabetes, two series were performed (10 rats each), in one of which, after administering a dose of streptozotocin of 60 mg/kg, the experiments were performed after 1 week, and in the other, the dose was halved (30 mg/kg) but the period was increased to 2 weeks [56]. At the same time, in most experiments (2/3) with echocardiography, diastolic dysfunction was detected. In an invasive study of this group, it was found that LV ejection fraction was normal, despite a reduced maximum ejection rate of 34%, probably due to increased arterial elasticity. But LV end-diastolic volume was significantly smaller compared to the systolic dysfunction group and the control group (0.36+ 0.02 ml, 0.46 + 0.03 ml, and 0.43 + 0.02 ml, respectively, $p < 0.05$). Reducing the LV diastolic volume with a lower stroke volume ensures the preservation of the normal ejection fraction even under conditions of a reduced LV maximal ejection rate. This circumstance allows us to think that the ejection fraction does not always characterize myocardial contractility, but rather reflects the relationship between the ventricle and arterial resistance. This opinion coincides with the recently expressed idea [65, 66], according to which the reduction of LV chamber in combination with moderate hypertrophy is the main structural characteristic of diastolic dysfunction in this type of diabetes.

Since myocardial contractility was maintained at a normal level in both forms of heart dysfunction, the question arises – can LV dysfunction in type 1 diabetes be considered cardiomyopathy? After all, a decrease in the pumping function of the heart can be observed with preserved myocardial contractility with various valvular defects, limited venous inflow to the heart, etc., but these conditions are not considered cardiomyopathy. There is currently no universally accepted definition of diabetic cardiomyopathy, with several definitions used that cover the entire spectrum of diabetic heart disease from subclinical changes to outright heart failure [67].

5. Conclusion

The presented data indicate that in all types of cardiomyopathy considered, the CHF formation passes through the stage of diastolic dysfunction. Its main signs are delayed myocardial relaxation and endothelial dysfunction. Myocardial relaxation is a complex process that has active and passive components. The active component is due to volatile transport of Ca^{++} from myofibrils into SR against a high concentration gradient. Both Ca^{++} uptake into SR and exit from SR to myoplasma are under constant mitochondrial control due to the fact that part of Ca^{++} ions enters mitochondria, where Ca^{++} acts as an activator of some key enzymes of the Krebs cycle [68]. Since Ca^{++} transport is energy dependent, any violation in ATP synthesis system will inevitably reduce Ca^{++} inflow into SR, and hence a Ca^{++} fraction released at next excitation. This process is carried out through a release of active oxygen species, a moderate amount of them activates Ca^{++} transport and an excessive one disrupts it [69, 70].

The passive component of relaxation is represented by connectin (titin). Its spring-like structure is stretched when the ventricle is filling, and after contraction completion, it participates in mechanical return of sarcomere length to the original value. The weightiest argument in favor of connectin participation in relaxation process is the phenomenon of elastic recoil, observed in isolated hearts [71–74]. A detailed study of connectin function made it possible to substantiate the idea of the "restorative force" [75–77], mobilized at enhanced compression of myofibrils. According to calculations, in rat cardiomyocytes within the length of sarcomeres of 1.6–2.1 μm, connectin is responsible for 90% of passive force and at least 60% of restorative force [75]. This is especially important for the hearts of small animals with a high heart rate and shortened diastolic pause. Our data showed that a change in the ratio of connectin isoforms to the direction of predominance of N2BA isoform favoring myocardial distensibility can reduce the degree of connectin participation in the relaxation process.

All types of cardiomyopathies considered are combined with an early change in the arterial tone. Isoproterenol and doxorubicin, the action of which is largely combined with the development of oxidative stress, suppressing the activity of endothelial NO synthase and increasing vascular tone, including coronary vessels. In diabetic cardiomyopathy, accompanied by hyperglycemia, the active factors of which are glucose glycation products, also increase the formation of reactive oxygen species and inhibit the activity of NO synthases, which leads to a stable increase in arterial rigidity.

The decreased myocardial contractility observed in isoproterenol and doxorubicin cardiomyopathy can be largely compensated by the inclusion of myocardial and systemic mechanisms. At the level of cardiomyocytes, the Starling mechanism is primarily included – an increase in myofibrillar stretching, largely realized by increasing the content of connectin N2BA isoform and phosphorylation of more elastic N2B isoform. An increased myofibrillar sensitivity to $Ca++$, usually occurring at decreased effective concentration, can also be mobilized. The systemic level of regulation aims to reduce peripheral resistance to facilitate LV ejection. As a result, at doxorubicin and isoproterenol cardiomyopathy, associated with decreased LV contraction, blood pressure decreases moderately, while at diabetic one it can remain normal. At the same time, to increase the inflow to the heart, the Parin reflex is mobilized – ("a decrease in peripheral resistance in the large circle is accompanied by a reciprocal increase in pressure in the small circle"). Systolic dysfunction is characterized by the same compensation mechanisms, but their mobilization is no longer sufficient to preserve the ejection fraction, and then the last compensation mechanisms are mobilized to maintain the cardiac output at an acceptable level – bradycardia, which prolongs the diastolic pause, and cardiac dilatation, which can further stretch the myofibrils. Each of these factors has a limited resource, used mainly by the autonomic nervous system. The degree of its mobilization, as well as the general condition of the body, largely predetermines the development of diastolic or systolic dysfunction in CHF.

Acknowledgements

This work has been supported by Russian Fund for Basic Research grant № 20-015-00027.

Conflict of interest

The author declares no conflict of interest.

Author details

Valeri Kapelko
Institute of Experimental Cardiology, E.I.Chazov National Medical Research Center of Cardiology, Moscow, Russia

*Address all correspondence to: valk69@yandex.ru

References

[1] Allawadhi P, Khurana A, Sayed N, Kumari P, Godugu C. Isoproterenol-induced cardiac ischemia and fibrosis: Plant-based approaches for intervention. Phytotherapy Research. 2018;**32**(10):1908-1932. DOI: 10.1002/ptr.6152

[2] Rona G. Catecholamine cardiotoxicity. Journal of Molecular and Cellular Cardiology. 1985;**17**(4):291-306. DOI: 10.1016/s0022-2828(85)80130-9

[3] Todd GL, Baroldi G, Pieper GM, Clayton FS, Eliot RS. Experimental catecholamine-induced myocardial necrosis. I.Morphology, quantification and regional distribution of acute contraction band lesions. Journal of Molecular and Cellular Cardiology. 1985;**17**(4):317-338. DOI: 10.1016/s0022-2828(85)80132-2

[4] Feng W, Li W. The study of ISO induced heart failure rat model. Experimental and Molecular Pathology. 2010;**88**:299-304. DOI: 10.1016/j.yexmp.2009.10.011

[5] Takaki M. Cardiac mechanoenergetics for understanding isoproterenol-induced rat heart failure. Pathophysiology. 2012;**19**(3):163-170. DOI: 10.1016/j.pathophys.2012.04.004

[6] Kapelko VI, Lakomkin VL, LukoshkovaEV,GramovichVV,VyborovON, Abramov AA, et al. A comprehensive study of the heart of rats at isoproterenol damage. Kardiologiia (in Russian). 2014;**54**(3):46-56

[7] Frederiksen JW, Weiss JL, Weisfeldt ML. Time constant of isovolumic pressure fall: Determinants in the working left ventricle. The American Journal of Physiology. 1978;**235**:H701-H706. DOI: 10.1152/ajpheart.1978.235.6.H701

[8] Grimm D, Elsner D, Schunkert H, Pfeifer M, Griese D, Bruckschlegel G, et al. Development of heart failure following isoproterenol administration in the rat: Role of the renin-angiotensin system. Cardiovascular Research. 1998;**37**:91-100. DOI: 10.1016/s0008-6363(97)00212-5

[9] Zhang Y, Wang WE, Zhang X, Li Y, Chen B, Liu C, et al. Cardiomyocyte PKA ablation enhances basal contractility while eliminates cardiac beta-adrenergic response without adverse effects on the heart. Circulation Research. 2019;**124**:1760-1777. DOI: 10.1161/CIRCRESAHA.118.313417

[10] Krestinina O, Baburina Y, Krestinin R. Mitochondrion as a target of astaxanthin therapy in heart failure. International Journal of Molecular Sciences. 2021;**22**:7964

[11] Nakajima-Takenaka C, Zhang GX, Obata K, Tohne K, Matsuyoshi H, Nagai Y, et al. Left ventricular function of isoproterenol-induced hypertrophied rat hearts perfused with blood: Mechanical work and energetics. American Journal of Physiology. Heart and Circulatory Physiology. 2009;**297**(5):H1736-H1743. DOI: 10.1152/ajpheart.00672.2009

[12] Bottone AE, Voest EE, de Beer EL. Impairment of the actin-myosin interaction in permeabilized cardiac trabeculae after chronic doxorubicin treatment. Clinical Cancer Research. 1998;**4**:1031-1037

[13] DeSantis CE, Lin CC, Mariotto AB, Siegel RL, Stein KD, Kramer JL, et al. Cancer treatment and survivorship

statistics 2014. CA: A Cancer Journal for Clinicians. 2014;**64**:252-271

[14] Yeh E, Tong A, Lenihan D, Wamique Yu S, Swafford J, Champion C, et al. Cardiovascular complications of cancer therapy: Diagnosis, pathogenesis, and management. Circulation. 2004;**109**:3122-3131. DOI: 10.1161/01.CIR.0000133187.74800.B9

[15] Olson RD, Mushlin PS. Doxorubicin cardiotoxicity: Analysis of prevailing hypotheses. The FASEB Journal. 1990;**4**:3076-3086

[16] Gille L, Nohl H. Analyses of the molecular mechanism of adriamycin-induced cardiotoxicity. Free Radical Biology & Medicine. 1997;**23**:775-782. DOI: 10.1016/s0891-5849(97)00025-7

[17] Sarvazyan N. Visualization of doxorubicin-induced oxidative stress in isolated cardiac myocytes. The American Journal of Physiology. 1996;**271**:H2079-H2085. DOI: 10.1152/ajpheart.1996.271.5.H2079

[18] Clementi ME, Giardina B, Di Stasio E, Mordente A, Misiti F. Doxorubicin-derived metabolites induce release of cytochrome C and inhibition of respiration on cardiac isolated mitochondria. Anticancer Research. 2003;**23**:2445-2450

[19] Hershko C, Pinson A, Link G. Prevention of anthracycline cardiotoxicity by iron chelation. Acta Haematologica. 1996;**95**:87-92. DOI: 10.1159/000203954

[20] Nohl H, Gille L, Staniek K. The exogenous NADH dehydrogenase of heart mitochondria is the key enzyme responsible for selective cardiotoxicity of anthracyclines. Z Naturforsch [C]. 1998;**53**(3-4):279-285. DOI: 10.1515/znc-1998-3-419

[21] Green PS, Leeuwenburgh C. Mitochondrial dysfunction is an early indicator of doxorubicin-induced apoptosis. Biochimica et Biophysica Acta. 2002;**1588**:94-101. DOI: 10.1016/s0925-4439(02)00144-8

[22] Wallace KB. Doxorubicin-induced cardiac mitochondrionopathy. Pharmacology & Toxicology. 2003;**93**(3):105-112. DOI: 10.1034/j.1600-0773.2003.930301.x

[23] Kapelko VI, Lakomkin VL, Tsyplenkova VG. Adaptation of the heart to toxic action of adriamycin. In: Lukyanova L, Takeda N, Singal PK, editors. Adaptation Biology and Medicine (Volume 5: Health Potentials). New Delhi, India: Narosa Publishing House; 2007. pp. 93-104

[24] Lakomkin VL, Abramov AA, Gramovich VV, Vyborov ON, Lukoshkova EV, Ermishkin VV, et al. The time course of the formation of systolic dysfunction of the heart in doxorubicin cardiomyopathy. Kardiologiia (in Russian). 2017;**57**(1):59-64. DOI: 10.18565/cardio.2017.1.59-64

[25] Lakomkin VL, Abramov AA, Gramovich VV, Vyborov ON, Lukoshkova EV, Ermishkin VV, et al. The ratio of diastolic and systolic myocardial dysfunction in doxorubicin cardiomyopathy. Cardiology Bulletin (in Russian). 2018;**2**:49-54. DOI: 10.17116/Cardiobulletin201813248

[26] Studneva IM, Lakomkin VL, Prosvirnin AV, Abramov AA, Veselova OM, Pisarenko OI, et al. Energy status of the myocardium in systolic dysfunction. Cardiology Bulletin. 2018;**3**:31-34. DOI: 10.17116/Cardiobulletin201813331

[27] Lygate CA, Neubauer S. Metabolic flux as a predictor of heart failure prognosis. Circulation Research.

2014;**114**(8):1228-1230. DOI: 10.1161/CIRCRESAHA.114.303551

[28] Meyer M, Schillinger W, Pieske B, Holubarsch C, Heilmann C, Posival H, et al. Alterations of sarcoplasmic reticulum proteins in failing human dilated cardiomyopathy. Circulation. 1995;**92**:778-784. DOI: 10.1161/01.cir.92.4.778 al

[29] Linke WA. Sense and stretchability: The role of titin and titin-associated proteins in myocardial stress-sensing and mechanical dysfunction. Cardiovascular Research. 2008;**77**:637-648. DOI: 10.1016/j.cardiores.2007.03.029

[30] Guo W, Sun M. RBM20, a potential target for treatment of cardiomyopathy via titin isoform switching. Biophysical Reviews. 2018;**10**:15-25. DOI: 10.1007/s12551-017-0267-5

[31] Bell SP, Nyland L, Tischler MD, McNabb M, Granzier H, Le Winter MM. Alterations in the determinants of diastolic suction during pacing tachycardia. Circulation Research. 2000;**87**:235-240. DOI: 10.1161/01.res.87.3.235

[32] Cazorla O, Freiburg A, Helmes M, Centner T, McNabb M, Wu Y, et al. Differential expression of cardiac titin isoforms and modulation of cellular stiffness. Circulation Research. 2000;**86**:59-67. DOI: 10.1161/01.res.86.1.59

[33] Wu Y, Bell SP, Trombitas K, Witt CC, Labeit S, LeWinter MM, et al. Changes in titin isoform expression in pacing-induced cardiac failure give rise to increased passive muscle stiffness. Circulation. 2002;**106**(11):1384-1389. DOI: 10.1161/01.cir.0000029804.61510.02

[34] Lakomkin VL, Abramov AA, Studneva IM, Ulanova AD, Vikhlyantsev IM, Prosvirnin AV, et al. Early changes in energy metabolism and isoform composition and level of titin phosphorylation in diastolic dysfunction. Kardiologiia (in Russian). 2020;**60**(2):4-9. DOI: 10.18087/cardio.2020.3.n531

[35] Granzier HL, Labeit S. The giant protein titin: A major player in myocardial mechanics, signaling, and disease. Circulation Research. 2004;**94**:284-295. DOI: 10.1161/01.RES.0000117769.88862.F8

[36] Kapelko VI, Lakomkin VL, Konovalova GG, Tsyplenkova VG, Tikhaze AK, Lankin VZ. Acute and prolonged effect of Adriamycin on the contractile function and antioxidant status of the myocardium. Kardiologiia (in Russian). 2010;**50:(12)**:53-61. https://elibrary.ru/item.asp?id=23054333

[37] Hrelia S, Fiorentini D, Maraldi T, Angeloni C, Bordoni A, Biagi PL, et al. Doxorubicin induces early lipid peroxidation associated with changes in glucose transport in cultured cardiomyocytes. Biochimica et Biophysica Acta. 2002;**1567**:150-156. DOI: 10.1016/s0005-2736(02)00612-0

[38] Pelikan PC, Weisfeldt ML, Jacobus WE, Miceli MV, Bulkley BH, Gerstenblith G. Acute doxorubicin cardiotoxicity: Functional, metabolic, and morphologic alterations in the isolated, perfused rat heart. Journal of Cardiovascular Pharmacology. 1986;**8**(5):1058-1066

[39] Kapelko VI, Tsyplenkova VG, Khatkevich AN, Beskrovnova NN. Morphological and functional estimation of acute and protracted cardiomyocyte alterations caused by adriamycin in varied doses. Experimental and Clinical Cardiology. 1999;**4**:35-42

[40] Vasquez-Vivar J, Martasek P, Hogg N, Masters BS, Pritchard KA Jr,

Kalyanaraman B. Endothelial nitric oxide synthase-dependent superoxide generation from adriamycin. Biochemistry. 1997;**36**:11293-11297. DOI: 10.1021/bi971475e

[41] Li T, Danelisen I, Singal PK. Early changes in myocardial antioxidant enzymes in rats treated with adriamycin. Molecular and Cellular Biochemistry. 2002;**232**(1-2):19-26

[42] Dziegiel P, Murawska-Cialowicz E, Jethon Z, Januszewska L, Podhorska-Okołów M, Surowiak P, et al. Melatonin stimulates the activity of protective antioxidative enzymes in myocardial cells of rats in the course of doxorubicin intoxication. Journal of Pineal Research. 2003;**35**:183-187. DOI: 10.1034/j.1600-079x.2003.00079.x

[43] Lakomkin VL, Lukoshkova EV, Kapelko VI. The reaction of the heart to high-frequency load in the acute action of doxorubicin. Bulletin of Experimental Biology and Medicine. 2020;**169**(5):619-622. DOI: 10.1007/s10517-020-04940-4

[44] Sarvazyan NA, Askari A, Huang WH. Effects of doxorubicin on cardiomyocytes with reduced level of superoxide dismutase. Life Sciences. 1995;**57**(10):1003-1010. DOI: 10.1016/0024-3205(95)02036-i

[45] Luo X, Evrovsky Y, Cole D, Trines J, Benson LN, Lehotay DC. Doxorubicin-induced acute changes in cytotoxic aldehydes, antioxidant status and cardiac function in the rat. Biochimica et Biophysica Acta. 1997;**1360**:45-52. DOI: 10.1016/s0925-4439(96)00068-3

[46] Skulachev VP, Anisimov VN, Antonenko YN, Bakeeva LE, Chernyak BV, Korshunova GA, et al. An attempt to prevent senescence: A mitochondrial approach. Biochimica et Biophysica Acta. 2009;**1787**(5):437-461. DOI: 10.1016/j.bbabio.2008.12.008

[47] Abramov AA, Lakomkin VL, Prosvirnin AV, Kapelko VI. The mitochondrial antioxidant plastomitin improves heart function in doxorubicin cardiomyopathy. Kardiologiia (in Russian). 2019;**59**:35-41. DOI: 10.18087/cardio.2019.6.2649

[48] Lakomkin VL, Abramov AA, Lukoshkova EV, Prosvirnin AV, Kapelko VI. Prevention of diastolic dysfunction caused by doxorubicin by mitochondrial antioxidant Plastomitin. Kardiologiia (in Russian). 2020;**60**(7):98-102. DOI: 10.18087/cardio.2020.7.n1157

[49] An D, Rodrigues B. Role of changes in cardiac metabolism in development of diabetic cardiomyopathy. American Journal of Physiology. Heart and Circulatory Physiology. 2006;**291**:H1489-H1506. DOI: 10.1152/ajpheart.00278.2006

[50] Joffe II, Travers KE, Perreault-Micale CL, Hampton T, Katz SE, Morgan JP, et al. Abnormal cardiac function in the streptozotocin-induced non-insulin-dependent diabetic rat: Noninvasive assessment with doppler echocardiography and contribution of the nitric oxide pathway. Journal of the American College of Cardiology. 1999;**34**:2111-2119. DOI: 10.1016/s0735-1097(99)00436-2

[51] Cosson S, Kevorkian JP. Left ventricular diastolic dysfunction: An early sign of diabetic cardiomyopathy? Diabetes & Metabolism. 2003;**29**:455-466. DOI: 10.1016/s1262-3636(07)70059-9

[52] Dillmann WH. Diabetic cardiomyopathy what is it and can it Be fixed? Circulation Research.

2019;**124**:1160-1162. DOI: 10.1161/CIRCRESAHA.118.314665

[53] Severson DL. Diabetic cardiomyopathy: Recent evidence from mouse models of type 1 and type 2 diabetes. Canadian Journal of Physiology and Pharmacology. 2004;**82**:813-823. DOI: 10.1139/y04-065

[54] Zhang L, Cannell MB, Phillips AR, Cooper GJ, Ward ML. Altered calcium homeostasis does not explain the contractile deficit of diabetic cardiomyopathy. Diabetes. 2008;**57**:2158-2166. DOI: 10.2337/db08-0140

[55] Lakomkin VL, Abramov AA, Lukoshkova EV, Prosvirnin AV, Kapelko VI. Systolic dysfunction of the heart in type 1 diabetes mellitus. Bulletin of Experimental Biology and Medicine. 2021;**172**(1):14-17. DOI: 10.1007/s10517-021-05321-1

[56] Lakomkin VL, Abramov AA, Studneva IM, Lukoshkova EV, Prosvirnin AV, Kapelko VI. Normalization of the pumping function of the diabetic heart with a decrease in functional load. Kardiologiia (in Russian). 2022;**62**(3):34-39. DOI: 10.18087/cardio.2022.3.n1761

[57] Rider OJ, Apps A, Miller J, Lau JYC, Lewis AJM, Peterzan MA, et al. Noninvasive in vivo assessment of cardiac metabolism in the healthy and diabetic human heart using hyperpolarized (13)C MRI. Circulation Research. 2020;**126**:725-736. DOI: 10.1161/CIRCRESAHA.119.316260

[58] Cieluch A, Uruska A, Zozulinska-Ziolkiewicz D. Can we prevent mitochondrial dysfunction and diabetic cardiomyopathy in type 1 diabetes mellitus? Pathophysiology and treatment options. International Journal of Molecular Sciences. 2020;**21**:2852. DOI: 10.3390/ijms21082852

[59] Bugger H, Chen D, Riehle C, Soto J, Theobald HA, Hu XX, et al. Tissue-specific remodeling of the mitochondrial proteome in type 1 diabetic Akita mice. Diabetes. 2009;**58**:1986-1997. DOI: 10.2337/db09-0259

[60] Pham T, Loiselle D, Power A, Hickey AJ. Mitochondrial inefficiencies and anoxic ATP hydrolysis capacities in diabetic rat heart. American Journal of Physiology. Cell Physiology. 2014;**307**:C499-C507. DOI: 10.1152/ajpcell.00006.2014

[61] Semaming Y, Kumfu S, Pannangpetch P, Chattipakorn SC, Chattipakorn N. Protocatechuic acid exerts a cardioprotective effect in type 1 diabetic rats. The Journal of Endocrinology. 2014;**223**:13-23. DOI: 10.1530/JOE-14-0273

[62] Baseler WA, Dabkowski ER, Williamson CL, Croston TL, Thapa D, Powell MJ, et al. Proteomic alterations of distinct mitochondrial subpopulations in the type 1 diabetic heart: Contribution of protein import dysfunction. American Journal of Physiology. Regulatory, Integrative and Comparative Physiology. 2011;**300**:R186-R200. DOI: 10.1152/ajpregu.00423.2010

[63] Croston TL, Shepherd DL, Thapa D, Nichols CE, Lewis SE, Dabkowski ER, et al. Evaluation of the cardiolipin biosynthetic pathway and its interactions in the diabetic heart. Life Sciences. 2013;**93**:313-322. DOI: 10.1016/j.lfs.2013.07.005

[64] Kapelko VI, Lakomkin VL, Abramov AA, Lukoshkova EV. Compensatory changes of the diastole under conditions of inflow restriction

to the heart. Bulletin of Experimental Biology and Medicine. 2021;**171**:15-18. DOI: 10.1007/s10517-021-05162-y

[65] Jensen MT, Fung K, Aung N, Sanghvi MM, Chadalavada S, Paiva JM, et al. Changes in cardiac morphology and function in individuals with diabetes mellitus: The UK biobank cardiovascular magnetic resonance substudy. Circulation. Cardiovascular Imaging. 2019;**12**:e009476. DOI: 10.1161/CIRCIMAGING.119.009476

[66] Seferovic PM, Paulus WJ. Clinical diabetic cardiomyopathy: A two-faced disease with restrictive and dilated phenotypes. European Heart Journal. 2015;**36**:1718-1727. DOI: 10.1093/eurheartj/ehv134

[67] Heather LC, Hafstad AD, Halade GV, Harmancey R, Mellor KM, Mishra PK, et al. Guidelines on models of diabetic heart disease. American Journal of Physiology. Heart and Circulatory Physiology. 2022;**323**:H176-H200. DOI: 10.1152/ajpheart.00058.2022

[68] Gunter TE, Yule DI, Gunter KK, Eliseev RA, Salter JD. Calcium and mitochondria. FEBS Letters. 2004;**567**(1):96-102. DOI: 10.1016/j.febslet.2004.03.071

[69] Yan Y, Liu J, Wei C, Li K, Xie W, Wang Y, et al. Bidirectional regulation of Ca2+ sparks by mitochondria-derived reactive oxygen species in cardiac myocytes. Cardiovascular Research. 2008;**77**:432-441

[70] Terentyev D, Györke I, Belevych AE, Terentyeva R, Sridhar A, Nishijima Y, et al. Redox modification of ryanodine receptors contributes to sarcoplasmic reticulum Ca2+ leak in chronic heart failure. Circulation Research. 2008;**103**(12):1466-1472. DOI: 10.1161/CIRCRESAHA.108.184457

[71] Katz LN. The role played by the ventricular relaxation process in filling the ventricle. The American Journal of Physiology. 1930;**95**:542-553

[72] Brecher GA. Experimental evidence of ventricular diastolic suction. Circulation Research. 1956;**4**:513-518. DOI: 10.1161/01.res.4.5.513

[73] Suga H, Goto Y, Igarashi Y, Yamada O, Nozava T, Yasamura Y. Ventricular suction under zero source pressure for filling. American Journal of Physiology. Heart and Circulatory Physiology. 1986;**251**:H47-H55. DOI: 10.1152/ajpheart.1986.251.1.H47

[74] Yellin EL, Hori M, Yoran C, Sonnenblick EH, Gabbay S, Frater RWM. Left ventricular relaxation in the filling and non–filling intact canine heart. American Journal of Physiology. Heart and Circulatory Physiology. 1986;**250**:H620-H629. DOI: 10.1152/ajpheart.1986.250.4.H620

[75] Helmes M, Trombitas K, Granzier H. Titin develops restoring force in rat cardiac myocytes. Circulation Research. 1996;**79**:619-626. DOI: 10.1161/01.res.79.3.619

[76] Granzier H, Helmes M, Trombitas K. Nonuniform elasticity of titin in cardiac myocytes: A study using immunoelectron microscopy and cellular mechanics. Biophysical Journal. 1996;**70**:430-442. DOI: 10.1016/S0006-3495(96)79586-3

[77] Preetha N, Yiming W, Helmes M, Norio F, Siegfried L, Granzier H. Restoring force development by titin/connectin and assessment of Ig domain unfolding. Journal of Muscle Research and Cell Motility. 2005;**26**:307-317. DOI: 10.1007/s10974-005-9037-2

Section 2

Metabolic Syndromes and Cardiomyopathy

Chapter 2

Biomarkers of Metabolic Syndrome in Cardiomyopathy: A Leading Cause of Heart Failure

Saima Sharif, Saira Rafaqat and Shagufta Naz

Abstract

Cardiomyopathy is a disease of the heart muscle, which makes the muscles harder to pump blood to the rest of the body leading to heart failure. The main types of cardiomyopathies include dilated cardiomyopathy, hypertrophic cardiomyopathy, ischemic cardiomyopathy, arrhythmogenic right ventricular dysplasia, restrictive cardiomyopathy, and Takotsubo cardiomyopathy. On the other hand, Metabolic syndrome (MetS) is the clustering of different medical conditions, which requires at least three of the five following diseases. These diseases are high blood sugar, high blood pressure, high serum triglycerides, low serum high-density lipoprotein, and central obesity. The risk of developing type 2 diabetes and cardiovascular disease associated with metabolic syndrome. In MetS, many different biomarkers are used in the early detection and risk stratification of MetS patients. It includes adiponectin, leptin, interleukin 6, tumor necrosis factor-alpha, uric acid, interleukin 10, ghrelin, adiponectin, paraoxonase, oxidized low-density lipoprotein, and plasminogen activator inhibitor-1. This chapter provides an overview and focuses on the basic role of major biomarkers of metabolic syndrome in the pathogenesis of different types of cardiomyopathies, which mainly highlights recent pathophysiological aspects in the development and progress of cardiomyopathy which is the leading cause of heart failure. In conclusion, biomarkers of metabolic syndrome play a significant role in the development and progress of cardiomyopathy which is the leading cause of heart failure.

Keywords: cardiomyopathy, types of cardiomyopathies, metabolic syndrome, biomarkers, heart failure

1. Introduction

Metabolic syndrome (MetS) is known by other names such as dysmetabolic syndrome, syndrome X, insulin resistance syndrome, and deadly quartet. It is a fast-growing health problem worldwide [1]. Metabolic syndrome is the clustering of different medical conditions, which requires at least three of the five following diseases. These diseases are high blood sugar, high blood pressure, high serum triglycerides, low serum high-density lipoprotein, and central obesity. The risk of developing type 2 diabetes and cardiovascular disease associated with metabolic syndrome [2].

A biomarker is a quantifiable sign of a certain biological state or condition. It is used to evaluate or measure the normal biological process, pharmacologic response, and pathogenic processes of a therapeutic intervention. In MetS, many different biomarkers are used in the early detection and risk stratification of MetS patients. It includes adiponectin, leptin, interleukin 6, tumor necrosis factor-alpha, uric acid, interleukin 10, ghrelin, adiponectin, paraoxonase, oxidized low-density lipoprotein (Ox-LDL), and plasminogen activator inhibitor-1 [3].

Cardiomyopathy is a disease of the heart muscle which makes the muscles harder to pump blood to the rest of the body leading to heart failure. The main types of cardiomyopathies include restricted cardiomyopathy, dilated cardiomyopathy, hypertrophic cardiomyopathy, ischemic cardiomyopathy, arrhythmogenic right ventricular dysplasia, and Takotsubo cardiomyopathy. The pathogenesis of dilated cardiomyopathy is complicated and includes myocardial fibrosis as well as myocyte injury induced by abnormal immune responses after viral infection are considered to be critical factors in the progress of dilated cardiomyopathy [4, 5]. Viral myocarditis-triggered dilated cardiomyopathy is a common cause of heart failure and is characterized by systolic dysfunction as well as left ventricular dilation [6]. Heart failure is a complex progressive pathology in which phenotype is reflective of end-organ damage as a result of insulin/injuries such as post-partum cardiomyopathy, dyslipidemia, congenital disorders, hypertension, ischemic heart disease, and diabetes [7–10].

This chapter will give the recent development of major biomarkers of metabolic syndrome (adiponectin, leptin, uric acid, TNF-α, interleukin-6) in the development and progress of cardiomyopathy which includes the different types of cardiomyopathies such as dilated cardiomyopathy, ischemic cardiomyopathy, hypertrophic cardiomyopathy, arrhythmogenic right ventricular dysplasia, and so on, and also emphasized their contribution in the heart failure patients.

2. Major biomarkers of metabolic syndrome in cardiomyopathy which is the leading cause of heart failure

According to the literature, there are many biomarkers of metabolic syndrome. However, this chapter has discussed only major biomarkers of metabolic syndrome such as adiponectin, leptin, uric acid, TNF-α, and interleukin-6 in the development and progress of cardiomyopathy which includes the different types of cardiomyopathies such as dilated cardiomyopathy, ischemic cardiomyopathy, hypertrophic cardiomyopathy, arrhythmogenic right ventricular dysplasia, and so on, and also emphasized their contribution in the heart failure patients as explained in **Figure 1** and **Table 1**.

2.1 Adiponectin

Adiponectin is an adipokine that adipocytes manufacture and release. Adiponectin's biological activities are mediated by interactions with receptor subtypes: adiponectin receptor 1 (AdipoR1), adiponectin receptor 2 (AdipoR2), and T-cadherin. Adiponectin has a variety of protective effects on different cell types, including insulin sensitization, anti-inflammation, anti-proliferation, anti-atherosclerosis, and carcinogenesis suppression. In humans, Adiponectin is a relatively prevalent serum protein. Insulin resistance, type 2 diabetes mellitus, obesity, metabolic syndrome, and cardiovascular diseases all cause a reduction in their levels.

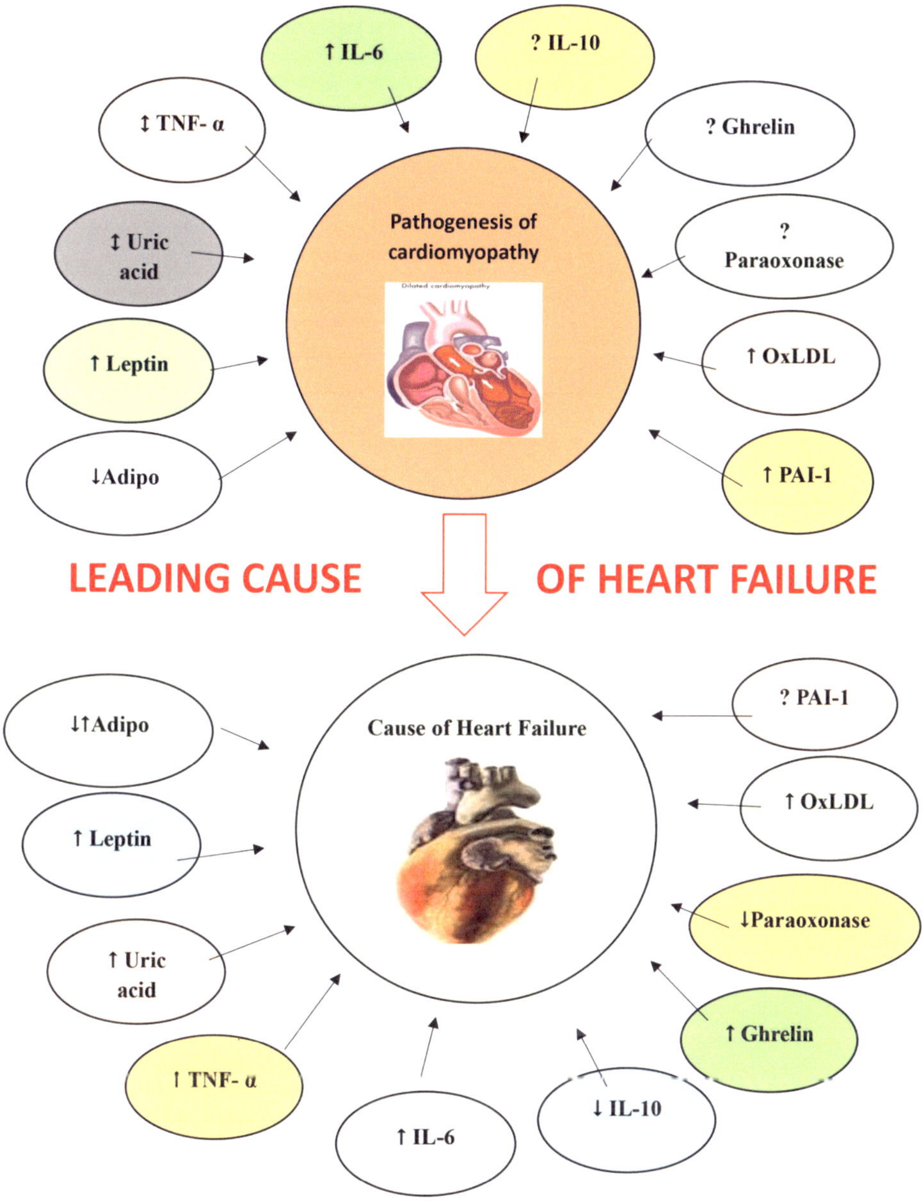

Figure 1.
Overview presentation of major biomarkers of metabolic syndrome in the pathogenesis of cardiomyopathy which is also a leading cause of heart failure. Source: Designed by the authors with the help of articles. Signs show further information, for example, ↑ (increased levels), ↓ (decreased levels), ? (No study still reported), ↕ (not sure if increased or decreased levels).

Adiponectin's preventive impact on obesity-related diseases and cancer has been demonstrated in numerous research. To carry out its physiological and defensive roles, adiponectin regulates many signaling pathways [39].

The pathogenesis of cardiovascular disease is closely linked with obesity-associated disorders. Adiponectin is a circulating adipose tissue-derived hormone that is down-regulated in obese patients. The independent risk of hypertension, type 2 diabetes, and coronary artery disease are linked with hypoadiponectinemia. In the

First author	Year of publication	Biomarkers of metabolic syndrome	The main finding of major biomarkers of metabolic syndrome in the development of heart failure and the prognostic implications of each biomarker	References
George et al.	2006	Adiponectin	Reported the elevated concentration of adiponectin in chronic heart failure patients and predicts mortality and morbidity	[11]
Won et al.	2012	Adiponectin	Decreased concentration of adiponectin in heart failure subjects with metabolic syndrome	[12]
Baldasseroni et al.	2012	Adiponectin	In the presence of diabetes, the progressive increase of adiponectin in the severity of left ventricular dysfunction was hampered and becomes evident only in overt heart failure	[13]
Bobbert et al.	2012	Leptin	Elevated expression of leptin and resistin in non-ischemic dilated patients and inflammatory cardiomyopathy was connected with chronic heart failure progression including independent of immune responses as well as severe cardiac dysfunction	[14]
Toth et al.	1997	Leptin	Leptin could contribute to the regulation of body energy stores as well as energy expenditure in heart failure subjects	[15]
Barbosa-Ferreira et al.	2013	Leptin	Leptin was important as a diagnostic and prognostic marker for heart failure patients and should be included in the routine investigation of heart failure patients	[16]
Wannamethee et al.	2014	Leptin	Decreased mortality risk linked with excess weight in men with CHD without heart failure could be due to elevated muscle mass, leptin (possibly reflecting cachexia) represents the inverse linked in men with heart failure	[17]
Wannamethee et al.	2011	Leptin	The link between obesity and heart failure may be mediated by plasma leptin in the absence of established coronary heart disease. Obesity seems to raise the risk of heart failure in those with coronary heart disease independently of leptin	[18]
Filippatos et al.	2000	Leptin	More prospective studies clarify the contribution of leptin in the pathophysiology of heart failure cachexia	[19]

First author	Year of publication	Biomarkers of metabolic syndrome	The main finding of major biomarkers of metabolic syndrome in the development of heart failure and the prognostic implications of each biomarker	References
Schulze et al.	2003	Leptin	Indicated that the participation of leptin in the catabolic state leads to the progress of cardiac cachexia in the context of CHF	[20]
Murdoch et al.	1999	Leptin	Leptin did not contribute to the cachexia of CHF	[21]
Lieb et al.	2009	Leptin	Elevated risk of chronic heart failure as well as cardiovascular disease was linked with elevated circulating levels of leptin, therefore, leptin did not give incremental prognostic information beyond body mass index	[22]
Anker et al.	2003	Uric acid	Elevated serum uric acid concentrations were strong as well as an independent marker of impaired prognosis in moderate to severe chronic heart failure patients	[23]
Cicoira et al.	2002	Uric acid	In chronic heart failure, elevated uric acid levels are linked to diastolic dysfunction. Theoretically, the diastolic function could be improved in patients with chronic heart failure by inhibiting xanthine oxydase	[24]
Wannamethee et al.	2018	Uric acid	The serum uric acid as a marker of increased xanthine oxidase activity may be a useful prognostic marker for heart failure risk in older men on antihypertensive treatment	[25]
Hamaguchi et al.	2011	Uric acid	In heart failure patients, hyperuricemia was common in clinical practice and elevated uric acid was independently linked with long-term adverse outcomes	[26]
Krishnan et al.	2009	Uric acid	The elevated uric acid level was a novel as well as an independent risk factor for heart failure in a group of young general community residents. This has implications for the development of preventive strategies for heart failure	[27]
Huang et al.	2014	Uric acid	Elevated serum uric acid was related to an increased risk of incident heart failure and adverse outcomes in heart failure patients	[28]
Doehner et al. Xu et al.	2002 2008	Uric acid	Individuals with heart failure have shown therapeutic benefits from serum uric acid-lowering medication with xanthine oxidase inhibitors such as allopurinol or febuxostat	[29, 30]

First author	Year of publication	Biomarkers of metabolic syndrome	The main finding of major biomarkers of metabolic syndrome in the development of heart failure and the prognostic implications of each biomarker	References
Dunlay et al.	2008	Tumor necrosis factor-alpha	Heart failure had elevated tumor necrosis factor-alpha, which was also associated with a significant decline in survival and provided a significant incremental increase in risk assessment over baseline signs. When determining risk in patients with heart failure with both preserved and lowered ejection fractions, tumor necrosis factor-alpha was helpful	[31]
Chia et al.	2021	Interleukin-6	The authors suggested whether interleukin-6 could be a novel treatment target to prevent heart failure with preserved ejection fraction	[32]
Markousis-Mavrogenis et al.	2019	Interleukin-6	Further studies were required to identify interleukin-6 as a potential therapeutic target in specific heart failure subpopulations	[33]
Deokar et al.	2018	Interleukin-6	Increased levels of interleukin-6 in heart failure patients played an important role as a pro-inflammatory marker in the development of cardiovascular disease including heart failure	[34]
Hudzik et al.	2011	Interleukin-6	The elevated level of interleukin-6 might be in the earlier manifestation of heart failure symptoms	[35]
MacGowan et al.	1997	Interleukin-6, TNF-α	Elevated concentrations of TNF-α and IL-6 could be present even in the absence of cachexia in heart failure patients	[36]
Meléndez et al. Rauchhaus et al.	2010 2000	Interleukin-6	Elevated IL-6 could be used as a predictive biomarker in HF and be considered a significant independent predictor for HF	[37, 38]

Table 1.
Summary of major biomarkers of metabolic syndrome in the pathogenesis of heart failure.

same way, adiponectin has a protective role in the development of inflammation, insulin resistance as well as atherosclerosis. The regulation of acute cardiac injury, as well as myocardial remodeling, is due to the role of adiponectin [40].

The presence of a local cardiac adiponectin system which is regulated independently of adiponectin as well as tumor necrosis factor-α serum concentrations also disturbed the cardiac pathology. Moreover, endomyocardial biopsies by immunohistological analysis revealed significant downregulation of cardiac adiponectin protein expression independent of serum tumor necrosis factor-α levels or serum adiponectin levels. Neither adiponectin receptor 1 nor adiponectin receptor 2 was deregulated in early dilated cardiomyopathy. Adiponectin mRNA and protein down-regulation were confirmed in the explanted hearts of patients with advanced dilated cardiomyopathy (LVEF <25%, $n = 8$). Neonatal rat ventricular myocytes incubated with adiponectin activated the pro-survival protein kinase B or PKB/Akt, enhanced eNOS-phosphorylation, and inhibited stress-induced cardiomyocyte apoptosis in an Akt-dependent manner in vitro. Additionally, the expression of the cytokine and its receptors increased along with the suppression of adiponectin release. The scientists also speculated that adiponectin may have a role in the pathophysiology of dilated cardiomyopathy (DCM) and identified adipocytokines as a potential new treatment target for dilated cardiomyopathy [41].

Oppositely, other studies reported that adiponectin expression in dilated cardiomyopathy subjects has been inconclusive partly because of the survival benefit of a high body mass index which was inversely correlated with adiponectin expression [42, 43].

New insights in variants of adiponectin receptor 1 are the risk factor for hypertrophic cardiomyopathy (HCM) in which adiponectin receptor 1 variant dysregulate lipid as well glucose metabolism which causes cardiac hypertrophy through the extracellular signal-regulated kinase pathways as well as the p38/mammalian target of rapamycin. In the same way, a transgenic mouse model representing an adiponectin receptor 1 variant displayed cardiomyopathy which recapitulated the cellular discoveries and these features were rescued by rapamycin [44]. These results collectively imply that the adiponectin-AMP-activated protein kinase (AMPK) regulatory axis controls intracellular signaling and metabolic alterations that were connected to the development of cardiac hypertrophy [40].

According to recent investigations, Adiponectin impacts heart remodeling in pathologic situations. Pressure overload causes increased concentric cardiac hypertrophy and worse mortality in adiponectin knockout (APN-KO) mice [45, 46]. On the other hand, in APN-KO, wild-type, and diabetic db/db mice, adenovirus-mediated administration of adiponectin reduces ventricular hypertrophy in response to pressure overload. Additionally, adiponectin overexpression reduces angiotensin II-induced cardiac hypertrophy, indicating that adiponectin has a broader role in suppressing pathological cardiac development. These results imply that in obese people, decreased adiponectin levels may play a role in the development of hypertrophic cardiomyopathy [40].

In the same way, Tamariz et al. reported the prevalence of the metabolic syndrome was elevated in indigent heart failure and also increased the risk of death. Moreover, physicians treating heart failure patients need to address the current metabolic syndrome epidemic in heart failure [47]. In contrast, Frankel et al. demonstrated that heart failure was not linked with concentrations of adiponectin [48].

Moreover, George et al. stated the elevated concentration of adiponectin in chronic heart failure patients predicts mortality and morbidity [11]. In contrast, decreased concentration of adiponectin in heart failure subjects with metabolic syndrome, and that relationship between adiponectin, abnormal diastolic function, and inflammation possibly leads to the progression of heart failure [12]. Additionally, adiponectin levels were raised throughout the stages of chronic heart failure; however, type 2 diabetic individuals show less of this tendency. Diabetes hinders the gradual rise in adiponectin, which revealed the extent of left ventricular dysfunction (LVD), and it only becomes visible in overt heart failure [13].

2.2 Leptin

The white adipocytes produced most abundantly leptin hormone which is act in the hypothalamus of the brain to lower the appetite and elevate energy expenditure. In the early 1990s, leptin was discovered after genetic mapping of the mutation in the gene which was observed in a specific strain of obese mice, the *ob/ob* mouse, which was originally represented in the 1950s [49, 50].

Additionally, leptin was linked with cardiovascular complications resulting from obesity including heart disease as well as hypertension. Obese patients have elevated concentrations of circulating leptin due to increased fat mass. Various clinical, as well as population studies, reported the elevated concentration of leptin with the development of cardiac hypertrophy in obesity. Increased growth of cultured cardiomyocytes was due to leptin. It also regulates cardiac metabolism which helps the oxidation of fatty acids as well as glucose [51]. Leptin could contribute to vascular stiffness as well as endothelial dysfunction which might also contribute to cardiac hypertrophy [52].

Bobbert et al., the study reported for the first time, In the incidence of chronic heart failure, the expression of leptin as well as resistin were positively correlated which was also implicated in cardiac remodeling and immunomodulation. Furthermore, elevated expression of leptin and resistin in non-ischaemic dilated patients and inflammatory cardiomyopathy was connected with chronic heart failure progression including independent of immune responses as well as severe cardiac dysfunction [14]. In the same context, Toth et al. concluded the relationship between energy expenditure and plasma leptin levels in heart failure patients, but not in healthy controls. Therefore, leptin could contribute to the regulation of body energy stores as well as energy expenditure in heart failure subjects [15]. Another study reported the finding which explains that leptin is important as a diagnostic and prognostic marker for heart failure patients and should be included in the routine investigation of heart failure patients [16]. Furthermore, Wannamethee's study concluded the decreased mortality risk linked with excess weight in men with coronary heart disease (CHD) without heart failure could be due to elevated muscle mass, leptin (possibly reflecting cachexia) represents the inverse linked in men with heart failure [17].

The relationship between heart failure and obesity could be mediated by plasma leptin concentration in the absence of established CHD. On the other side, for those with CHD, obesity appears to elevate the risk of heart failure independently of leptin levels [18]. Oppositely, Filippatos' study indicated a need for more prospective studies which clarify the contribution of leptin in the pathophysiology of heart failure cachexia [19]. Also, elevated serum concentration of leptin in advance CHF and its soluble receptor. Moreover, the authors indicated that the participation of leptin in the catabolic state leads to the progress of cardiac cachexia in the context of CHF [20]. In contrast, another study reported that leptin does not contribute to the cachexia of CHF [21].

Lieb et al., reported in the moderate-sized community-based elderly sample, elevated risk of chronic heart failure as well as a cardiovascular disease were linked with elevated circulating levels of leptin, therefore, leptin did not give incremental prognostic information beyond body mass index. So, the authors required more investigation which elucidates the U-shaped link of leptin to mortality [22].

2.3 Uric acid

The uric acid is the end product of an external purine pool and endogenous purine metabolism. Animal proteins contribute significantly to the exogenous purine pool, which varies significantly with diet. The liver, intestines, and other tissues such as muscles, kidneys, and the vascular endothelium are the main sources of endogenous uric acid synthesis. Uric acid synthesis and metabolism are complicated processes involving several variables that control the hepatic, renal, and gastrointestinal excretion of this molecule [53]. The association between uric acid and metabolic syndrome was explored, and it was discovered that increasing uric acid causes a gradual increase in the prevalence of metabolic syndrome in both sexes, although there were differences in levels between males and females [54].

Various clinical and experimental studies explain the numerous mechanisms through which elevated uric acid levels exert deleterious effects on cardiovascular health such as insulin resistance, reduced availability of nitric oxide, elevated oxidative stress, promotion of local and systemic inflammation as well as vasoconstriction, reduced endothelial dysfunction, the proliferation of vascular smooth muscle cells, and metabolic dysregulation [55].

Elevated serum uric acid concentrations were strong as well as an independent marker of impaired prognosis in moderate to severe chronic heart failure patients. The authors graded the relationship between serum uric acid and survival in chronic heart failure. The metabolic, hemodynamic, and functional staging of patients with chronic heart failure was feasible [23].

Another study investigated the potential relationship between left ventricular systolic, diastolic dysfunction, and serum uric acid, a marker of altered oxidative metabolism, in chronic heart failure. In chronic heart failure, elevated uric acid levels were linked to diastolic dysfunction. Theoretically, the diastolic function could be improved in patients with chronic heart failure by inhibiting xanthine oxidase [24].

The serum uric acid as a marker of increased xanthine oxidase activity may be a useful prognostic marker for heart failure risk in older men on antihypertensive treatment [25]. In heart failure patients, hyperuricemia was common in clinical practice and elevated uric acid was independently linked with long-term adverse outcomes in these patients [26]. Krishnan et al. described that elevated uric acid level was a novel as well as an independent risk factor for heart failure in a group of young general community residents. This has implications for the development of preventive strategies for heart failure [27]. Huang et al. also demonstrated that Elevated serum uric acid was related to an increased risk of incident heart failure and adverse outcomes in heart failure patients [28].

Based on these presumptions, individuals with heart failure have shown therapeutic benefits from serum uric acid-lowering medication with xanthine oxidase inhibitors such as allopurinol or febuxostat [29, 30]. Further research was required because some trials have not found any notable advantages of uric acid-lowering therapy with xanthine oxidase inhibitors in heart failure patients with hyperuricemia [56, 57].

2.4 TNF-α

Tumor necrosis factor-α (TNFα) is an inflammatory cytokine produced by macrophages/monocytes during acute inflammation. It is responsible for a variety of signaling events within cells, including necrosis and apoptosis. The protein is also necessary for infection resistance and cancer resistance [58]. The early identification of a patient's inflammatory status, including TNF-α and IL-6, could be effective in metabolic syndrome and its comorbidities monitoring and early intervention [59].

The overwhelming inflammatory reactions caused by viral myocarditis, which are mediated by CD4+ T lymphocytes, cause myocardial fibrosis in people with dilated cardiomyopathy. Recently, a small number of researchers found that B cells also possess an aberrant pro-inflammatory potential in addition to producing autoantibodies. First, the authors proposed that TNF-secreting B cells were involved in cardiac fibrosis, revealing a novel pathogenic mechanism of B cells in dilated cardiomyopathy and suggesting potential therapeutic options against these cells [60].

A considerable number of patients with community-acquired heart failure elevated tumor necrosis factor-α which was also associated with a significant decline in survival and provided a significant incremental increase in risk assessment over baseline signs. When determining risk in patients with heart failure with both preserved and lowered ejection fractions, Tumor necrosis factor-α was helpful [31]. Tumor necrosis factor-α contributes to adverse left ventricular remodeling during pressure overload through regulation of cardiac repair as well as remodeling which leads to ventricular dysfunction [61]. Numerous studies have found a persistent relationship between circulating TNFα and soluble TNF receptors and mortality in patients with heart failure [62]. Schumacher et al. explained the understanding of how tumor necrosis factor-α, as well as interleukin-6, contribute to cardiac failure and cardiac dysfunction [63].

2.5 Interleukin-6

IL-6 is a soluble mediator that affects inflammation, immunological response, and hematopoiesis in a pleiotropic manner. The human IL-6 gene has been localized to chromosome 7p21 and has 212 amino acids, including a 28-amino-acid signal peptide. Although the core protein is only about 20 kDa, glycosylation accounts for the size of natural IL-6, which is between 21 and 26 kDa [64].

The initiation as well as the development of heart failure contributes to immune activation and inflammation. Interleukin-6 was not only a sign of inflammatory activation but also could induce ventricular dilatation, apoptosis, systolic dysfunction, and cardiomyocyte hypertrophy through various mechanisms that directly act on the pathological process of heart failure, assisting the progression and deterioration, which is the primary pathophysiological mechanism of heart failure. Interleukin-6, a potent inflammatory cytokine inducer, alters heart failure patients' hemodynamic and oxidative stress status [65].

Elevated serum levels of IL-6 were linked with lower ejection fraction, elevated incidence of functional class III to IV and worse prognosis in idiopathic dilated cardiomyopathy [66]. In the same way, Santoro et al. hypothesized that systemic inflammation is the possible mechanism of Takotsubo cardiomyopathy (TTC) in which authors aimed to assess the role of interleukin-6 and interleukin-10 in subjects with an episode of Takotsubo cardiomyopathy. The authors concluded that serum interleukin-6 as well as interleukin-10 admission levels related to an elevated risk of adverse events during follow-up [67].

The interleukin-6 was linked with a new onset of heart failure with preserved ejection fraction (HFrEF) individuals, independent of potential confounders. Moreover, the authors suggested whether interleukin-6 could be a novel treatment target to prevent heart failure with preserved ejection fraction [32].

Similarly, a higher level of interleukin-6 was determined in more than 50% of heart failure patients. Interleukin-6 was linked with reduced left ventricular ejection fraction, iron deficiency, atrial fibrillation, and poor clinical outcomes.

Additionally, the authors investigated those further studies that were required to identify interleukin-6 as a potential therapeutic target in specific heart failure subpopulations [33].

The significantly increased serum interleukin-6 (median [IQR] 14.3[26.2] pg/mL) in heart failure patients as compared to age and sex-matched controls (median [IQR] 0[2.4] pg/mL). The authors showed an increased level of interleukin-6 in heart failure patients played an important role as a pro-inflammatory marker in the development of cardiovascular disease including heart failure [34].

In the severity of chronic heart failure, interleukin-6 spillover was increased in the peripheral circulation and mainly linked with the activation of the sympathetic nervous system. Elevation levels of interleukin-6 could provide prognostic information in chronic heart failure patients which was independent of left ventricular ejection fraction as well as plasma norepinephrine (NE) which was suggesting an important contribution to the interleukin-6 in the pathophysiology of chronic heart failure [68]. In the same context, the elevated level of interleukin-6 might be in the earlier manifestation of heart failure symptoms [35]. Additionally, elevated concentrations of TNF-α and IL-6 could be present even in the absence of cachexia in heart failure patients [36].

The data was overwhelming in demonstrating that individuals with HF had higher levels of IL-6 in their blood circulation as well as myocardium and these levels were correlated with the progression of their condition. A key factor in the development and progression of HF is ventricular remodeling, which was mediated by inflammation. IL-6 controls the entire inflammatory process and encourages the development of ventricular remodeling [28].

The IL-6 induced cardiac interstitial fibrosis, which in turn produced ventricular wall sclerosis and HF, by encouraging cardiac fibroblasts to produce collagen. IL-6 can also make cardiomyocytes stiffer by decreasing actin phosphorylation. In conclusion, elevated IL-6 could be used as a predictive biomarker in HF and be considered a significant independent predictor for HF [37, 38].

3. Conclusion

In conclusion, biomarkers of metabolic syndrome play a significant role in the development and progress of cardiomyopathy which is the leading cause of heart failure. Also, major biomarkers of metabolic syndrome such as adiponectin, leptin, uric acid, TNF-α, and interleukin-6 played their pathophysiological role in different types of cardiomyopathies as well as in heart failure. However, future studies are also required to control metabolic diseases in cardiomyopathy patients which ultimately prevents heart failure which in turn does not increase the prevalence of cardiovascular diseases.

Conflict of interest

The authors declare that they have no competing interests.

List of abbreviations

AdipoR1	adiponectin receptor 1
AdipoR2	adiponectin receptor 2

CHD	coronary heart disease
DCM	dilated cardiomyopathy
IL-10	interleukin 10
IL-6	interleukin 6
MetS	metabolic syndrome
Ox-LDL	oxidized low-density lipoprotein or oxidized LDL
TNF alpha or TNF-α	tumor necrosis factor-alpha

Author details

Saima Sharif*, Saira Rafaqat and Shagufta Naz
Department of Zoology, Lahore College for Women University, Lahore, Punjab

*Address all correspondence to: ssharif1978@yahoo.com

References

[1] Varanasi VK. Metabolic syndrome: The genetic aspect. Endocrinology & Metabolic Syndrome. 2011;**1**(S1):1-2

[2] Kaur J. A comprehensive review on metabolic syndrome. Cardiology research and practice. 2014;**2014**:1-21; 943162

[3] Srikanthan K, Feyh A, Visweshwar H, Shapiro JI, Sodhi K. Systematic review of metabolic syndrome biomarkers: A panel for early detection, management, and risk stratification in the West Virginian population. International Journal of Medical Sciences. 2016;**13**(1):25

[4] Sagar S, Liu PP, Cooper LT Jr. Myocarditis. The Lancet. 2012 Feb 25;**379**(9817):738-747

[5] Schwarz F, Mall G, Zebe H, Blickle J, Derks H, Manthey J, et al. Quantitative morphologic findings of the myocardium in idiopathic dilated cardiomyopathy. The American Journal of Cardiology. 1983 Feb 1;**51**(3):501-506

[6] Jefferies JL, Towbin JA. Dilated cardiomyopathy. The Lancet. 2010 Feb 27;**375**(9716):752-762

[7] Chung MW, Tsoutsman T, Semsarian C. Hypertrophic cardiomyopathy: From gene defect to clinical disease. Cell Research. 2003;**13**:9-20

[8] Yndestad A, Damas JK, Oie E, Ueland T, Gullestad L, Aukrust P. Role of inflammation in the progression of heart failure. Current Cardiology Reports. 2007;**9**:236-241

[9] Francis GS, Tang WH. Pathophysiology of congestive heart failure. Reviews in Cardiovascular Medicine. 2003;**4**(Suppl 2):S14-S20

[10] Lefkowitz RJ, Willerson JT. Prospects for cardiovascular research. JAMA. 2001;**285**:581-587

[11] George J, Patal S, Wexler D, Sharabi Y, Peleg E, Kamari Y, et al. Circulating adiponectin concentrations in patients with congestive heart failure. Heart. 2006 Oct 1;**92**(10):1420-1424

[12] Won H, Kang SM, Shin MJ, Oh J, Hong N, Park S, et al. Plasma adiponectin concentration and its association with metabolic syndrome in patients with heart failure. Yonsei Medical Journal. 2012 Jan 1;**53**(1):91-98

[13] Baldasseroni S, Antenore A, Di Serio C, Orso F, Lonetto G, Bartoli N, et al. Adiponectin, diabetes and ischemic heart failure: A challenging relationship. Cardiovascular Diabetology. 2012 Dec;**11**(1):1-8

[14] Bobbert P, Jenke A, Bobbert T, Kühl U, Rauch U, Lassner D, et al. High leptin and resistin expression in chronic heart failure: Adverse outcome in patients with dilated and inflammatory cardiomyopathy. European Journal of Heart Failure. 2012 Nov;**14**(11):1265-1275

[15] Toth MJ, Gottlieb SS, Fisher ML, Ryan AS, Nicklas BJ, Poehlman ET. Plasma leptin concentrations and energy expenditure in heart failure patients. Metabolism. 1997 Apr 1;**46**(4):450-453

[16] Barbosa-Ferreira JM, Fernandes F, Dabarian A, Mady C. Leptin in heart failure. Expert Opinion on Medical Diagnostics. 2013 Jan 1;7(1):113-117

[17] Wannamethee SG, Shaper AG, Whincup PH, Lennon L, Papacosta O, Sattar N. The obesity paradox in men with coronary heart disease and heart

failure: The role of muscle mass and leptin. International Journal of Cardiology. 2014 Jan 15;**171**(1):49-55

[18] Wannamethee SG, Shaper AG, Whincup PH, Lennon L, Sattar N. Obesity and risk of incident heart failure in older men with and without pre-existing coronary heart disease: Does leptin have a role? Journal of the American College of Cardiology. 2011 Oct 25;**58**(18):1870-1877

[19] Filippatos GS, Tsilias K, Venetsanou K, Karambinos E, Manolatos D, Kranidis A, et al. Leptin serum levels in cachectic heart failure patients: Relationship with tumor necrosis factor-α system. International Journal of Cardiology. 2000 Nov 1;**76**(2-3):117-122

[20] Schulze PC, Kratzsch J, Linke A, Schoene N, Adams V, Gielen S, et al. Elevated serum levels of leptin and soluble leptin receptor in patients with advanced chronic heart failure. European Journal of Heart Failure. 2003 Jan;**5**(1):33-40

[21] Murdoch DR, Rooney E, Dargie HJ, Shapiro D, Morton JJ, McMurray JJ. Inappropriately low plasma leptin concentration in the cachexia associated with chronic heart failure. Heart. 1999 Sep 1;**82**(3):352-356

[22] Lieb W, Sullivan LM, Harris TB, Roubenoff R, Benjamin EJ, Levy D, et al. Plasma leptin levels and incidence of heart failure, cardiovascular disease, and total mortality in elderly individuals. Diabetes Care. 2009 Apr 1;**32**(4):612-616

[23] Anker SD, Doehner W, Rauchhaus M, Sharma R, Francis D, Knosalla C, et al. Uric acid and survival in chronic heart failure: Validation and application in metabolic, functional, and hemodynamic staging. Circulation. 2003 Apr 22;**107**(15):1991-1997

[24] Cicoira M, Zanolla L, Rossi A, Golia G, Franceschini L, Brighetti G, et al. Elevated serum uric acid levels are associated with diastolic dysfunction in patients with dilated cardiomyopathy. American Heart Journal. 2002 Jun 1;**143**(6):1107-1111

[25] Wannamethee SG, Papacosta O, Lennon L, Whincup PH. Serum uric acid as a potential marker for heart failure risk in men on antihypertensive treatment: The British Regional Heart Study. International Journal of Cardiology. 2018 Feb 1;**252**:187-192

[26] Hamaguchi S, Furumoto T, Tsuchihashi-Makaya M, Goto K, Goto D, Yokota T, et al. Hyperuricemia predicts adverse outcomes in patients with heart failure. International Journal of Cardiology. 2011 Sep 1;**151**(2):143-147

[27] Krishnan E. Hyperuricemia and incident heart failure. Circulation: Heart Failure. 2009 Nov 1;**2**(6):556-562

[28] Huang H, Huang B, Li Y, Huang Y, Li J, Yao H, et al. Uric acid and risk of heart failure: A systematic review and meta-analysis. European Journal of Heart Failure. 2014 Jan;**16**(1):15-24

[29] Doehner W, Schoene N, Rauchhaus M, Leyva-Leon F, Pavitt DV, Reaveley DA, et al. Effects of xanthine oxidase inhibition with allopurinol on endothelial function and peripheral blood flow in hyperuricemic patients with chronic heart failure: Results from 2 placebo-controlled studies. Circulation. 2002 Jun 4;**105**(22):2619-2624

[30] Xu X, Hu X, Lu Z, Zhang P, Zhao L, Wessale JL, et al. Xanthine oxidase inhibition with febuxostat attenuates systolic overload-induced left ventricular hypertrophy and dysfunction in mice. Journal of Cardiac Failure. 2008 Nov 1;**14**(9):746-753

[31] Dunlay SM, Weston SA, Redfield MM, Killian JM, Roger VL. Tumor necrosis factor-α and mortality in heart failure: A community study. Circulation. 2008 Aug 5;**118**(6):625-631

[32] Chia YC, Kieneker LM, van Hassel G, Binnenmars SH, Nolte IM, van Zanden JJ, et al. Interleukin 6 and development of heart failure with preserved ejection fraction in the general population. Journal of the American Heart Association. 2021 Jun 1;**10**(11):e018549

[33] Markousis-Mavrogenis G, Tromp J, Ouwerkerk W, Devalaraja M, Anker SD, Cleland JG, et al. The clinical significance of interleukin-6 in heart failure: Results from the BIOSTAT-CHF study. European Journal of Heart Failure. 2019 Aug;**21**(8):965-973

[34] Deokar SA, Dandekar SP, Shinde GA, Prabhu SS, Patawardhan M. Role of serum interleukin-6 in heart failure. International Journal of Advances in Medicine. 2018;**5**:936-940

[35] Hudzik B, Szkodzinski J, Romanowski W, Danikiewicz A, Wilczek K, Lekston A, et al. Serum interleukin-6 concentration reflects the extent of asymptomatic left ventricular dysfunction and predicts progression to heart failure in patients with stable coronary artery disease. Cytokine. 2011 Jun 1;**54**(3):266-271

[36] MacGowan GA, Mann DL, Kormos RL, Feldman AM, Murali S. Circulating interleukin-6 in severe heart failure. The American Journal of Cardiology. 1997 Apr 15;**79**(8):1128-1131

[37] Meléndez GC, McLarty JL, Levick SP, Du Y, Janicki JS, Brower GL. Interleukin 6 mediates myocardial fibrosis, concentric hypertrophy, and diastolic dysfunction in rats. Hypertension. 2010 Aug 1;**56**(2):225-231

[38] Rauchhaus M, Doehner W, Francis DP, Davos C, Kemp M, Liebenthal C, et al. Plasma cytokine parameters and mortality in patients with chronic heart failure. Circulation. 2000 Dec 19;**102**(25):3060-3067

[39] Nguyen TM. Adiponectin: Role in physiology and pathophysiology. International Journal of Preventive Medicine. 2020;**11**:136

[40] Ouchi N, Shibata R, Walsh K. Cardioprotection by adiponectin. Trends in Cardiovascular Medicine. 2006 Jul 1;**16**(5):141-146

[41] Skurk C, Wittchen F, Suckau L, Witt H, Noutsias M, Fechner H, et al. Description of a local cardiac adiponectin system and its deregulation in dilated cardiomyopathy. European Heart Journal. 2008 May 1;**29**(9):1168-1180

[42] Kistorp C, Faber J, Galatius S, Gustafsson F, Frystyk J, Flyvbjerg A, et al. Plasma adiponectin, body mass index, and mortality in patients with chronic heart failure. Circulation. 2005 Sep 20;**112**(12):1756-1762

[43] Anker SD, Ponikowski P, Varney S, Chua TP, Clark AL, Webb-Peploe KM, et al. Wasting as independent risk factor for mortality in chronic heart failure. The Lancet. 1997 Apr 12;**349**(9058):1050-1053

[44] Dhandapany PS, Kang S, Kashyap DK, Rajagopal R, Sundaresan NR, Singh R, et al. Adiponectin receptor 1 variants contribute to hypertrophic cardiomyopathy that can be reversed by rapamycin. Science Advances. 2021 Jan 6;**7**(2):eabb3991

[45] Liao Y, Takashima S, Maeda N, Ouchi N, Komamura K, Shimomura I, et al. Exacerbation of heart failure in adiponectin-deficient mice due to impaired regulation of AMPK and

glucose metabolism. Cardiovascular Research. 2005 Sep 1;**67**(4):705-713

[46] Shibata R, Ouchi N, Ito M, Kihara S, Shiojima I, Pimentel DR, et al. Adiponectin-mediated modulation of hypertrophic signals in the heart. Nature Medicine. 2004 Dec;**10**(12):1384-1389

[47] Tamariz L, Hassan B, Palacio A, Arcement L, Horswell R, Hebert K. Metabolic syndrome increases mortality in heart failure. Clinical Cardiology. 2009 Jun;**32**(6):327-331

[48] Frankel DS, Vasan RS, D'Agostino RB, Benjamin EJ, Levy D, Wang TJ, et al. Resistin, adiponectin, and risk of heart failure: The Framingham offspring study. Journal of the American College of Cardiology. 2009 Mar 3;**53**(9):754-762

[49] Lane PW, Dickie MM. The effect of restricted food intake on the life span of genetically obese mice. The Journal of Nutrition. 1958;**64**:549-554

[50] Zhang Y, Proenca R, Maffei M, Barone M, Leopold L, Friedman JM. Positional cloning of the mouse obese gene and its human homologue. Nature. 1994;**372**:425-432

[51] Hall ME, Harmancey R, Stec DE. Lean heart: Role of leptin in cardiac hypertrophy and metabolism. World Journal of Cardiology. 2015 Sep 26;**7**(9):511-524

[52] Singhal A, Farooqi IS, Cole TJ, O'Rahilly S, Fewtrell M, Kattenhorn M, et al. Influence of leptin on arterial distensibility: A novel link between obesity and cardiovascular disease? Circulation. 2002;**106**:1919-1924

[53] Chaudhary K, Malhotra K, Sowers J, Aroor A. Uric acid-key ingredient in the recipe for cardiorenal metabolic syndrome. Cardiorenal Medicine. 2013;**3**(3):208-220

[54] Ishizaka N, Ishizaka Y, Toda E, Nagai R, Yamakado M. Association between serum uric acid, metabolic syndrome, and carotid atherosclerosis in Japanese individuals. Arteriosclerosis, Thrombosis, and Vascular Biology. 2005;**25**:1038-1044

[55] Ndrepepa G. Uric acid and cardiovascular disease. Clinica Chimica Acta. 2018 Sep 1;**484**:150-163

[56] Givertz MM, Anstrom KJ, Redfield MM, Deswal A, Haddad H, Butler J, et al. Effects of xanthine oxidase inhibition in hyperuricemic heart failure patients: The xanthine oxidase inhibition for hyperuricemic heart failure patients (EXACT-HF) study. Circulation. 2015 May 19;**131**(20):1763-1771

[57] Hare JM, Mangal B, Brown J, Fisher C, Freudenberger R, Colucci WS, et al. Impact of oxypurinol in patients with symptomatic heart failure: Results of the OPT-CHF study. Journal of the American College of Cardiology. 2008 Jun 17;**51**(24):2301-2309

[58] Idriss HT, Naismith JH. TNF alpha and the TNF receptor superfamily: Structure-function relationship(s). Microscopy Research and Technique. 2000 Aug 1;**50**(3):184-195

[59] Balasoiu M, Balasoiu AT, Stepan AE, Dinescu SN, Avramescu CS, Dumitrescu D, et al. Proatherogenic adipocytokines levels in metabolic syndrome. Romanian Journal of Morphology and Embryology [Revue roumaine de morphologie et embryologie]. 2014;**55**:29-33

[60] Yu M, Wen S, Wang M, Liang W, Li HH, Long Q, et al. TNF-α-secreting B cells contribute to myocardial

fibrosis in dilated cardiomyopathy. Journal of Clinical Immunology. 2013 Jul;**33**(5):1002-1008

[61] Sun M, Chen M, Dawood F, Zurawska U, Li JY, Parker T, et al. Tumor necrosis factor-α mediates cardiac remodeling and ventricular dysfunction after pressure overload state. Circulation. 2007 Mar 20;**115**(11):1398-1407

[62] Mann DL. Inflammatory mediators and the failing heart: Past, present, and the foreseeable future. Circulation Research. 2002 Nov 29;**91**(11):988-998

[63] Schumacher SM, Naga Prasad SV. Tumor necrosis factor-α in heart failure: An updated review. Current Cardiology Reports. 2018 Sep 26;**20**(11):117. DOI: 10.1007/s11886-018-1067-7 PMID: 30259192; PMCID: PMC6311126

[64] Tanaka T, Narazaki M, Kishimoto T. IL-6 in inflammation, immunity, and disease. Cold Spring Harbor Perspectives in Biology. 2014 Sep 4;**6**(10):a016295

[65] Gullestad L, Ueland T, Vinge LE, Finsen A, Yndestad A, Aukrust P. Inflammatory cytokines in heart failure: Mediators and markers. Cardiology. 2012;**122**(1):23-35

[66] Roig E, Orús J, Paré C, Azqueta M, Filella X, Perez-Villa F, et al. Serum interleukin-6 in congestive heart failure secondary to idiopathic dilated cardiomyopathy. The American Journal of Cardiology. 1998 Sep 1;**82**(5):688-690

[67] Santoro F, Tarantino N, Ferraretti A, Ieva R, Musaico F, Guastafierro F, et al. Serum interleukin 6 and 10 levels in Takotsubo cardiomyopathy: Increased admission levels may predict adverse events at follow-up. Atherosclerosis. 2016 Nov 1;**254**:28-34

[68] Tsutamoto T, Hisanaga T, Wada A, Maeda K, Ohnishi M, Fukai D, et al. Interleukin-6 spillover in the peripheral circulation increases with the severity of heart failure, and the high plasma level of interleukin-6 is an important prognostic predictor in patients with congestive heart failure. Journal of the American College of Cardiology. 1998 Feb;**31**(2):391-398

Chapter 3

Effects of Diabetes Mellitus on the Conduction System of the Heart: Mini-Review

Manal Smail, Sunil Rupee, Khemraj Rupee, Abla Mohammed Ahmed Ismail, Sara Sultan, Frank Christopher Howarth, Ernest A. Adeghate and Jaipaul Singh

Abstract

Diabetes mellitus can induce substantial damage to the conduction system of the heart, especially the sinoatrial node. This is due to hyperglycemia leading to bradyarrhythmia. DM, via the elevation of HG, generates the production of a number of insulting agents in the myocardium known as reactive oxygen species and reactive carbonyl species, which elicit direct damage to neuro-filament-M and β_2-adrenergic receptors in the conducting system as well as a number of cardiac contractile, cation transporting and channel proteins. One cation channel protein is the hyperpolarization-activated cyclic nucleotide-gated potassium channel. It encodes the protein responsible for the hyperpolarizing-activated current or the "funny current" that participates in spontaneous diastolic membrane depolarization in sinoatrial node cells. Gene expression of these proteins and their physiological functions are decreased in the diabetic heart, which affects the generation of electrical impulses or action potentials resulting in increases in RR and PR intervals and QRS complex duration of the electrocardiogram. The heart rate and force of contraction of the myocardium are decreased leading to bradyarrhythmia and sudden cardiac death. This review attempts to explain the cellular mechanism(s) involved in diabetes-induced bradyarrhythmia with emphasis on cation-transporting proteins, especially the hyperpolarization-activated cyclic nucleotide-gated channels pacemaker current channels.

Keywords: diabetes mellitus, sinoatrial node (SAN), heart, cardiac conduction system, arrhythmias

1. Introduction

Diabetes mellitus (DM) is a serious global disease that currently affects more than 480 million people, and its number is growing rapidly. DM results from hyperglycemia (HG) and it is responsible for many long-term complications [1]. Cardiovascular diseases (CVDs) account for more than half of the observed mortality in the diabetic population [2]. Nodal myocytes spontaneously generate APs in the absence of hormonal and neural stimulation [3]. Decreased heart rate (HR) is a common finding in patients with type 1 diabetes mellitus (T1DM) [4] indicating that many of these patients are likely to have impaired pacemaker function [5]. Cardiovascular defects are the major cause of morbidity and mortality in diabetic patients [6]. The cause of cardiac conduction disorders (CCDs) in DM patients is not fully understood. It remains unclear whether autonomic neuropathy or CVDs play a role [7]. This review addresses the effects of DM on the cardiac conduction system (CCS) which in turn can lead to arrhythmias and subsequently, sudden cardiac death (SCD). But first, it is important to understand the normal physiology of the conduction system before considering the mechanism(s) that might underlie the pathophysiology of DM-induced electrical conduction defects in the heart and its treatment.

2. Conduction system of the heart

2.1 Sinoatrial node action potential

The human SAN is composed of specialized cardiomyocytes. SAN cells spontaneously generate APs [8]. SAN cells are smaller than the surrounding atrial muscle cells and have fewer mitochondria and myofilaments. Atrial myocytes interdigitate with the SAN cells and assist in the conduction of APs from SAN to atrial myocytes. The SAN is the primary pacemaker center of the heart, and it is necessary to describe the normal function of the SAN before considering the effects of DM [8]. In a normal heart, pacemaker cells in the SAN control the rate of contraction of the heart. APs generated by the SAN cells are conducted and spread rapidly through the atria leading to the contraction of the atrial myocardium and the passage of blood into the ventricles [9]. There is a short delay in the atrioventricular node (AVN) before the APs are conducted and spread rapidly through the ventricles leading to contraction of the ventricles and pumping of blood into the pulmonary and systemic circulations. The atria and ventricles are electrically isolated from each other by what is known as the skeleton of the heart [10]. It consists of connective tissue that insulates the atria from the ventricles and provides a framework to support the heart valves [11]. The AVN is connected to the bundle of His. The bundle of His is an effective cable for conducting APs and distributing them to the ventricles. Conduction through the AVN is rather slow (about 100 ms) to prevent ventricular stimulation before the atria have finished contracting. **Figure 1** illustrates the physiological events involved in cardiac muscle contraction (systole) and relaxation (diastole) starting with the initiation of electrical impulses in the SAN and spreading throughout the myocardium [12].

The APs of the SAN occur in three phases. Phase 4 involves a period of gradual depolarization, which is unique to pacemaker cells, that participates in spontaneous diastolic membrane depolarization in SAN cells. Pacemaker currents are generated by the slow influx of Na^+ ions through the HCN channels [13]. The passage of electrical currents through L-type and T-type Ca^{2+} channels and reduced K^+ conductance also contribute to SAN phase 4 depolarization. This pacing current changes the membrane potential from −60 mV to a threshold potential of −40 mV. The Phase 4 gradient determines HR and varies from region to region and from pacemaker cell to pacemaker cell. The SAN pacemaker cells depolarize at a rate from 60 to 100 per minute, and the AVN depolarizes at a rate from 40 to 60 per minute [14].

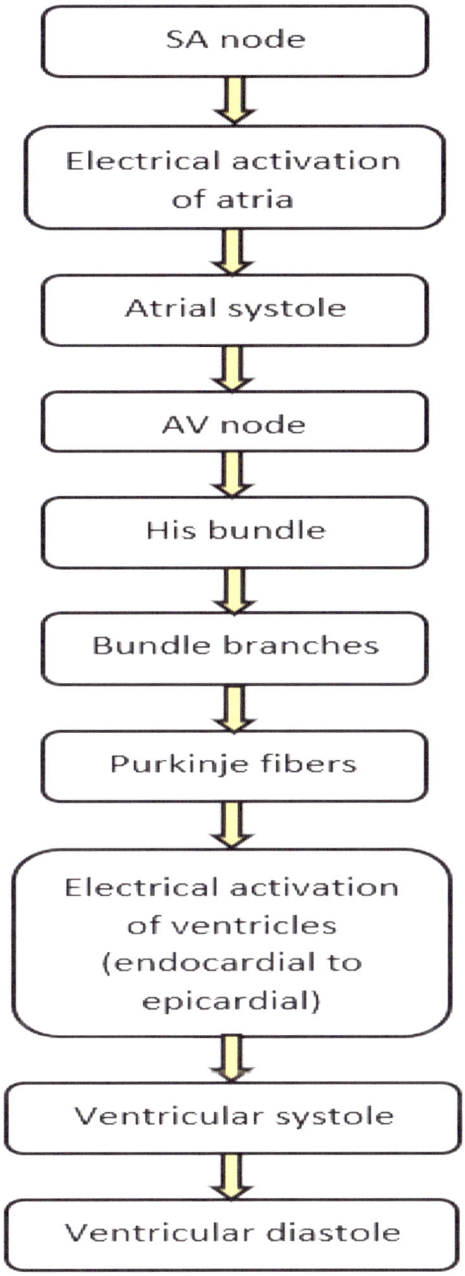

Figure 1.
Flow diagram showing the different physiological events of excitation-contraction-coupling (ECC) in the heart starting from the initiation of an electrical impulse in the SAN, and then transmission of the impulse to the different parts of the conduction system to initiate contraction (ejection of blood) and relaxation (filling) of the myocardium.

Since the SAN has the highest depolarization rate, it is normally the primary pacemaker center of the heart. Phase 0 is the depolarization phase of the AP. This stage begins when the membrane potential reaches the threshold potential. L-type Ca^{2+} current is the major ionic conductance responsible for phase 0 [15]. This influx of Ca^{2+} increases the membrane potential from −40 mV to +10 mV. Calcium channels are slow channels (compared to sodium channels), so the depolarizing upstrokes are not as steep as those observed in cardiomyocytes. During repolarization (phase 3), the Ca^{2+} channels close, and the voltage-gated K^+ channels open, allowing the outflow of K^+. This cation outflow reduces the membrane potential from +10 to −60 mV. Phases 1 and 2 do not exist in pacemaker cells [14]. The slope of phase 4 determines the HR, and it is different for pacemaker cells in different regions of the heart. The rate of AP generation by the SAN is limited by the rate at which Na^+ enters through the HCN channel (funny current) [16]. The more HCN channels open, the faster Na^+ enters the cell and the steeper the pacemaker potential allowing the cell membrane to reach threshold sooner, thereby shortening the time between APs as illustrated in **Figure 2** [14].

The sympathetic and parasympathetic branches of the autonomic nervous system (ANS) have the opposite effects on HR by opening and closing HCN channels as illustrated in **Figure 3**. Norepinephrine (NEP) released from the sympathetic nerves binds to the β1-adrenergic receptor. The β1-adrenergic receptor binds via the G protein or Gs (stimulation) and stimulates the enzyme adenylate cyclase to increase the production of the second messenger, cyclic adenosine monophosphate (cAMP) [17]. The epinephrine (EPI) that circulates in the blood also binds to β1-adrenergic receptors. HCN channels are sensitive to cAMP, which, in turn, increases HCN "funny current," thereby decreasing the time between APs in the SAN. On the other hand, acetylcholine (ACh), released by the parasympathetic nerves, has the opposite effect because it binds to M2 muscarinic receptors, which are linked to the generation of

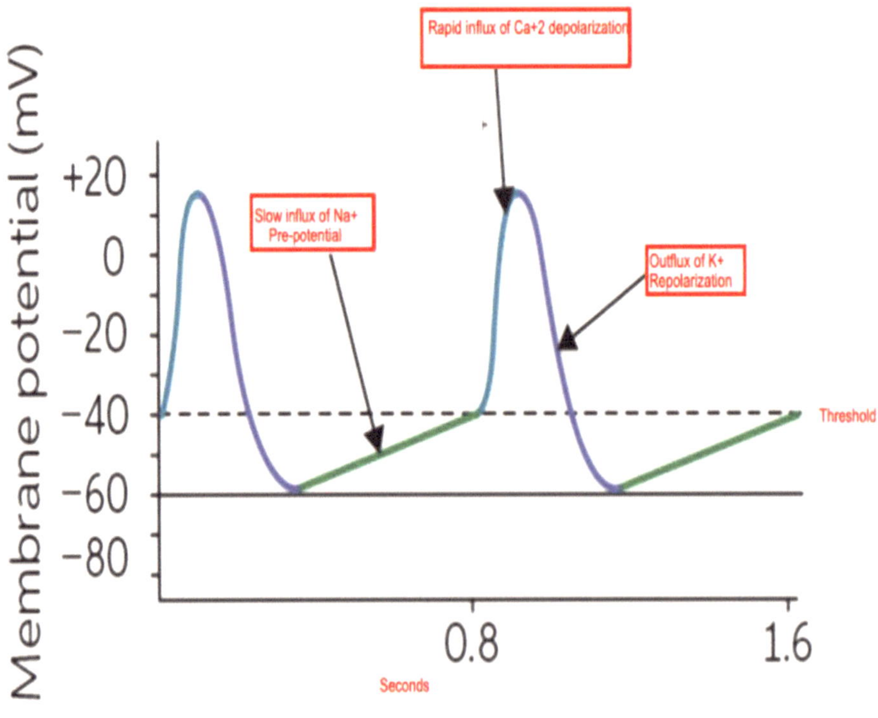

Figure 2.
Different phases of the SAN action potential.

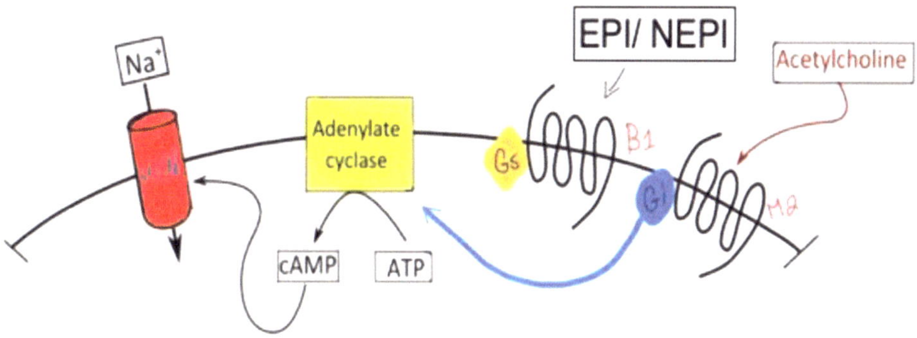

Figure 3.
The opening and closing of HCN channels are regulated by the intracellular second messenger cAMP. Increased cAMP occurs when either norepinephrine or epinephrine binds to Gs-coupled β1 receptors, whereas acetylcholine has the opposite effect when bound to Gi-coupled M2 receptors (ATP = adenosine triphosphate); NEP = norepinephrine; EPI = epinephrine.

cyclic guanosine monophosphate (cyclic GMP) via the activation of guanylate cyclase and at the same time inhibiting adenylate cyclase; thereby, reducing HCN "funny current" [18].

2.2 Automaticity of the sinoatrial node

The spontaneous excitation of pacemaker cells of SAN is responsible for the generation of automaticity in the heart. The presence of diastolic depolarization (DD) is what causes spontaneous activity. This depolarization brings the membrane voltage from the end of the repolarization phase to the threshold of the action potential that will follow. As a reflection of the complex nature of this physiological process, there has been a long-standing and significant amount of debate regarding the ionic mechanisms that are underlying DD [14]. DD in the SAN is caused by the opening of hyperpolarization-activated cyclic nucleotide-gated (HCN) channels, which pass an inward cation current known as the "funny" current (If) [14]. There are two types of voltage-gated Ca^{2+} channels: T-type and L-type. Subtypes of the T-type include Cav3.1, Cav3.2, and Cav3.3. And the L-type subtypes are Cav1.2 and Cav1.3; Cav1.3 is highly expressed in SAN. As Vm becomes more positive, HCN channels begin to close, and voltage-gated Ca^{2+} channels 3.1 (CaV3.1) and 1.3 (CaV1.3) begin to open, generating the depolarizing transient (T-type) current (ICa,T) and the CaV1.3 component of the long-lasting (L-type) Ca^{2+} current (ICa,L) that result in the continuation of DD [19].

Ryanodine receptors (RyRs) regulate Ca^{2+} release from the sarcoplasmic reticulum (SR) during late diastolic depolarization. This has been shown to be another important factor in regulating APs in pacemaker cells [20]. The sarco/endoplasmic reticulum Ca^{2+}-ATPase (SERCA) recycles some of this Ca^{2+} back into the SR, but the Na^{+}-Ca^{2+} exchanger pumps the rest out of the cell via an electrogenic, depolarizing current [20]. At a voltage of 40 mV, the CaV1.2 channel opens, producing more ICa, L and stimulating the SAN. By repolarizing Vm, K^{+} currents from both fast and slow delayed rectifiers reactivate If and kick off a new cycle of DD [21].

The autonomic nervous system (ANS) is a major regulator of SAN automaticity and sinoatrial conduction [17]. Autonomic dysfunction is a common cause of SAN dysfunction. Adrenergic or cholinergic dysregulation may contribute to pacemaker and conduction abnormalities within the SAN [18]. Tachycardia-bradycardia syndrome is the extreme manifestation of a continuum characterized by a significant loss of SAN function integrity [18, 19]. It has been reported that a high concentration (30 mol/L) of ryanodine, which blocks the SR Ca^{2+} release channel, eliminates the spontaneous activity of isolated SA node cells from rabbits, which led them to hypothesize that SR Ca^{2+} release is essential for pace-making. Because of the observation of the chronotropic effect in isolated SA node cells from rabbits is abolished or greatly reduced after the suppression of the Ca^{2+} transient by a submaximal concentration of ryanodine (3 mol/L), another study reported that the positive chronotropic effect of β-adrenergic stimulation is the result of the increase in the Ca^{2+} transient caused by β-adrenergic stimulation [18].

2.3 Atrioventricular node action

The atrioventricular node (AVN) is a complex structure that performs various functions in the heart and works primarily as an electrical gatekeeper between the atria and the ventricles. It introduces a delay between atrial and ventricular excitation; thereby, facilitating the emptying of the atria and filling of the ventricles. This delay prevents simultaneous ventricular excitation and ensures one-way blood flow through the heart chambers [22]. The AVN transmits electrical stimulation from the atria to the ventricles via fast or slow pathways. Many electrophysiological differences between these pathways predispose the atrioventricular junction to arrhythmias [23]. These different electrophysiological properties of fast and slow signaling pathways are due to their unique structural and molecular composition (tissue and cellular geometry, ion channels, and gap junctions). Similar to SAN cells, AVN cells spontaneously depolarize. In a normal heart, the rate of spontaneous depolarization of the AVN is slower than that of the SAN; and thus, the rate of AVN cell depolarization is controlled by impulses generated by the SAN [21].

The depolarization phase 0 of the AP in AVN cells is due to voltage-gated Ca^{2+} channels, and most of the current is due to Ca^{2+} influx through L-type Ca^{2+} channels. These voltage-gated ion channels are closed in the resting state and become either active or open when the threshold voltage is reached. When active, these channels allow Ca^{2+} ions to flow into the cell [24]. The influx of Ca^{2+} into the cell causes the release of additional Ca^{2+} from the SR. This is called calcium-induced calcium release (CICR) and occurs through a specific channel in the SR membrane known as the ryanodine receptor (RyR). Over time, L-type Ca^{2+} channels undergo a conformational change to an inactive, closed, or non-conductive state, even if the cell membrane potential remains above the threshold voltage [14]. At this time, the SR ryanodine receptor channel also closes, stopping the influx of Ca^{2+} into the cytoplasm. Thereafter, Ca^{2+} released into the cytoplasm of AV node cells is removed from the cytoplasm by two mechanisms. They include the sodium-calcium exchanger (NCX), which transports Ca^{2+} from inside the cell in exchange for Na^+ entering the cell. During phase 3 of action potentials, the AVN cell membrane is repolarized by the outflow of K^+ from the cell due to the activation of voltage-gated K^+ channels. The relative gradient of Na^+ and K^+ and the electrical gradient across the cell membrane are finally restored by the action of the Na^+/K^+ ATPase pump, and the AV nodule cells are ready for depolarization again [25].

Gap junctions are important in impulse conduction in the heart. Over the last decade, research has revealed that gap junctions are encoded by the connexins, a multigene family [22]. There are at least 15 connexin genes in the vertebrate genome. Connexins have been classified into two groups based on their molecular weight or their class as determined by protein sequence. There are three major connexin isotypes expressed in the heart: connexin (Cx)43 (1 connexin), Cx45 (6 connexin), and Cx40 (5 connexin). Each of these connexins has distinct channel properties and is regulated by distinct gating mechanisms. The distribution of Cx channels varies within the SAN. Electrical coupling is weak in the center of the SAN because Cx40 and Cx43, which form large and medium conductance channels, are only sparingly expressed or absent. However, Cx45, which forms small-conductance channels, is expressed in the SAN's center. Cx40, Cx43, and Cx45 are all present at the SAN's periphery; however, the strong electrical coupling is required to drive the atrial myocardium [22].

3. Diabetes mellitus induces changes in the conduction system of the heart

DM is a major risk factor for the development of cardiovascular complications, including cardiac arrhythmias, prolonged QT intervals, and SCD [26]. AVN blockade and bradycardic arrhythmia [27] are significantly higher in DM patients. There is considerable evidence for cardiac remodeling and altered ion channel activity/expression which are involved in HR and rhythm regulation [28]. In particular, Type 1 diabetes mellitus (T1DM) affects a range of cardiac ion channel currents, including L-type calcium currents (ICaL) and fast and slow delayed rectifier potassium currents (IKr and IKs) [29], as well as transient outward potassium current (Ito) [30].

Insulin treatment of rat ventricles and human atrial cardiomyocytes has been reported to increase ICaL density with significant upregulation of mRNA and protein expression of L-type calcium channels [31]. Altered SR-Ca^{2+} content and RyR2 binding, as well as altered RyR2 mRNA protein levels [32], are normalized after insulin treatment in STZ-induced T1DM animals. In addition, decreased SR Ca-ATPase (SERCA2a) activity in rats with STZ-induced T1DM can be reversed by insulin treatment [33]. Insulin therapy has also been shown to restore decreased levels of NCX1 protein and mRNA in the ventricles [34]. Taken together, these findings suggest a direct stimulatory effect of insulin on cell contractility, mediated by Ca^{2+} signaling proteins and membrane ion channels. Therefore, insulin treatment may be an important approach that reverses the QT interval and QRS complex prolongation in T1DM.

Among the diabetes induced electrical disorders is nodular dysfunction, which is due to alterations in HCN channels. Four alpha subunit isoforms have been described, including HCN1, HCN2, HCN3, and HCN4 (encoded by HCN14). HCN channels are mainly expressed in the myocytes of the cardiac conduction system. Genetic studies have characterized the functional role of HCN4 in cardiac physiology. Mice subjected to heart-specific HCN4 ablation showed bradycardia and atrioventricular block [35]. In addition, patch-clamp analysis of SAN cells showed a 70% reduction in the "funny" current (IF) and a 60% reduction in spontaneous beat rate [35]. These results confirm that HCN4 is important in maintaining the molecular mechanism of pacemaker function. Previously, Howarth et al. identified reduced expression of HCN4 mRNA in rats with STZ-induced T1DM. Some diabetics have shown slow depolarization of the ventricles [36]. This is shown in the ECG as an increase in QRS duration. Reduced expression of HCN4, connexin, and ion channels was also identified in various regions of the cardiac conduction system (CCS) in the STZ model of T1DM [37]. Moreover, in a study on hearts of T1DM rats, it was reported that the dysfunction of the CCS plays an integral role in developing cardiac arrhythmias due to increases in RR interval, PR interval and QRS complex duration of the ECG [38]. These alterations were due to decreases in rate of SAN and HCN4 (pacemaker current) as well as downregulation of the gene expression for HCN4 channels, neuro-filament-M and β2-adrenergic receptor within the SAN of the myocardium during T1DM. It is possible that changes in the expression of these different cardiac proteins within the SAN are closely associated with the regulation of the electrical signaling of the myocardium. In turn, this can adversely affect cardiac AP generation and propagation, leading to arrhythmia [38].

4. Pathological effect of diabetes on sinoatrial node activity

Both basic and clinical research studies have shown that diabetes can impair the autonomic control of heart rate (HR) [39]. According to McDowell et al. [40], diabetic rabbits have a significant impairment in the parasympathetic-mediated baroreceptor control of HR. This impairment has been linked to impaired parasympathetic control of the heart in diabetes. The parasympathetic control of HR is also significantly impaired in diabetic rats, as shown by lower heart rate variability (HRV) [41]. Zhang et al. [42] reported that the negative chronotropic response to carbachol (a parasympathomimetic agonist) was blunted in Akita diabetic mice versus wild-type mice. These findings are consistent with results obtained in human T1DM patients who had significant impairments in parasympathetic control of heart rate [43].

Diabetes may also be associated with an increase in harmful arrhythmias due to impaired SAN activity. SAN function is evaluated *in vivo* using intracardiac programmed electrical stimulation and sinus node recovery time (SNRT) [44]. Experimental studies have used both animal and human models to study changes in SNRT. Depending on the conditions in which these alterations take place, sinus node prolongation and shortening of the SNRT can both be pathological and indicative of sinus node dysfunction [44]. This response may reflect the impaired ability of the SAN to correct for physiological changes in heart rate following the development of diabetes [45]. Experimental and clinical studies showed that a diseased or failing heart is prone to develop ventricular fibrillation (VF), which is the main cause of sudden cardiac death, particularly during a heart attack. Slow conduction and fractionated electrocardiograms were recorded in the infarcted human heart [46, 47]. Atrial tachyarrhythmias caused by rapid pacing were more likely to occur in RCx40-deficient mice [48]. As well as a reduction in Cx40 was found in humans with chronic atrial fibrillation (AF) [49]. As a result, it suggests that connexin down-regulation may also be a factor in the persistence of AF. It should be stressed that aging and CVDs are, in addition to structural and gap junction remodeling, characterized by abnormal Ca^{2+} handling [50]. Myocardial conduction in Cx43-deficient mice was noticeably slowed, which encourages re-entrant arrhythmias and sudden arrhythmic death (SAD) [51]. In rats with diabetes mellitus, down-regulation and/or abnormal distribution of myocardial Cx43-positive gap junctions have been linked with increased susceptibility to ventricular arrhythmia. Diabetes was linked to myocardial fibrosis. Reduced gap junction coupling in fibrosis-affected regions of the myocardium may disrupt wave-front propagation and thereby obstruct synchronized and uniform cardiomyocyte function [50]. Given the importance of gap junction connexin channels in cardiac arrhythmogenesis, it appears that aimed modulation of intercellular communication to prevent spatial electrical heterogeneities in viable myocardium is a promising way to combat life-threatening arrhythmias and SCD in humans. Nonetheless, more detailed analysis and research are required to address this issue in search of novel therapeutic approaches.

5. Conclusion

Figure 4 summarizes the various events leading to a decreased HR or bradyarrhythmia and subsequently, SCD. It is postulated that DM, via an elevation in HG, can initiate the production of ROS and RCS to induce cardiac muscle damage, apoptosis, fibrosis, and subsequently cardiac remodeling. These pathophysiological changes are associated with severe damage to nerves and β1-adrenergic receptors as well as electrical and mechanical dysfunction of the myocardium leading to a decrease in HR, cardiac arrhythmias, and subsequently SCD. Experiments with animal models have consistently shown that diabetes can alter the expression and regulation of cardiac ion channels and contractile proteins, which impair impulse generation, conduction,

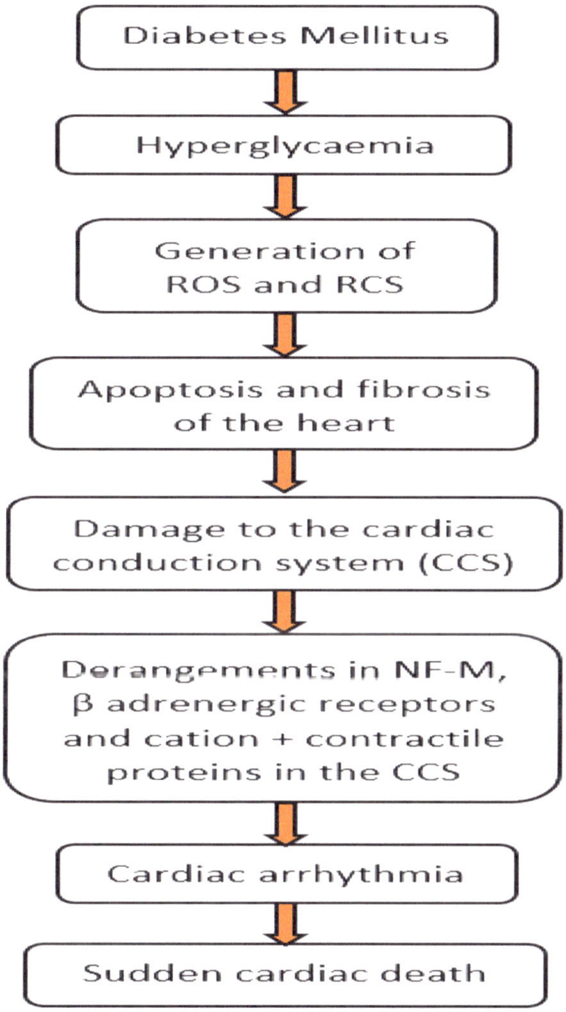

Figure 4.
A flow diagram summarizes the effects of DM on the myocardium starting with hyperglycemia to the generation of ROS and RCS followed by apoptosis, fibrosis, and subsequent damage to the cardiac conduction system and β2-adrenergic nerves and receptors leading to arrhythmias and sudden cardiac death (CCS = cardiac conduction system; ROS = reactive oxygen species; RCS = reactive carbonyl species; NF-M = neuro-filament M). Note that both ROS and RCS exert lethal damage to the different parts of the cardiac conduction system as well as cation and contractile proteins in the myocardium.

ECC, and subsequently, myocyte contractility. Prolonged QTc intervals persist in many treated diabetic patients, suggesting that glycemic control has to be adequate to normalize electrophysiological and mechanical disorders in the myocardium. Available hypoglycemic agents that can improve cardiovascular prognosis are important for the management of patients with type 2 diabetes (T2DM) who have existing CVDs and high cardiovascular risk. More research is required to understand the exact pathophysiological mechanisms at subcellular, cellular, and molecular levels, which can lead to cardiac conduction disorders in DM patients. In turn, this will help in the development of novel hypoglycemic drugs to treat the condition.

Conflict of interest

None.

Authors' participation

Manal Smail, Jaipaul Singh, Sunil Rupee, and Frank Christopher Howarth initiated the idea, and wrote and revised the review. Sunil Rupee, Khemraj Rupee, Abla Mohammed Ahmed Ismail, and Sara Sultan helped with the literature search and drew all the figures.

Ethical clearance

None since this is a review article.

Abbreviations

DM	diabetes mellitus
SAN	sinoatrial node
HG	hyperglycemia
ROS	reactive oxygen species
NFM	neuro-filament-M
HCN	hyperpolarization-activated cyclic nucleotide-gated
APs	action potentials
ECG	electrocardiogram
SCD	sudden cardiac death
CVDs	cardiovascular diseases
HR	decreased heart rate
T1DM	type 1 diabetes mellitus
CCDs	cardiac conduction disorders
AVN	atrioventricular node
ECC	excitation-contraction-coupling
ANS	autonomic nervous system
NEP	norepinephrine
ACh	acetylcholine
EPI	epinephrine

cyclic GMP	cyclic-guanosine monophosphate
DD	diastolic depolarization
ICa,T	transient (T-type) current
ICa,L	long-lasting (L-type) Ca^{2+} current
RyRs	ryanodine receptors
SR	sarcoplasmic reticulum
SERCA	sarco/endoplasmic reticulum Ca^{2+}-ATPase
CICR	calcium-induced calcium release
NCX	sodium-calcium exchanger
Cx	connexin
IKr and IKs	slow delayed rectifier potassium currents
Ito	transient outward potassium current
CCS	cardiac conduction system
HRV	heart rate variability
SNRT	Sinus node recovery time
SAD	sudden arrhythmic death

Author details

Manal Smail[1*], Sunil Rupee[1], Khemraj Rupee[1], Abla Mohammed Ahmed Ismail[2], Sara Sultan[3], Frank Christopher Howarth[4], Ernest A. Adeghate[4] and Jaipaul Singh[1]

1 School of Natural Sciences, College of Science and Technology, University of Central Lancashire, Preston, England, UK

2 Corniche Hospital, United Arab Emirates

3 Sheikh Shakhbout Medical City, United Arab Emirates

4 Department of Physiology, College of Medicine and Health Sciences, United Arab Emirates

*Address all correspondence to: farawla-9@hotmail.com

References

[1] Yaras N, Ugur M, Ozdemir S, Gurdal H, Purali N, Lacampagne A, et al. Effects of diabetes on ryanodine receptor Ca release channel (RyR2) and Ca^{2+} homeostasis in rat heart. Diabetes. 2005;**54**:3082-3088

[2] Haffner SM, Lehto S, Ronnemaa T, Pyorala K, Laakso M. Mortality from coronary heart disease in subjects with type 2 diabetes and in nondiabetic subjects with and without prior myocardial infarction. The New England Journal of Medicine. 1998;**339**:229-234

[3] Dobrzynski H, Anderson RH, Atkinson A, Borbas Z, D'Souza A, Fraser JF, et al. Structure, function and clinical relevance of the cardiac conduction system, including the atrioventricular ring and outflow tract tissues. Pharmacology & Therapeutics. 2013;**139**(2):260-288

[4] Hasslacher C, Wahl P. Diabetes prevalence in patients with bradycardiac arrhythmias. Acta Diabetologica. 1977;**14**:229-234

[5] Movahed MR. Diabetes as a risk factor for cardiac conduction defects: A review. Diabetes, Obesity & Metabolism. 2007;**9**:276-281

[6] Linnemann B, Janka HU. Prolonged QTc interval and elevated heart rate identify the type 2 diabetic patient at high risk for cardiovascular death. The Bremen Diabetes Study. Experimental and Clinical Endocrinology & Diabetes. 2003;**111**:215-222

[7] Softeland E, Brock C, Frokjaer JB, Brogger J, Madacsy L, Gilja OH, et al. Association between visceral, cardiac and sensorimotor polyneuropathies in diabetes mellitus. Journal of Diabetes and its Complications. 2014;**28**:370-377

[8] Dobrzynski H, Boyett MR, Anderson RH. New insights into pacemaker activity: Promoting understanding of sick sinus syndrome. Circulation. 2007;**115**:1921-1932

[9] Irisawa H, Brown HF, Giles W. Cardiac pacemaking in the sinoatrial node. Physiological Reviews. 1993;**73**:197-227

[10] Weinhaus AJ, Roberts KP. Anatomy of the human heart. In: Handbook of Cardiac Anatomy, Physiology, and Devices. New York: Humana Press; 2005

[11] Padala SK, Cabrera JA, Ellenbogen KA. Anatomy of the cardiac conduction system. Pacing and Clinical Electrophysiology. 2021;**44**(1):15-25

[12] Dobrzynski H, Anderson RH, Atkinson A, Borbas Z, D'Souza A, Fraser JF, et al. Structure, function and clinical relevance of the cardiac conduction system, including the atrioventricular ring and outflow tract tissues. Pharmacology. 2013;**139**:260-288

[13] Maltsev VA, Vinogradova TM, Bogdanov KY, Lakatta EG, Stern MD. Diastolic calcium release controls the beating rate of rabbit sinoatrial node cells: Numerical modeling of the coupling process. Biophysical Journal. 2004;**86**(4):2596-2602

[14] Stoyek MR, MacDonald EA, Mantifel M, Baillie JS, Selig BM, Croll RP, et al. Drivers of sinoatrial node automaticity in zebrafish: Comparison with mechanisms of mammalian pacemaker function. Frontiers in Physiology. 2022;**13**(1):1-12

[15] Bristow DG, Clark JW. A mathematical model of primary pacemaking cell in SA node of the

heart. American Journal of Physiology-Heart and Circulatory Physiology. 1982;**243**(2):207-218

[16] Kennedy A, Finlay D, Guldenring D, Bond R, Moran K, McLaughlin J. The cardiac conduction system: Generation and conduction of the cardiac impulse. Critical Care Nursing Clinics. 2016;**28**(3):269-279

[17] Brodde OE, Michel MC. Adrenergic and muscarinic receptors in the human heart. Pharmacological Reviews. 1999;**51**:651-690

[18] Honjo H, Inada S, Lancaster MK, et al. Sarcoplasmic reticulum Ca^{2+} release is not a dominating factor in sinoatrial node pacemaker activity. Circulation Research. 2003;**92**:41-44

[19] Vinogradova TM, Lyashkov AE, Zhu W, Ruknudin AM, Sirenko S, Yang D, et al. High basal protein kinase A-dependent phosphorylation drives rhythmic internal Ca^{2+} store oscillations and spontaneous beating of cardiac pacemaker cells. Circulation Research. 2006;**98**:505-514

[20] Ginneken V. MinK: A double-hearted partner in cardiac repolarization. Cardiovascular Research. 2009;**82**:390-391

[21] Berecki G, Wilders R, de Jonge B, van Ginneken AC, Verkerk AO. Re-evaluation of the action potential upstroke velocity as a measure of the Na+ current in cardiac myocytes at physiological conditions. PLoS One. 2010;**5**:1-10

[22] Lo CW. Role of gap junctions in cardiac conduction and development. Circulation Research. 2000;**87**:346-348

[23] George SA, Faye NR, Murillo-Berlioz A, Lee KB, Trachiotis GD, Efimov IR. At the atrioventricular crossroads: Dual pathway electrophysiology in the atrioventricular node and its underlying heterogeneities. Arrhythmia & Electrophysiology Review. 2017;**6**:100-179

[24] Nerbonne JM, Kass RS. Molecular physiology of cardiac repolarization. Physiological Reviews. 2005;**85**(4): 1205-1253

[25] Al Kury L, Sydorenko V, Smail MM, Qureshi MA, Shmygol A, Papandreou D, et al. Calcium signaling in endocardial and epicardial ventricular myocytes from streptozotocin-induced diabetic rats. Journal of Diabetes Investigation. 2021;**12**(4):493-500

[26] Nobe S, Aomine M, Arita M, Ito S, Takaki R. Chronic diabetes mellitus prolongs action potential duration of rat ventricular muscles: Circumstantial evidence for impaired Ca^{2+} channel. Cardiovascular Research. 1990;**24**:381-389

[27] Grimm W, Langenfeld H, Maisch B, Kochsiek K. Symptoms, cardiovascular risk profile and spontaneous ECG in paced patients: A five-year follow-up study. Pacing and Clinical Electrophysiology. 1990;**13**:2086-2090

[28] Casis O, Echevarria E. Diabetic cardiomyopathy: Electromechanical cellular. Current Vascular Pharmacology. 2004;**2**:237-248

[29] Lengyel C, Virag L, Biro T, Jost N, Magyar J, Biliczki P, et al. Diabetes mellitus attenuates the repolarization reserve in mammalian heart. Cardiovascular Research. 2007;**73**: 512-520

[30] Shimoni Y, Firek L, Severson D, Giles W. Short-term diabetes alters K+ currents in rat ventricular myocytes. Circulation Research. 1994;**74**:620-628

[31] Aulbach F, Simm A, Maier S, Langenfeld H, Walter U, Kersting U, et al. Insulin stimulates the L-type Ca^{2+} current in rat cardiac myocytes. Cardiovascular Research. 1999;**42**:113-120

[32] Bidasee KR, Nallani K, Besch HR Jr, Dincer UD. Streptozotocin-induced diabetes increases disulfide bond formation on cardiac ryanodine receptor (RyR2). The Journal of Pharmacology and Experimental Therapeutics. 2003;**305**(3):989-998

[33] Zhong Y, Ahmed S, Grupp IL, Matlib MA. Altered SR protein expression associated with contractile dysfunction in diabetic rat hearts. American Journal of Physiology-Heart and Circulatory Physiology. 2001;**281**(3):1137-1147

[34] Hattori Y, Matsuda N, Kimura J, Ishitani T, Tamada A, Gando S, et al. Diminished function and expression of the cardiac Na^{+}-Ca^{2+} exchanger in diabetic rats: Implication in Ca^{2+} overload. Journal of Physiology. 2000;**527**:85-94

[35] Baruscotti M, Bucchi A, Viscomi C, Mandelli G, Consalez G, Gnecchi-Rusconi T, et al. Deep bradycardia and heart block caused by inducible cardiac-specific knockout of the pacemaker channel gene Hcn4. Proceedings of the National Academy of Sciences of the United States of America. 2011;**108**(4):1705-1710

[36] Howarth FC, Al-Sharhan R, Al-Hammadi A, Qureshi MA. Effects of streptozotocin-induced diabetes on action potentials in the sinoatrial node compared with other regions of the rat heart. Molecular and Cellular Biochemistry. 2007;**3**(1/2):39-46

[37] Watanabe H, Makita N, Tanabe N, Watanabe T, Aizawa Y. Electrocardiographic abnormalities and risk of complete atrioventricular block. International Journal of Cardiology. 2012;**155**:462-464

[38] Zhang Y, Wang Y, Yanni J, Qureshi MA, Logantha SJRJ, Kassab S, et al. Electrical conduction system remodeling in streptozotocin-induced diabetes mellitus rat heart. Frontiers in Physiology. 2019;**10**:820-826

[39] Vinik AI, Ziegler D. Diabetic cardiovascular autonomic neuropathy. Circulation. 2007;**115**:387-397

[40] McDowell TS, Hajduczok G, Abboud FM, Chapleau MW. Baroreflex dysfunction in diabetes mellitus. II. Site of baroreflex impairment in diabetic rabbits. American Journal of Physiology. 1994;**266**:244-249

[41] Fazan R Jr, Ballejo G, Salgado MC, Moraes MF, Salgado HC. Heart rate variability and baroreceptor function in chronic diabetic rats. Hypertension. 1997;**3**:632-635

[42] Zhang Y, Welzig CM, Picard KL, Du C, Wang B, Pan JQ, et al. Glycogen synthase kinase-3beta inhibition ameliorates cardiac parasympathetic dysfunction in type 1 diabetic Akita mice. Diabetes. 2014;**63**:2097-2113

[43] Javorka M, Javorkova J, Tonhajzerova I, Javorka K. Parasympathetic versus sympathetic control of the cardiovascular system in young patients with type 1 diabetes mellitus. Clinical Physiology and Functional Imaging. 2005;**25**(5):270-274

[44] Chadda KD, Banka VS, Bodenheimer MM, Helfant RH. Corrected sinus node recovery time. Experimental physiologic and pathologic determinants. Circulation. 1975;**51**:797-801

[45] Narula OS, Samet P, Javier RP. Significance of the sinus-node recovery time. Circulation. 1972;**45**:140-158

[46] De Bakker JM, van Capelle FJ, Janse MJ, et al. Slow conduction in the infarcted human heart. "Zigzag" course of activation. Circulation. 1993;**88**:915-926

[47] Gardner PI, Ursell PC, Fenoglio JJ, et al. Electrophysiologic and anatomic basis for fractionated electrograms recorded from healed myocardial infarcts. Circulation. 1985;**72**:596-611

[48] Hagendorff A, Schumacher B, Kirchhoff S, et al. Conduction disturbances and increased atrial vulnerability in Connexin40-deficient mice analyzed by transesophageal stimulation. Circulation. 1999;**99**:1508-1515

[49] Polontchouk L, Haefliger J-A, Ebelt B, et al. Effects of chronic atrial fibrillation on gap junction distribution in human and rat atria. Journal of the American College of Cardiology. 2001;**38**:883-891

[50] Dhalla N. Subcellular remodeling and heart dysfunction in chronic diabetes. Cardiovascular Research. 1998;**40**:239-247

[51] Gutstein DE, Morley GE, Tamaddon H. Conduction slowing and sudden arrhythmic death in mice with cardiac-restricted inactivation of Connexin43. Circulation Research. 2001;**88**:333-339

Section 3

Hypertrophic Cardiomyopathy

Chapter 4

Hypertrophic Cardiomyopathy: Surgical Perspectives

Sameh M. Said, Eduard Quintana and Khaled F. Salhab

Abstract

Hypertrophic cardiomyopathy is a unique myocardial disorder that can present in all ages from neonate to adults and has strong genetic basis. Several key features characterize hypertrophic cardiomyopathy. These include: the presence of left ventricular hypertrophy that can not be explained by another etiology, and left ventricular outflow tract obstruction secondary to systolic anterior motion of the anterior mitral valve leaflet with varying degrees of mitral valve regurgitation. Surgical septal myectomy continues to be the standard line of treatment when medical therapy fails or become intolerable. We summarize in the current chapter the technical tips and pitfall of septal myectomy, its alternatives/adjuncts and its outcomes.

Keywords: hypertrophic cardiomyopathy, septal reduction, septal myectomy, subaortic stenosis, left ventricular outflow tract obstruction

1. Introduction: history

Brock and Teare in 1958 reported the first pathological case that drew the attention to HCM, while the first surgical procedure to address HCM was credited to Cleland and colleagues in the same year [1]. The "Morrow" operation was the main surgical procedure for years since it was initially reported by Morrow and Brockenbrough in 1960 [2].

Mitral valve replacement has been historically considered a way of eliminating the LVOTO by eliminating SAM, however with appropriate and complete septal myectomy, this is rarely considered an option in the current era except in the presence of unrepairable concomitant mitral valve disease.

Surgical septal myectomy; however, has evolved over the years from the traditional "Morrow" operation to the current "extended left ventricular septal myectomy" to ensure complete elimination of recurrence or residual LVOTO as will be discussed in the current chapter.

2. Background

Hypertrophic cardiomyopathy (HCM) is a unique myocardial disorder that is characterized by the presence of dynamic left ventricular outflow tract (LVOT) obstruction (LVOTO) and systolic anterior motion (SAM) of the anterior mitral valve leaflet with resultant various degrees of mitral regurgitation. HCM was previously known as idiopathic hypertrophic subaortic stenosis (IHSS) or asymmetric septal hypertrophy which is due to the presence of left ventricular hypertrophy that can not be explained by other pathology. Another key feature in this unique disease.

HCM has been one of the main causes of sudden death in young adults and athletes. Patients may present with a variety of clinical pictures that range from completely asymptomatic to exertional fatigue, chest pain, and/or shortness of breath.

The first line treatment in HCM continued to be medical therapy especially in those symptomatic with LVOTO [3]. Septal reduction therapy should be considered for those who failed or became intolerant to medical therapy [4].

3. Morphological variants of hypertrophic cardiomyopathy

HCM is characterized by varying degree of septal hypertrophy and this led to the emergence of several morphological variants of HCM. These variants include basal septal hypertrophy, apical, midventricular or combination of any [5]. A key feature in the basal variant is the presence of SAM of the anterior mitral valve leaflet, while a key feature in the apical variant is the presence of small left ventricular cavity and absence of SAM.

Recognition of these variants is critical especially when considering patients for septal reduction therapy to ensure delivering the right modality and decrease the chance of persistence or recurrence of the LVOT obstruction.

4. Current indications for septal myectomy

Surgical septal myectomy should be considered for those symptomatic patients who failed medical treatment or for those who are intolerant to medical therapy. Morphological variants may play a role in proceeding with surgery as well. Variants like apical and midventricular level of obstruction are difficult to manage medically and do not respond to Alcohol septal ablation.

5. Surgical approaches for septal myectomy

Understanding the different morphological variants of HCM is critical in selecting the right surgical approach for the patient. This ensures elimination of the LVOT obstruction and minimizes if not prevents any residual/recurrent significant gradient/obstruction.

The procedure is done through a standard median sternotomy with central aortic and single venous (right atrial) cannulation. Although septal myectomy has been reported via a minimally invasive approaches such as endoscopic [6] and robotic [7], we do believe median sternotomy should be considered the gold standard for these cases as it provides adequate exposure to the heart and mediastinal structures and facilitates performing all maneuvers that are needed to facilitate exposure to the interventricular septum and performance of an adequate septal myectomy.

Prior to venous cannulation, we measure the gradient across the LVOT directly by placing a needle in the distal ascending aorta and another one in the left ventricular cavity (via the right ventricle free wall) simultaneously (**Figure 1A** and **B**).

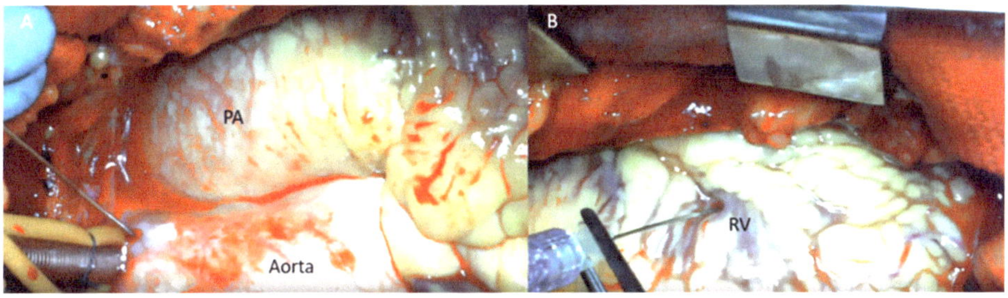

Figure 1.
Intraoperative photos showing the technique of direct pressure measurement of the left ventricular outflow tract gradient prior to initiation of cardiopulmonary bypass. In (A), a needle is placed in the distal ascending aorta, and in (B) the second needle is placed into the left ventricular cavity indirectly via the free wall of the right ventricle (RV) and the interventricular septum. PA: Pulmonary artery; RV: Right ventricle.

This measures the resting LVOT gradient (**Figure 2**) and then provocative maneuvers are performed. These maneuvers are important to evaluate the LVOT gradient as it occurs with exercise. A variant of HCM is known as "Latent obstruction" will be discussed later but patients with this variant do not have any significant gradient at rest but they do with exercise. These provocative maneuvers can be either an induction of a premature ventricular contraction (Brockenbrough-Braunwald-Morrow) (**Figure 3**) or administration of isoproterenol.

This will be repeated after coming off cardiopulmonary bypass to document elimination of any significant gradient across the LVOT. Based on the variant of septal hypertrophy and the level of obstruction, the technique of myectomy may differ or be a combination of the following:

5.1 Trans-aortic myectomy

This is the most common approach and is used for the most common variant which is basal or subaortic obstruction. The technical details have been described

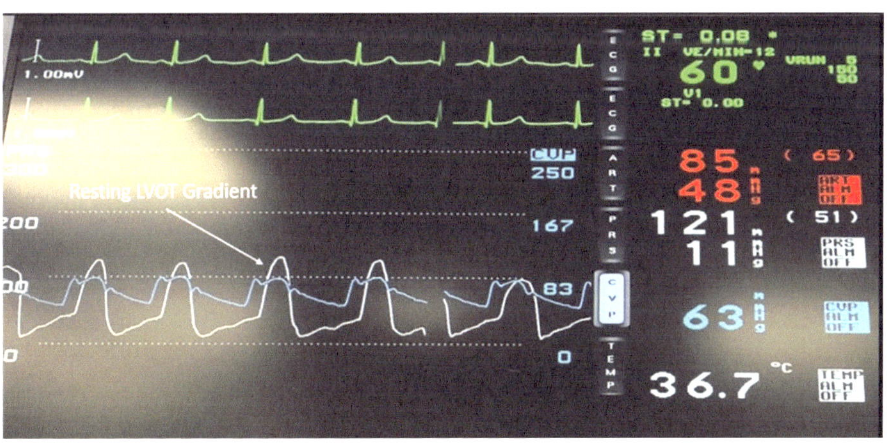

Figure 2.
Intraoperative pressure tracing showing the resting left ventricular outflow tract gradient by direct needle pressures. The left ventricular pressure is in white, while the aortic pressure is in light blue colors. LVOT: Left ventricular outflow tract.

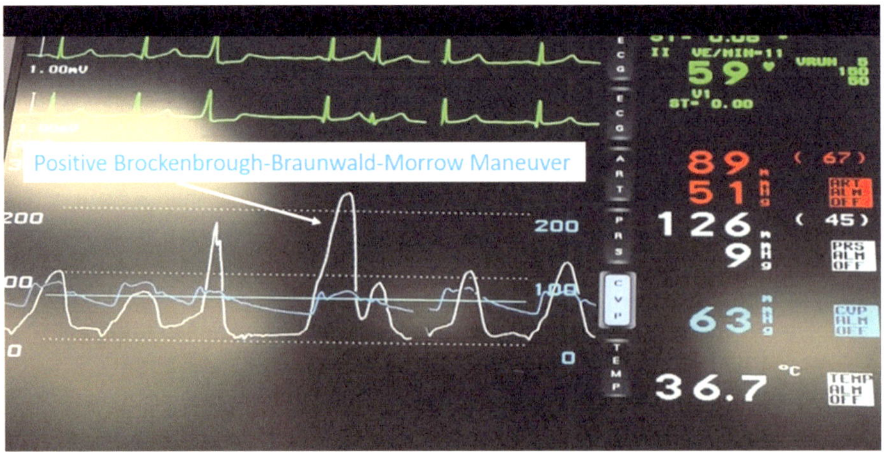

Figure 3.
Intraoperative pressure tracing from the same patient showing positive Brockenbrough-Braunwald-Morrow maneuver by induction of premature ventricular contraction. The left ventricular pressure (white color) increased, while the aortic pressure (light blue) decreased, resulting in significant left ventricular outflow tract gradient.

before [8]. Once the heart is arrested with antegrade cardioplegia, a hockey-stick aortotomy is performed down to the base of the non-coronary sinus of Valsalva. The aortotomy in these cases has to be a bit lower than standard aortotomy for aortic valve replacement to provide adequate exposure to the LVOT.

Stay sutures are then applied and the LVOT is assessed. This is a 360-degree visual assessment of the LVOT and the mitral apparatus prior to performing any resection (**Figure 4**). The result of this assessment determines the degree of septal bulge, how far down in the left ventricular cavity the resection has to extend, the abnormalities that may coexist in the mitral subvalvular apparatus such as anomalous chordae (**Figure 5**) and/or papillary muscles. These all can lead to persistent or recurrent LVOT gradient. A variety of instruments – seen in **Figure 6**- are needed to perform the myectomy.

The resection then starts below the nadir of the right coronary cusp (**Figure 7**) and extends in an anti-clockwise direction towards the commissure between the left and non-coronary cusps. Scissors are then used to complete the resection. This is the initial resection which serves to widen the subaortic area and facilitates further access to the left ventricular cavity. Further resection has to be performed along the interventricular septum and towards the left ventricular apex to ensure complete elimination of any residual gradient. Some maneuvers can help with exposing that part of the septum such as placing a sponge stick on the free wall of the right ventricle that helps bringing the interventricular septum in view (**Figure 8**). The area of resection is further widened as we go deeper into the ventricular cavity which what makes this "extended" in comparison to the initial "Morrow" operation.

A proper septal myectomy is a 3-dimensional operation in regards to the extent of resection [9], and all other potential causes of recurrent/residual LVOT obstruction have to be addressed such as resection of anomalous papillary muscles and/or chordae (**Figure 9**). The aortotomy is then closed in two-layers and the heart is de-aired and the aortic cross clamp is removed.

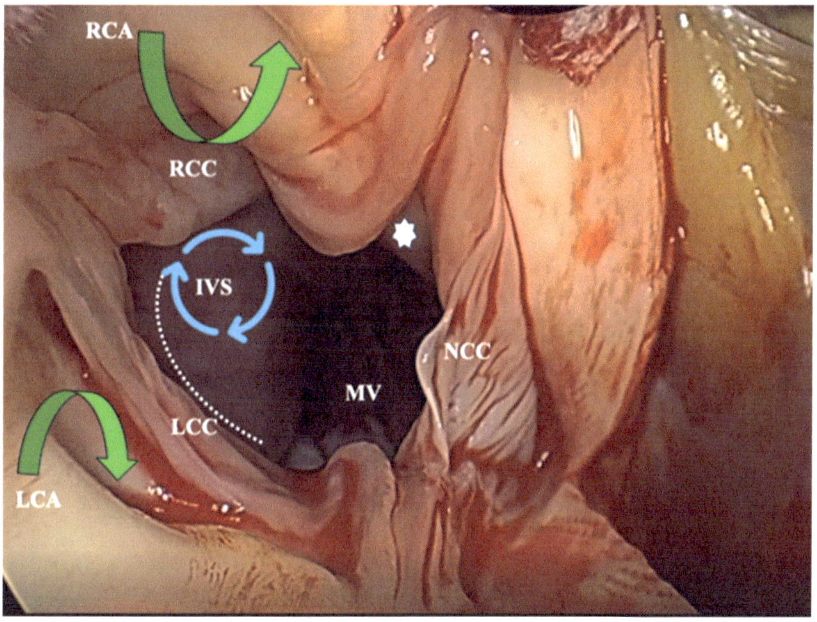

Figure 4.
The anatomic landmarks of the left ventricular outflow tract after performing the aortotomy and prior to the myectomy. The area of the interventricular septum (IVS) is visualized, as well as the membranous septum (*) where resection should be avoided. The mitral valve (MV) is visualized deep in the left ventricle. RCA: Right coronary artery ostium; RCC: Right coronary cusp; LCA: Left coronary artery ostium; LCC: Left coronary cusp; NCC: Non-coronary cusp; MV: Mitral valve; IVS: Interventricular septum.

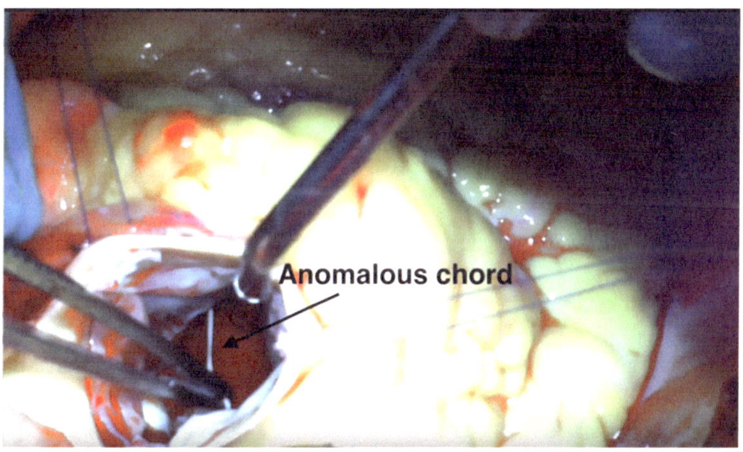

Figure 5.
An intraoperative view through the aortotomy showing an anomalous mitral valve chord in the left ventricular outflow tract. These chordae can result in persistent or recurrence of gradient after an initial myectomy as it limits the mobility of the anterior mitral valve leaflet and can result in persistence of systolic anterior motion (SAM).

5.2 Trans-apical myectomy

Trans-apical approach can be done for one of three main indications: (1) mid-ventricular variant, where the transaortic approach may not be adequate, (2) apical

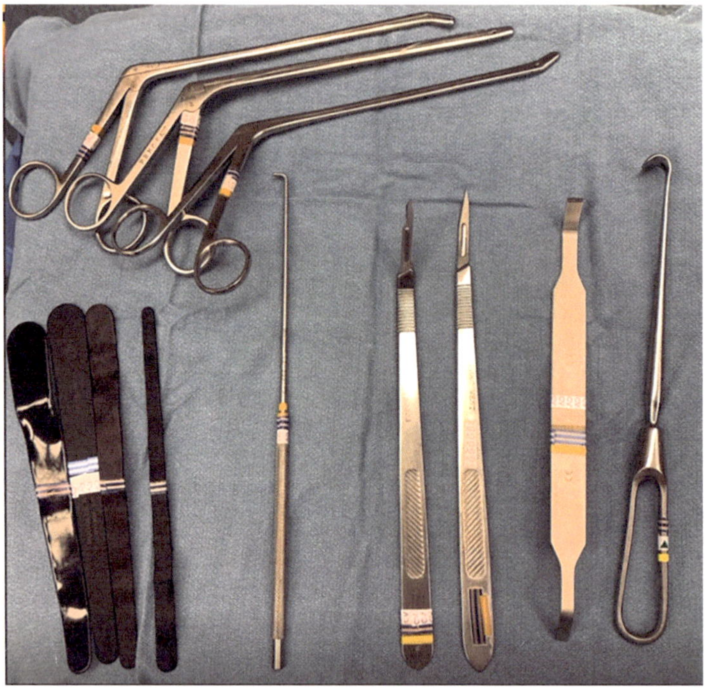

Figure 6.
The variety of surgical instruments that are useful during the myectomy procedure. Different types of surgical blades, aortic cusp retractors, pituitary Rongeurs to help with removal of the muscle pieces.

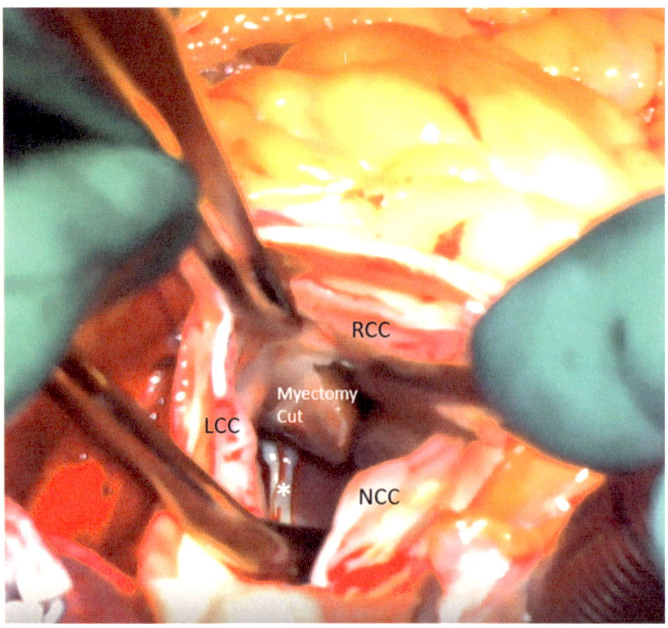

Figure 7.
The resection starts below the nadir of the right coronary cusp (RCC) and goes into anti-clockwise direction towards the anterior mitral valve leaflet and chordal structures (*). RCC: Right coronary cusp; LCC: Left coronary cusp; NCC: Non-coronary cusp.

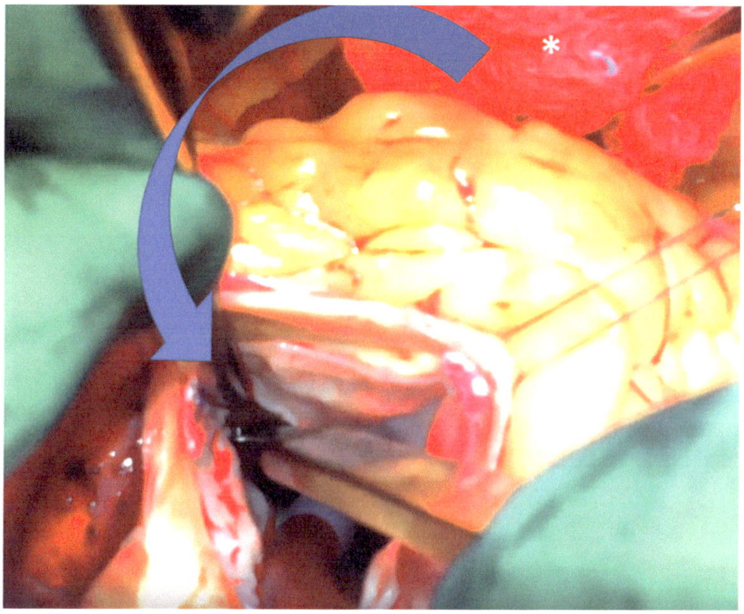

Figure 8.
One of the helpful maneuvers to facilitate exposure of the lower part of the interventricular septum is using a sponge stick (*) to depress the free wall of the right ventricular and rotate the septum, thus bringing it in view to the surgeon.

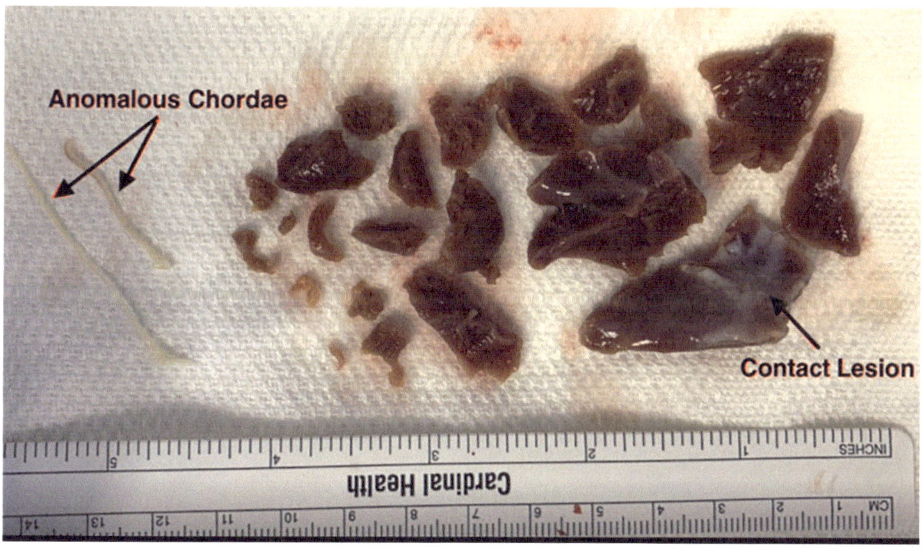

Figure 9.
The completed myectomy specimen with two anomalous chordae. Notice the contact lesion (white scar) on the resected specimen. This occurs as a result of the anterior mitral vale leaflet hitting the septum during systole (systolic anterior motion).

variant, and (3) in those patients who do not have adequate left ventricular cavity and non-obstructive variant of HCM where left ventricular enlargement can be performed to improve their left ventricular end-diastolic volume.

We have described the technique previously [10], but briefly, after the cardioplegic arrest, the left ventricular apex is delivered into the field and the left anterior descending (LAD) coronary artery is identified. An apical incision is done 1 cm to the left and parallel of the LAD (**Figure 10**). In the apical variant, the left ventricular apex is quite obliterated with muscles and it is critical to stay on the interventricular septum side (**Figure 11**) to avoid risk of injury of the mitral valve papillary muscles

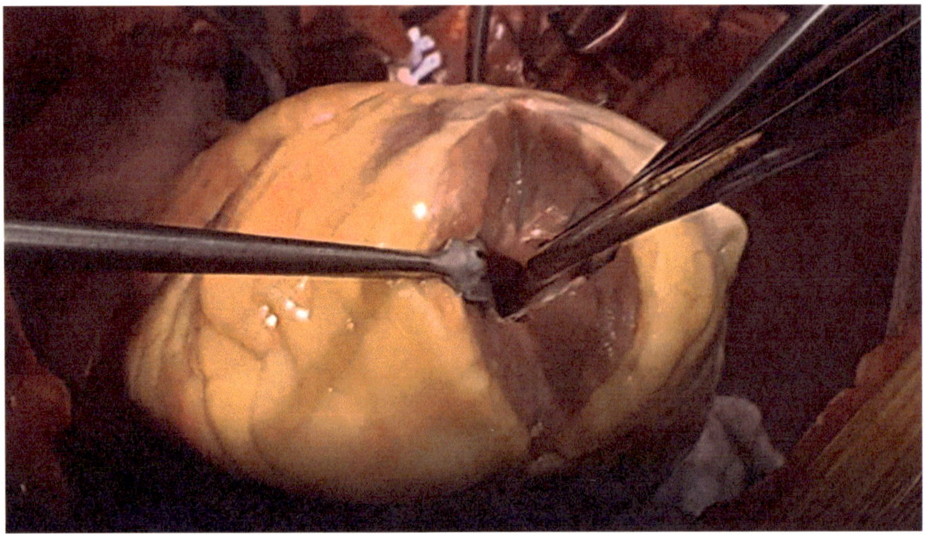

Figure 10.
An apical incision is made in the left ventricular apex which facilitates myectomy in patients with midventricular and apical hypertrophic cardiomyopathy.

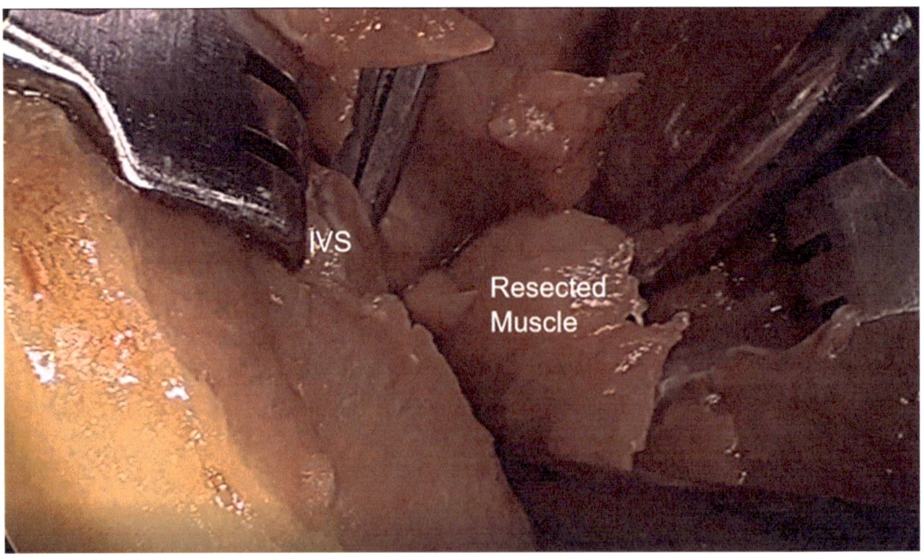

Figure 11.
A view through the opened left ventricular apex showing the resected muscle specimen-in progress- and the interventricular septum (IVS). It is important for the surgeon to stay on the IVS side during resection till he/she able to visualize the papillary muscles of the mitral valve to avoid inadvertent injury to the mitral subvalvular structures. IVS: Interventricular septum.

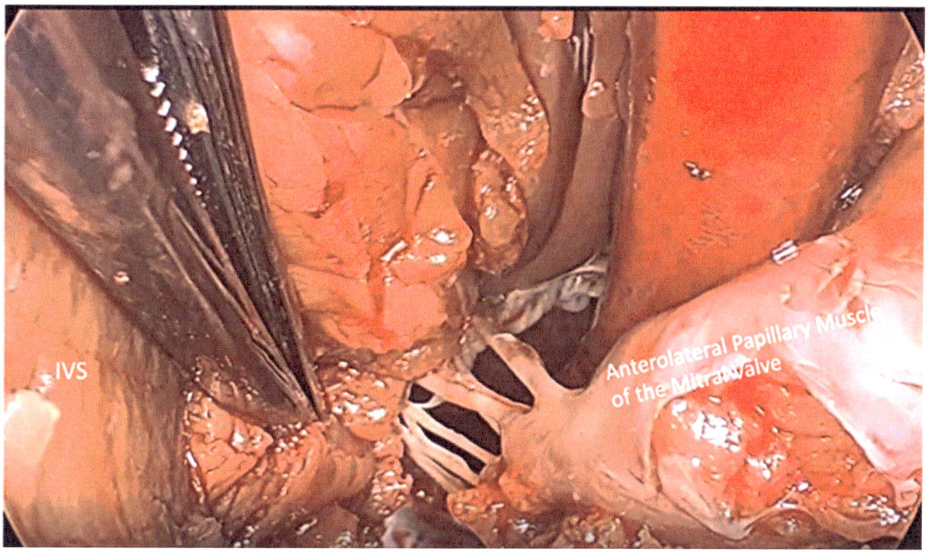

Figure 12.
After the resection, the left ventricular cavity now is widened and the mitral valve subvalvular structures can be easily visualized.

which are usually apical displaced and hypertrophied in these cases (**Figure 12**). Once the left ventricular cavity is entered, further resection is performed and the cavity is further widened. The apex is then closed in two layers and suture line is supported with Teflon felt.

5.3 Trans-mitral myectomy

This is a left atrial approach to the interventricular septum through the mitral valve. It has been used by some authors as an alternative to the transaortic approach but it requires detachment of the anterior leaflet of the mitral valve followed most likely by patch augmentation after completing the resection [11]. One has to be familiar with this approach as the anatomy of the interventricular septum differs through this approach compared to the trans-aortic exposure.

We believe this may be more of value in children and those with small aortic root where the trans-aortic approach may not be adequate. Another potential advantage is that it helps addressing the mitral valve pathology and performing the myectomy through one incision.

6. Adjuncts to septal myectomy

6.1 Abnormalities of the mitral subvalvular apparatus

6.1.1 Papillary muscle abnormalities

Detection of papillary muscle abnormalities on preoperative echocardiogram can be challenging, therefore, it is important for the surgeon to evaluate the mitral subvalvular apparatus as part of the overall thorough evaluation of the LVOT. Anomalous papillary muscle can be a cause of persistent/recurrent gradient after an initial-what it seems like- a complete myectomy [12].

It is critical to differentiate these anomalous muscles from the true papillary muscles of the mitral valve. A key difference is the insertion of the anomalous papillary muscle into the body of the leaflet, rather than the free edge and therefore, it can be excised safely.

6.1.2 Anomalous chordae

These anomalous chordae are attached to the body of the anterior mitral valve leaflets and not to the free edge which helps differentiating these chordae from primary chordal structures of the mitral valve. These can limit the mobility of the anterior mitral leaflet and result in SAM as well.

Some anomalous chordae can cause adherence of the papillary muscles to the septum and cutting this helps mobilizing these papillary muscles and minimize the gradient and the chance of SAM after septal myectomy. In general, there should be no chordal attachment between the mitral valve apparatus and the interventricular septum.

6.2 Management of concomitant atrial fibrillation

Due to the elevated left ventricular end-diastolic pressure and subsequently left atrial pressure secondary to the significant LVOTO, it is not uncommon for patients with HCM to present with atrial fibrillation (AFib). Losing the atrial kick in those with HCM and diastolic dysfunction results in significant drop in their cardiac output and symptoms, therefore, it is important to maintain normal sinus rhythm in these patients [13].

Our strategy is to offer biatrial Cox-maze IV procedure using a combination of radiofrequency and cryoablation for those with chronic persistent AFib, while in those with paroxysmal AFib, bilateral pulmonary vein isolation is sufficient. Routine excision or exclusion of the left atrial appendage is part of either procedures.

6.3 Mitral valve surgery

Historically, mitral valve replacement was one of the proposed solutions to LVOTO in patients with HCM, however this is not currently the case. With adequate extended left ventricular septal myectomy, all SAM is eliminated and the mitral regurgitation-even if severe- is significantly improved if not completely eliminated.

Our approach is to perform mitral valve surgery in the settings of septal myectomy only in the presence of intrinsic mitral valve pathology and mitral regurgitation that is not the result of SAM and the dynamic nature of the LVOTO in HCM. Repair is preferred over replacement in all cases due to the long-term survival benefit of mitral repair that is documented across multiple studies in the literature. Mitral valve repair techniques may also need to be modified in these cases to avoid recreating SAM after the repair such as if a ring to be used, a one size larger may be preferred.

In some cases, when there is a question about the need for mitral valve repair or if the mechanism of regurgitation is unclear, we will perform a complete myectomy, and then come off cardiopulmonary bypass and re-evaluate the mitral valve and make the decision if interventions on the mitral valve is necessary at this stage.

If mitral valve replacement is necessary, then it is important to choose a mechanical or a low profile bioprosthesis that does not project into the LVOT and results in LVOT gradient.

6.4 Myocardial bridging

Myocardial bridging (MB) is a challenging problem in the presence of HCM. It can cause significant symptoms (chest pain) after an initial septal myectomy and at the same time not all patients with MB requires unroofing of their MB. A challenging task is to identify those who will benefit from concomitant unroofing of MB and septal myectomy. Currently no guidelines or recommendations regarding the optimal management of these patients.

Wang and colleagues reported their midterm results of different treatment methods for MB in patients with HCM after their septal myectomy [14]. A total of 823 patients were included, where the authors identified 31 events with mortality in 24 patients and nonfatal myocardial infarction (MI) in 7. The three-year cumulative event-free survival of all cause-death was 100% for both those who underwent coronary artery bypass grafting, and unroofing, however, the 3-year cumulative event-free survival of non-fatal MI and the combined endpoints were significantly lower in the un-treated group. The authors concluded that surgical treatment of MB at the time of septal myectomy is beneficial.

We do perform coronary angiography in the majority of these patients especially when the presentation is of a chest pain. If a MB is identified, a hemodynamic evaluation of the bridge is performed to determine its significance and help making the decision for concomitant unroofing.

We have described the technique previously [15] and we prefer performing the unroofing procedure on the arrested heart to avoid inadvertent injury of the coronary artery. A combination of sharp and electrocautery dissection is used to unroof the entire bridged segment (**Figure 13**). It is critical to remember that the bridged segment of the coronary artery is always fragile and the unroofing process has to be done with extreme caution.

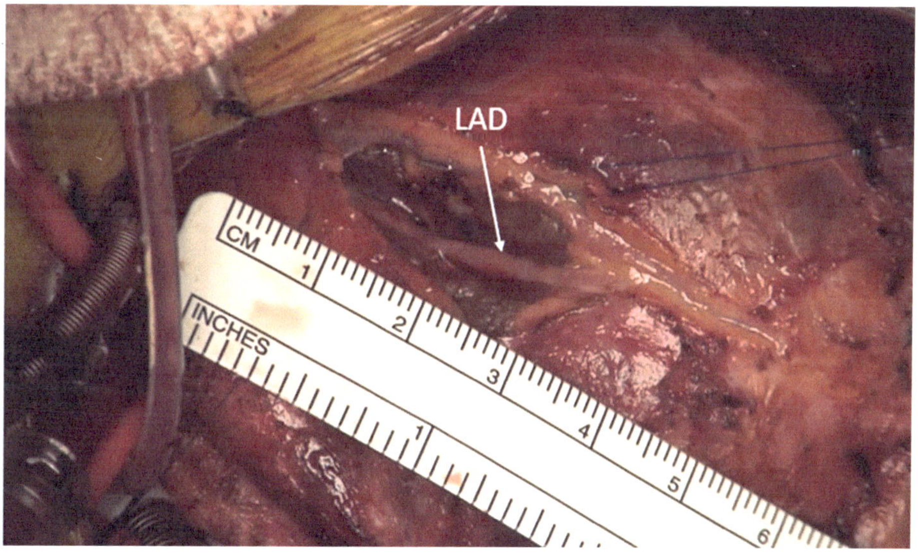

Figure 13.
Intraoperative photo of a patient with hypertrophic cardiomyopathy who underwent repeat operation with unroofing of a long segment of the left anterior descending coronary artery due to missed diagnosis of myocardial bridge after his initial septal myectomy. LAD: Left anterior descending coronary artery.

6.5 Left ventricular apical aneurysm

These are outpouchings that appear at the left ventricular apex and can occur in those with HCM. The aneurysms are usually thin-walled and either dyskinetic or akinetic on echocardiographic images. It has been reported to occur in 15–30% of patients with the apical and midventricular variants of HCM [16], however detection of these aneurysms is not always straightforward. In the study by Yang and colleagues, the authors analyzed 1332 patients with apical HCM with cardiac magnetic resonance imaging (cMRI), and 31 patients had an apical aneurysm (2.3%). The rate of missed diagnosis of apical aneurysms by echocardiogram was 64.5% [17].

Several adverse events have been reported with apical aneurysms such as ventricular arrhythmias, heart failure and up to sudden cardiac death. These apical aneurysms are not amenable to medical treatment and in many cases, surgical resection is recommended at the time of septal myectomy [18]. In those with midventricular obstruction, access to the left ventricular cavity can be facilitated through the aneurysm with less risk of injury to the mitral valve apparatus. Small aneurysms can be plicated, while larger ones should be resected.

6.6 Internal cardioverter defibrillator (ICD) placement

Those with risk factors of sudden cardiac death and history of sustained ventricular tachycardia/fibrillation benefit from placement of internal cardioverter defibrillator (ICD) [19].

Several strategies and techniques have been proposed for placement of ICD such as endovenous, subcutaneous [20] and epicardial (**Figure 14A** and **B**). If the patient did not have ICD prior to surgery, and meets the criteria, our practice is to place the ICD prior to hospital discharge after septal myectomy. In children, the preference has been to perform concomitant myectomy with epicardial ICD placement through the sternotomy incision.

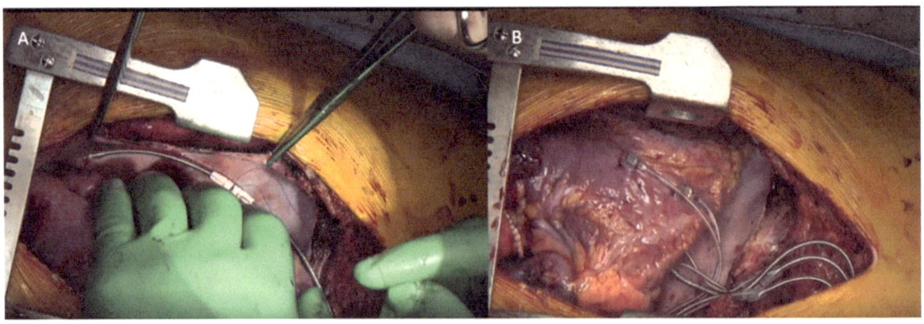

Figure 14.
In children who needed an internal cardioverter defibrillator placement, the procedure is usually done after completion of the myectomy where an epicardial system is placed and the defibrillator coil (visualized in figure A) is secured to the pericardium below the phrenic nerve, while the sensing epicardial leads are secured to the epicardial surface of the right ventricle (seen in figure B) and the device is placed in the epigastric area behind the rectus abdominis muscle.

7. Alterantive surgical options to septal myectomy

7.1 Mobilization of the right and left fibrous trigones

Yacoub et al. has pioneered this technique as an alternative to septal myectomy in those with obstructive type of HCM [21]. It is based on the role of the right and left fibrous trigones in the functional anatomy of the LVOT. The authors proposed that LVOTO is secondary to connection of the both the right and left fibrous trigones by a complete fibromuscular ring which is needed to be excised and both trigones be mobilized to ensure complete relief of the LVOT gradient.

After resection of a fibromuscular wedge of tissue from the interventricular septum, the left fibrous trigone is mobilized be extending the incision laterally to open the hinge mechanism between the septum and the subaortic curtain. Mobilization of the right fibrous trigone is done by excision of a wedge of abnormal tissue in the angle between the membranous septum and the subaortic curtain.

7.2 Modified Konno procedure

While extended left ventricular septal myectomy is considered the gold standard surgery for HCM with obstruction, the procedure is quite challenging in young children and in those with right ventricular outflow tract (RVOT) obstruction.

Modified Konno emerged as an alternative and another tool in the box for some of these cases. The procedure is performed after cardioplegic arrest by making a transverse incision in the (RVOT) and through the aortotomy, a right-angled instrument is passed and used to perforate the interventricular septum. This provides the upper limit for the septal incision. The conal septum is then incised towards the apex and away from the conduction tissue. Myectomy is performed on both sides of the septum, followed by patch closure of the created ventricular septal defect.

The long-term results of modified Konno have been reported in 79 patients with 38% of them below the age of five years, and 25% had Noonan syndromes with RVOTO present in 28% of them. Survival without death or transplantation was 82% at 20 years [22].

8. Latent obstruction

A subgroup of HCM patients have symptoms despite what appears to be a low LVOT gradient at rest and it is important to differentiate between diastolic dysfunction and labile LVOT gradient as an etiology for their symptoms. It is critical in evaluating these patients, to perform provocative maneuvers such as exercise, amyl nitrite, and/or Valsalva maneuver. If provocative maneuvers revealed significant LVOT gradient, the patient should be offered septal myectomy as symptoms in these patients are related to a latent form of obstruction rather than to diastolic dysfunction.

A report of 249 patients with latent obstruction (gradient <30 mmHg at rest) was compared to those who had severe LVOT gradient at rest and both underwent septal myectomy. Early mortality was 1% with comparable long-term survival to that of an age-matched population [23].

9. Recurrent left ventricular outflow tract obstruction after septal myectomy

With complete and proper septal myectomy (**Figure 15**), recurrence is quite low, especially in adults. As discussed previously, anatomic causes of recurrence such as mitral subvalvular abnormalities (anomalous papillary muscles, and anomalous chordae) should be ruled out during the initial myectomy to avoid reoperation or persistence/recurrence of symptoms.

Other possible etiology includes unidentified midventricular obstruction which is being unmasked by the initial subaortic resection. Muscle growth is rare to occur in adults and is most likely to occur in those with congenital subaortic stenosis.

The following mechanisms were identified in more than 50 patients with redo myectomy: limited initial myectomy, midventricular obstruction, and anomalous papillary muscles [24]. The repeat septal myectomy remains safe and feasible and should be the main treatment for those with recurrent/persistent LVOT gradient after initial limited resection.

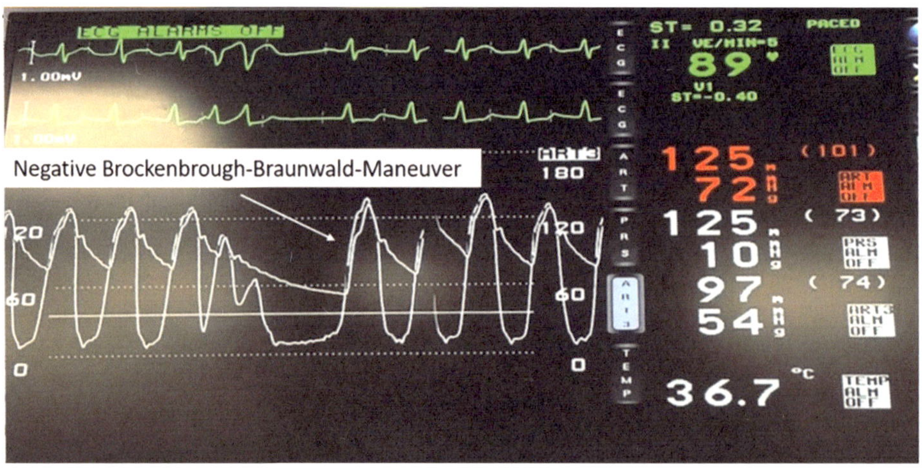

Figure 15.
Intraoperative tracing after a complete myectomy showing no resting gradient between the left ventricle and the aorta with negative Brockenbrough-Braunwald-maneuver.

10. Septal myectomy after alcohol septal ablation

Alcohol septal ablation (ASA) has been considered as an alternative to septal myectomy in suitable patients. It relies on septal artery ablation with subsequent reduction in the basal septal thickness. We do believe it is an alternative for high risk patients and those who deemed not suitable for standard surgical septal myectomy.

However, it is important to be aware that patients who require septal myectomy after ASA are at high risk for needing a permanent pacemaker and have lower survival compared with those who receive primary surgical septal myectomy [25]. ASA results in right bundle branch block and standard myectomy will result in left bundle branch block (**Figure 16**), thus increasing the chance for needing permanent pacing after surgery.

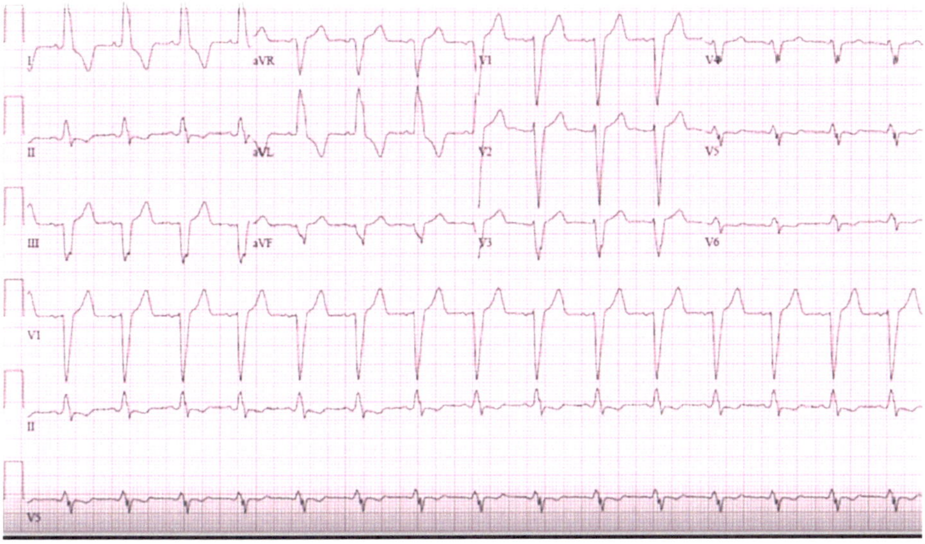

Figure 16.
It is not uncommon after septal myectomy to have a left bundle branch block as visualized on this patient postoperative electrocardiogram.

There are also some anatomic substrates that will not be suitable for ASA such as the midventricular and apical variants so as those with significant basal septal thickness (3 cm or more) where surgical septal myectomy would be considered the first line septal reduction modality.

11. Right ventricular myectomy

A subgroup of patients with HCM, particularly in association with genetic syndromes such as Noonan's, can present with biventricular outflow tract obstruction.

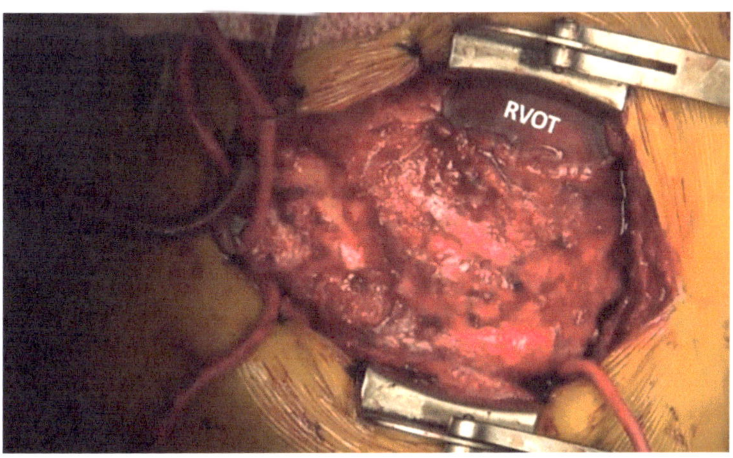

Figure 17.
Right ventricular septal myectomy is done through an incision in the right ventricular outflow tract (RVOT) followed by patch augmentation after completion of the myectomy. RVOT: Right ventricular outflow tract.

This is important to recognize during their evaluation and especially if they are being offered surgical myectomy on the left side.

Septal myectomy on the right side is a bit different from the left side. Shaving on the right side of the interventricular septum has to be done with caution to avoid injury to conduction tissue and/or the tricuspid valve apparatus which is different from the left side where there is no septal attachment to the mitral valve. This is usually done through an infundibular incision, followed by patch augmentation of the RVOT (**Figure 17**) [26].

12. Outcomes

12.1 Surgical outcomes in adults

In a report form Mayo Clinic, the risk of hospital death after isolated septal myectomy for obstructive HCM is less than 1%. Reported complications after septal myectomy such as need for permanent pacemaker secondary to complete heart block, and iatrogenic ventricular septal defect occur in about 2% of patients and are considered uncommon. Approximately 90% of patients reported significant improvement in their symptoms after extended left ventricular septal myectomy. Late survival after myectomy has been also reported to be equivalent to an age-matched population and the risk of ICD discharges decreased significantly with elimination of the LVOT obstruction [27].

The transapical approach has been reported in 113 patients with apical HCM. Early mortality was 4% and at late follow-up, 76% of these patients reported improvement in their symptoms. Three patients (3%) underwent heart transplantation due to recurrent heart failure. Survival of this group was superior in comparison to those waiting for heart transplantation [28].

12.2 Surgical outcomes in children

Children with HCM can present in a similar fashion to adults, with a wide variety of presentations. These symptoms are mostly related to a combination of diastolic dysfunction and significant mitral regurgitation. Sudden death as an initial presentation is more common in children compared to adults [29].

The operation is technically more challenging in children compared to adults due to the obvious anatomic barriers secondary to the small aortic annulus and LVOT. A report from Mayo Clinic included 127 patients who underwent septal myectomy with age ranging from 2 months to 21 years old. There was no early mortality, and the most common concomitant procedures were resection of accessory papillary muscles, mitral valve repair, and closure of an atrial level shunt. Complications included two patients with iatrogenic injury to the mitral valve and seven with aortic valve injury and all were repaired. One iatrogenic ventricular septal defect occurred. There were four late death but the remaining patients reported improvement of their symptoms with 96% being in NYHA class I or II. Repeat septal myectomy was needed in six patients [30].

12.3 Septal myectomy versus alcohol septal ablation

ASA as mentioned previously has emerged as an alternative to surgical septal myectomy. It can decrease the gradient in the LVOT and improve symptoms, however several studies confirmed the better long-term symptom relief by surgical septal myectomy.

The success rate for septal myectomy is higher and the complication rate is lower when it is performed with experienced hands. In a report of 138 patients who underwent ASA, mortality and morbidity were higher than that of age- and gender-matched population who underwent septal myectomy [31]. Survival with septal myectomy is also better in those 65 years of age or younger, in addition to the immediate relief of LVOT gradient and symptoms that is provided by proper septal myectomy.

As mentioned earlier patient selection is a key for either procedure and important to be aware with the risks inherent in those who will undergo septal myectomy after ASA prior to committing them to ASA.

Author details

Sameh M. Said[1*], Eduard Quintana[2] and Khaled F. Salhab[3]

1 Division of Pediatric Cardiovascular Surgery, Department of Surgery, Maria Fareri Children's Hospital, Westchester Medical Center, New York, United States

2 Cardiovascular Surgery Department, Hospital Clinic-IDIBAPS, University of Barcelona, Barcelona, Spain

3 Department of Cardiothoracic Surgery, New York University Langone Hospital, New York, United States

*Address all correspondence to: sameh.said@wmchealth.org

References

[1] Goodwin JF, Hollman A, Cleland WP, et al. Obstructive cardiomyopathy simulating aortic stenosis. British Heart Journal. 1960;**22**:403-414

[2] Morrow AG, Brockenbrough EC. Surgical treatment of idiopathic hypertrophic subaortic stenosis: Technique and hemodynamic results of subaortic ventriculomyotomy. Annals of Surgery. 1961;**154**:181-189

[3] Gersh BJ, Maron BJ, Bonow RO, et al. 2011 ACCF/AHA guideline for the diagnosis and treatment of hypertrophic cardiomyopathy: A report of the American College of Cardiology Foundation/American Heart Association task force on practice guidelines. The Journal of Thoracic and Cardiovascular Surgery. 2011;**142**(6):e153-e203

[4] Nishimura RA, Giuliani ER, Brandenburg RO, et al. Hypertrophic cardiomyopathy. In: Giuliani ER, Gersh BJ, McGoon MD, Hayes DL, Schaff HV, editors. Myocardial Disease: Mayo Clinic Practice of Cardiology. 3rd ed. St. Louis, MO: Mosby-Year Book; 1996. pp. 689-711

[5] Said SM, Schaff HV. Surgical treatment of hypertrophic cardiomyopathy. Semin Thoracic Surg. 2014;**25**:300-309

[6] Wang S, Wang Z, Zhou B, Liu Z, Mei F, Luo C, et al. Minimally invasive right infra-axillary thoracotomy for transaortic septal myectomy. Journal of Cardiac Surgery. 2022;**37**(7):2197-2201

[7] Cj AK, Marc Gillinov A, Smedira NG, Hodges K, DJP B, Wierup P. Robotic trans-mitral septal myectomy and papillary muscle reorientation for HOCM combined with or without mitral valve repair: Technical aspects - how we do it. Journal of Cardiac Surgery. 2020;**35**(11):3120-3124

[8] Said S, Marey G. Transaortic extended left ventricular septal myectomy in an adult with hypertrophic obstructive cardiomyopathy. Multimedia Manual of Cardiothoracic Surgery. 23 Dec 2020;**2020**. DOI: 10.1510/mmcts.2020.074

[9] Said SM. Commentary: Extended left ventricular septal myectomy for hypertrophic cardiomyopathy: The nuts and bolts. The Journal of Thoracic and Cardiovascular Surgery. 2020;**159**(5):e299-e300

[10] Said SM, Schaff HV, Abel MD, Dearani JA. Transapical approach for apical myectomy and relief of midventricular obstruction in hypertrophic cardiomyopathy. Journal of Cardiac Surgery. 2012;**27**(4):443-448

[11] Matsuda H, Nomura F, Kadoba K, et al. Transatrial and transmitral approach for left ventricular myectomy and mitral valve plication for diffuse-type hypertrophic obstructive cardiomyopathy: A novel approach. The Journal of Thoracic and Cardiovascular Surgery. 1996;**112**(1):195-196

[12] Klues HG, Roberts WC, Maron BJ. Anomalous insertion of papillary muscle directly into anterior mitral leaflet in hypertrophic cardiomyopathy; significance in producing left ventricular outflow tract obstruction. Circulation. 1991;**84**:1188-1197

[13] Chen MS, McCarthy PM, Lever HM, et al. Effectiveness of atrial fibrillation surgery in patients with hypertrophic cardiomyopathy. The American Journal of Cardiology. 2004;**93**(3):373-375

[14] Wang S, Wang S, Lai Y, et al. Midterm results of different treatment methods for myocardial bridging in patients after septal myectomy. Journal of Cardiac Surgery. 2021;**36**:501-508

[15] Said SM, Marey G, Hiremath GM. Unroofing of myocardial bridging after septal Myectomy in a child with Noonan syndrome. World J Pediatr Congenit Heart Surg. 2021;**12**(5):659-660

[16] Rowin EJ, Maron BJ, Haas TS, Garberich RF, Wang W, Link MS, et al. Hypertrophic cardiomyopathy with left ventricular apical aneurysm: Implications for risk stratification and management. Journal of the American College of Cardiology. 2017;**69**:761-773

[17] Yang K, Song YY, Chen XY, et al. Apical hypertrophic cardiomyopathy with left ventricular apical aneurysm: Prevalence, cardiac magnetic resonance characteristics, and prognosis. Eur Heart J-Cardiovasc Imaging. 2020;**21**:1341-1350

[18] Nguyen A, Schaff HV. Electrical storms in patients with apical aneurysms and hypertrophic cardiomyopathy with midventricular obstruction - a case series. The Journal of Thoracic and Cardiovascular Surgery. 2017;**154**:e101-e103. DOI: 10.1016/j.jtcvs.2017.06.002

[19] Maron BJ, Shen WK, Link MS, et al. Efficacy of implantable cardioverter-defibrillators for the prevention of sudden death in patients with hypertrophic cardiomyopathy. The New England Journal of Medicine. 2000;**342**:365-373

[20] Francia P, Adduci C, Palano F, et al. Eligibility for the subcutaneous implantable cardioverter-defibrillator in patients with hypertrophic cardiomyopathy. Journal of Cardiovascular Electrophysiology. 2015;**26**:893-899

[21] Yacoub M, Onuzo O, Riedel B, et al. Mobilization of the left and right fibrous trigones for relief of severe left ventricular outflow obstruction. The Journal of Thoracic and Cardiovascular Surgery. 1999;**117**(1):126-132

[22] Laredo M, Khraiche D, Raisky O, et al. Long-term results of the modified Konno procedure in high-risk children with obstructive hypertrophic cardiomyopathy. The Journal of Thoracic and Cardiovascular Surgery. 2018;**156**:2285-2294

[23] Schaff HV, Dearani JA, Ommen SR, et al. Expanding the indications for septal myectomy in patients with hypertrophic cardiomyopathy: Results of operation in patients with latent obstruction. The Journal of Thoracic and Cardiovascular Surgery. 2012;**143**(2):303-309

[24] Minakata K, Dearani JA, Schaff HV, et al. Mechanisms for recurrent left ventricular outflow tract obstruction after septal myectomy for obstructive hypertrophic cardiomyopathy. The Annals of Thoracic Surgery. 2005;**80**(3):851-856

[25] ElBardissi AW, Dearani JA, Nishimura RA, et al. Septal myectomy after previous septal artery ablation in hypertrophic cardiomyopathy. Mayo Clinic Proceedings. 2007;**82**(12):1516-1522

[26] Said SM. Unroofing of LAD myocardial bridge combined with right ventricular septal Myectomy in a child with Noonan syndrome and HCM. 13 May 2020. DOI: 10.25373/ctsnet.12275447

[27] McCully RB, Nishimura RA, Tajik AJ, et al. Extent of clinical improvement after surgical treatment of hypertrophic obstructive cardiomyopathy. Circulation. 1996;**94**:467-471

[28] Nguyen A, Schaff HV, Nishimura RA, Geske JB, Dearani JA, King KS, et al. Apical myectomy for patients with hypertrophic cardiomyopathy and advanced heart failure. The Journal of Thoracic and Cardiovascular Surgery. 5 Apr 2019;**5**:S0022-5223(1)30772-X. DOI: 10.1016/j.jtcvs.2019.03.088 [Online ahead of print]

[29] Maron BJ, Spirito P, Wesley Y, et al. Development and progression of left ventricular hypertrophy in children with hypertrophic cardiomyopathy. The New England Journal of Medicine. 1986;**315**:610-614

[30] Arghami A, Dearani JA, Said SM, O'Leary PW, Schaff HV. Hypertrophic cardiomyopathy in children. Ann Cardiothorac Surg. 2017;**6**(4):376-385

[31] Sorajja P, Valeti U, Nishimura RA, et al. Outcome of alcohol septal ablation for obstructive hypertrophic cardiomyopathy. Circulation. 2008;**118**(2):131-139

Section 4

Infiltrative Cardiomyopathy

Chapter 5

Cardiac Amyloidosis

Sonia Vicenty-Rivera and Ingrid Bonilla-Mercado

Abstract

Cardiac amyloidosis is a protein-folding disorder mostly caused by abnormal deposition of either transthyretin proteins or light chain (AL) proteins, into one or more organs, including the heart. The main cardiac manifestations are right ventricular heart failure and arrhythmias. Extracardiac symptoms usually precede cardiac symptoms and are evident several years before the development of symptomatic cardiac problems. The prognosis is poor without appropriate management. Non-invasive evaluation with multi-imaging modalities has allowed earlier diagnosis, particularly when used in combination with monoclonal gammopathy evaluation. Management will vary depending on the subtype of amyloidosis. It consists of supportive treatment of cardiac-related symptoms, pharmacological treatment that targets amyloid fibrils formation and deposition, thus attacking the underlying disease, and addressing the management of extracardiac symptoms to improve the patients' quality of life.

Keywords: cardiac amyloidosis (CA), transthyretin cardiomyopathy (ATTR-CM), wild type-ATTR (wtATTR), hereditary (variant, mutant) transthyretin cardiomyopathy (hATTR, vATTR), systemic (AL) cardiac amyloidosis (AL-CM), atrial fibrillation (AF), heart failure (HF)

1. Introduction

Amyloidosis is an infiltrative disorder primarily caused by extracellular tissue deposition of amyloid fibrils. It occurs when the misfolded protein assembles with similar proteins to form oligomers, which circulate in the blood and deposit as highly ordered fibrils, in the interstitial space of target organs [1]. These deposits are comprised of insoluble low molecular weight protein subunits ranging from 5 to 25 kD leading to the outlined systemic disease [2]. Up to date there are at least 25 different human and 8 different animal amyloidogenic proteins identified [1]. Tissue infiltration occurs in many organs such as kidney, liver, autonomic nervous system, and heart. However, >95% of cardiac amyloidosis is secondary to immunoglobulin light chain amyloidosis (AL) and transthyretin amyloidosis (ATTR) [3].

It was previously understood that cardiac amyloidosis was a rare and fatal disease. Nevertheless, with the emergence of advanced cardiac imaging studies as well as the availability of new pharmacological treatment for transthyretin amyloidosis and increased awareness of the disease among physicians, and better guidance for accurate diagnosis there has been a marked increase in diagnosis of this previously underrecognized medical condition. Nevertheless, despite increased awareness of the disease, sociodemographic disparities in diagnosis and management of cardiac amyloidosis exist, thus leading to a delay in treatment and increased disease severity at time of diagnosis within certain sociodemographic groups [4, 5].

In this chapter, we will discuss in detail the clinical presentation, identification process, and implications for early detection of cardiac amyloidosis to improve patient outcomes. Additionally, we will discuss new emerging therapeutic approaches and the importance of socioeconomic disparities within the disease.

2. Pathophysiology

Cardiac amyloidosis (CA) is also known as "stiff heart syndrome" because the amyloid protein infiltration leads to increased cardiac wall thickness and ventricular stiffness (**Figure 1**) [1]. The natural progression of amyloidosis includes involvement of other organs prior to its cardiac manifestation.

2.1 AL amyloidosis

In AL amyloidosis, the deposits are formed by accumulation of kappa or lambda light chain proteins. These proteins in normal conditions are produced by plasma cells. However, when the cells overproduce light chains, they become amyloidogenic

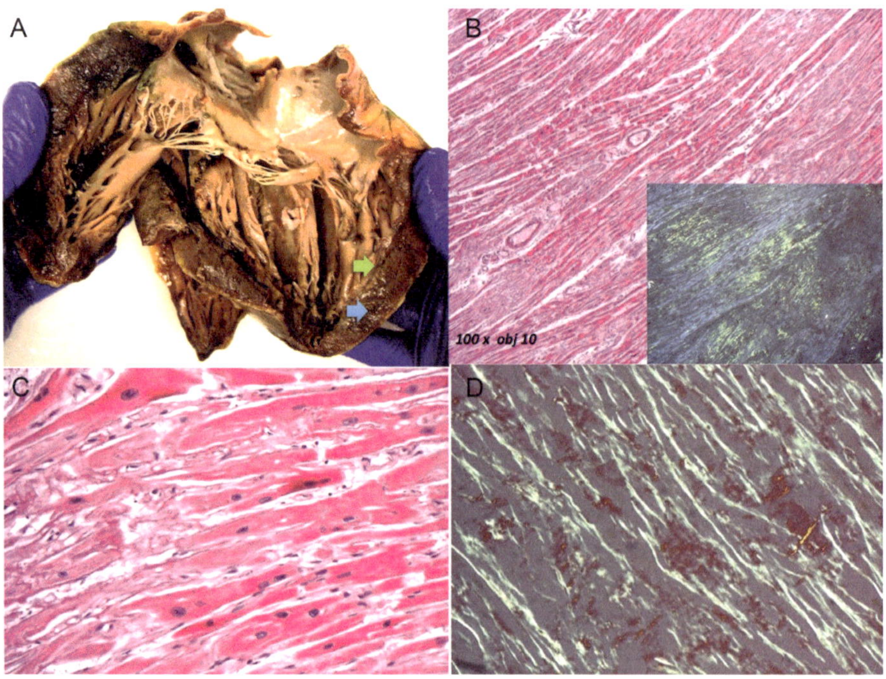

Figure 1.
Cardiac amyloidosis Pathophysiology. (A) Gross specimen inspection reveals a rubbery consistency of the myocardium. On some occasions, there can be evidence of intracardiac thrombi. The lighter-tan colored material is amyloid (green arrowhead) and the darker tissue represents normal myocardium (blue arrowhead). (B) Hematoxylin and eosin-stained (inset) microscopic sections with characteristic ring-like encircling of myofibers and the lack of the wavy fibrillar character of collagen. (C) 400× magnification and (D) is 400× magnification of the eosin-stained section with Congo Red staining microscopic sections, amyloid is red-orange, the protein is birefringent so that when Congo Red-stained tissue is viewed under polarized light it transmits an apple-green color.

and deposit in the autonomic and peripheral sensory nervous system, spleen, lungs, and heart. This process can happen spontaneously or because of certain blood or immune system cancers. The major conditions associated with AL amyloidosis are multiple myeloma, Waldenström's macroglobulinemia, and B-cell lymphomas [6].

In addition to mechanical and architectural damage mediated by cardiac AL-fibril deposition, the soluble AL protein has been proven to have directly toxic effects on myocardial tissue. In experimental mouse models, it was shown that the rapid progression of heart failure and left ventricular dysfunction seen in AL amyloidosis is caused by toxic effect of circulating light chains on the already diseased myocardium by the amyloid protein deposition [7]. Later another group demonstrated that this toxic effect was mediated by p38α mitogen-activated protein kinases (MAPK) signaling which can upregulate pro-BNP. In fact, increased pro-BNP can be indicative of both amyloid disease activity and the degree of cardiac injury [8, 9].

2.2 ATTR cardiomyopathy

ATTR cardiomyopathy is caused by a transthyretin protein (TTP), previously known as prealbumin. It is a 55 kD protein whose main function is to transport both thyroxine (T4) and retinol-binding protein. About 85% of the TTP protein is produced in the liver, with the rest being synthesized in the choroid plexus, the retinal and ciliary pigment epithelia of the eye, and the pancreas [10–12]. TTP normally circulates as a homotetramer, with a small amount of transthyretin circulating in monomeric form. The monomeric form of transthyretin is prone to misfolding leading to a gradual formation of amyloid deposits. There are two types of transthyretin amyloidosis, hereditary or variant (ATTRv) and wild or senile (ATTRwt), both of which are caused by a misfolding of TTR protein.

2.2.1 Hereditary ATTR (ATTRv)

The hereditary type is caused by a TTR gene missense mutation the patient is born with, that causes a decrease in the stability of the tetramer conformation of the protein, promoting its dissociation into monomers and consequent leading to misfolding. Following the dissociation and misfolding events, the aggregation and deposition of insoluble TTR and nonbranching amyloid fibers, typically with a diameter of 10 nm, occur in the extracellular spaces of many tissues and organs [11]. Currently, there are over 130 identified point mutations in the gene that encodes TTR synthesis, which is located on the long arm of chromosome 18 [10, 11]. Most of these point mutations can cause amyloidosis disease. In the US, the most common mutation is the V122I, found in 3–3.5% of individuals of African descent. Despite the prevalence of the mutation within the African American population, cardiac amyloidosis still represents a severely underdiagnosed form of heart failure within this population [13]. ATTRv phenotypic expression will vary depending on the type of transthyretin protein mutation with symptoms ranging from severe peripheral neuropathy (familial amyloidotic polyneuropathy) to cardiac amyloid cardiomyopathy and conduction abnormalities (familial amyloid cardiomyopathy) [9–11].

2.2.2 Wild-type or senile ATTR (ATTRwt)

In ATTRwt, it is believed the phenomenon occurs as part of an unknown aging-related mechanism, where TTR molecules misfold and deposit within the heart and other organs as amyloid fibrils. The most common clinical manifestations are motor and sensory neuropathy, gastrointestinal disturbances, and cardiomyopathy [14]. Both amyloid deposition and its effects on surrounding organs establish the phenotype of the disease [1]. Amyloid fibers can cause direct compression or obstruction in neighboring structures, which manifests as conditions such as carpal tunnel syndrome and vitreous opacities [14]. As amyloid fibers accumulate, patients experience progressive dysfunction with symptoms that may not start until years after the initial amyloid formation and deposition [11].

3. Epidemiology

About >95% of cases of cardiac amyloidosis are caused or related to light chain (AL) amyloidosis and transthyretin (ATTR) amyloidosis.

3.1 AL-amyloidosis

AL amyloidosis has an incidence of approximately 4000 new cases of amyloidosis annually in the United States. However, the actual incidence may be higher due to the disease under diagnosis. While the incidence is thought to be equal in males and females, about 60% of patients referred to amyloid centers are males [15]. However, only half of these patients present cardiac manifestations of systemic (AL) amyloidosis. Once heart failure symptoms ensue, prognosis is poor with a median survival of <6 months if plasma cell dyscrasia is left untreated [16]. In AL-cardiac amyloidosis, poor prognosis is associated with increased LV relative wall thickness, older age, NYHA class, elevated pro-BNP, and increased C-reactive proteins [16, 17].

3.2 ATTR amyloidosis

On the other hand, ATTR amyloidosis, which was thought to be a rare cause for CA, has recently been more frequently diagnosed. This is a result of the use of new cardiac imaging techniques and increased availability of imaging and diagnostic tools clinical practices, that have revolutionized the diagnosis of cardiac diseases. However, despite advances and availability in imaging techniques, this condition is still frequently underdiagnosed due its myriad of signs and symptoms, which are often associated with other diseases, leading to a poorly delineated prevalence of the disease. Earlier reports of patients undergoing noninvasive diagnosis with patients older than 60 years, Gonzalez et al. found a staggering 13% prevalence of CA in patients admitted with clinical diagnosis of decompensated heart failure with preserved ejection fraction [13]. Meanwhile, AbouEzzeddine et al. performed a community based-setting cohort study in which ATTR-CM was found in a substantial number of older male patients with heart failure with preserved ejection fraction (HFpEF) (2.5% with 95% CI, 1.4–4.0%). This study highlights the importance of systemic screening for CA in male patients with HFpEF and LV wall thickening [14].

3.2.1 ATTRwt

ATTRwt almost exclusively occurs in male patients 70 years or older with a median survival after the onset of heart failure of 7.5 years [18]. The average worldwide prevalence is estimated to be 1/6000 [19]. Interestingly autopsy studies on from patients with antemortem diagnosis of HFpEF demonstrated presence of fibrillar deposits within the heart in 25% of the patients older than 80 years of age [20]. Moreover several studies have shown that one in seven elderly patient with aortic stenosis also suffer from cardiac amyloidosis [5]. While the exact mechanism or reason behind the frequent coexistence of both diseases in such patients is not fully understood, several hypotheses have been drawn in aims to provide a plausible explanation. The coexistence of severe aortic stenosis with ATTRwt has been shown to not have a significant impact in patient survival; special considerations should be taken with these patients at the time of treatment and will be addressed in greater detail later in the chapter. In comparison to ATTRv, ATTRwt almost exclusively affects the heart with involvement of both atrial and ventricular chambers and frequent incidence of conduction disorder and arrhythmias [20]. However, patients with ATTRwt have been shown to have some extracardiac manifestations of the disease such as musculoskeletal involvement like carpal tunnel syndrome in up to 33–49%, traumatic bicep rupture 33%, and lumbar stenosis 37% [21–23]. Extracardiac symptoms can precede cardiac ones up 5–7 years before cardiac amyloidosis diagnosis [24].

3.2.2 ATTRv

ATTRv onset has been shown to occur earlier in males than in females. Interestingly, the age of onset is progressively earlier in successive generations [11]. From the hereditary subtypes, the mutations known to have cardiac effects are TTR V30M, t TTR V122I, and TTR T60A. Most of these mutations are found clustered into distinct ethnicity groups and/or within certain geographical areas. Its inheritance has an autosomal dominant pattern [25]. The V30M mutation is the most common mutation worldwide, especially in parts of Portugal, Japan, and northern Sweden. Nevertheless, it has also been identified in Spain, France, South America, and some nonendemic areas of Africa. It has a slight female predominance with a bimodal presentation with earlier onset of V30M ATTR symptoms being mostly neurological and late-onset symptoms that present with both cardiomyopathic and polyneuropathic involvement [26].

On the other hand, the most common mutation in the US associated with late-onset cardiomyopathy is V122I. It is frequently diagnosed among African Americans with an incidence of 3–4% compared to 0.44% among white individuals. Moreover, within African American population this mutation can be found in up to 10% of the patients over 65 years of age who have developed severe HF [27]. The T60A variant is the second-most-common TTR variant in the US and the most common in the UK and Ireland, affecting approximately 1% of the population of north-western Ireland. It has an unknown gender distribution which occurs in patients >60 years of age with cardiac involvement as well as autonomic and peripheral neuropathies [10, 11, 27]. However, even though there are no set gender distribution male patients tend to have a mean age of presentation of 60–65 years of age, while female patients tend to have a latter onset. ATTRv is an important cause of heart failure that disproportionately affects people of African descent. Despite the high burden of ATTRv among black individuals, just a few studies include African American patients and most of the clinical data, we have for ATTRv come from North America and Europe. Moreover, despite the known and well-established predisposition to cardiovascular diseases within other minority groups such as Hispanic/Latino population, the only minority group to be included and studied in clinical trials so far has been African American patients [28]. There is no known clinical data to describe epidemiological characteristics of ATTRv in the Hispanic/Latino population. Nevertheless, efforts to promote earlier identification of ATTRv in general practice will improve clinical outcomes for all groups.

4. Clinical manifestations and physical examination

As previously mentioned, amyloidosis is a systemic disease. Therefore, patients with cardiac amyloidosis have amyloid fibril affecting the cardiovascular system and involvement of the musculoskeletal system, peripheral nervous system, and autonomic nervous system. Since the systemic manifestation commonly precedes the cardiac manifestation, it often results in delayed diagnosis. Non-cardiac clinical manifestations are diverse and includes lumbar spinal stenosis, GI symptoms such as constipation or diarrhea, nausea or vomiting, unexplained nephrotic syndrome with some degrees of renal insufficiency, sensorimotor peripheral neuropathy, arrhythmias, autonomic and peripheral neuropathies, and bilateral carpal tunnel syndrome. The latter can be diagnosed up to 10 years before confirmation and diagnosis of ATTR amyloidosis [13, 14, 18, 19]. Therefore, by the time patient starts to develop cardiovascular symptoms, usually there is extensive systemic and myocardial infiltration. A survey of 533 people, including patients with ATTR and their family members, by Lousada et al. found that the correct diagnosis in patients with wild-type ATTR, was made within 6 months in up to 46% of patients and at times the correct diagnosis required >5 different physicians [29].

Cardiovascular manifestations can be four-fold, including congestive heart failure due to restrictive cardiomyopathy, vascular abnormalities, autonomic dysfunction, and conduction abnormalities. Dyspnea is the most common complaint associated with elevated right heart side pressure. Physical examination in advanced disease is noteworthy for prominent jugular venous distention associated with evident "x" and "y" descent, peripheral edema, hepatic congestion, and ascites [30]. The lower extremity edema is usually disproportionate to the degree of heart failure and is related to the degree of nephrotic syndrome. A right ventricular S3 is usually present and correlates with the degree of right ventricular dilatation and dysfunction. The S4 is always absent despite a decrease in left ventricular compliance due to atrial dysfunction secondary to amyloid infiltration. Lung field can reveal bilateral pleural effusion that tends to be diuretics resistant requiring in many cases frequent thoracentesis for fluid removal with high degree of recurrence [31].

Vascular involvement can be seen due to amyloid deposition leading to increase in vessel wall thickness or endothelial functional abnormalities (**Figure 1**). Autopsy studies have demonstrated amyloid infiltration of the small intramural coronary arteries in up to 88–90% of AL patients. Furthermore, the arterial abnormalities do not appear to be related to echocardiographic evidence of cardiac involvement [32]. Patients may present with atypical and typical angina pectoris due to small vessels involvement [33]. Persistent increase in troponin level may be present leading with misdiagnosis of non-ST elevation myocardial infarction [34]. Despite the presence or absence of at true ischemic event, this elevation of cardiac markers is a negative prognostic factor [35, 36].

A hallmark of CA is autonomic dysfunction and can be interpreted as an early symptom, thus patients should be carefully evaluated for dizziness, near syncope and syncopal events. However, many factors may contribute to syncope such as postural hypotension due to excessive diuresis or autonomic neuropathy and small ventricular cavities. Low blood pressure is a common finding and not necessarily accompanied by orthostatic hypotension. It has long been known that syncope is common in AL amyloid heart disease and mostly precipitated by physiologic stress. Stress-precipitated syncope is associated with a poor prognosis in such patients, both in terms of their median survival (2 months) and as a common precursor of sudden cardiac death [32]. Additionally, autonomic dysfunction in these patients is associated with decreased cardiac output. However, there is no evident association between syncopal events and mortality in ATTR patients despite frequent events and poor quality of life [37, 38].

5. Diagnostic evaluation

The diagnostic evaluation begins with a complete history and physical examination, mainly considering both cardiac and non-cardiac signs and symptoms or "red flags" that suggest high suspicion for the condition to delineate a diagnostic approach using a combination of serum biomarkers as well as imaging studies (**Table 1**).

Clinical findings	Imaging studies	Biomarkers
Cardiac symptoms • Heart Failure • Intolerance to standard HF treatment • Cardiac arrhythmias (CAVB, slow AF • Low flow low gradient or paradoxical Low flow low gradient AS	**Transthoracic echocardiogram** • Increase left ventricular wall width >1.2 cm in the absence of underlying cause • Phenotypical echocardiographic finding of infiltrative characteristics such as atrioventricular wall thickening, interatrial septum thickening, and thickening of the left ventricular free wall	• Persistent elevation of troponin in the absence of acute coronary events • Persistent elevation of N-Pro-BNP
Non-cardiac Symptoms • Musculoskeletal-> bilateral carpal tunnel, lumbar spinal stenosis, biceps tendon rupture • Symptoms of peripheral or sensorimotor neuropathy and dysautonomia • Gastrointestinal manifestations such as diarrhea, constipation, or unintentional weight loss • Renal impairment or cardiorenal syndrome	**CMR** • Global subendocardial late gadolinium enhancement • Elevated native T1 value • Expanded ECV	

HF, heart failure; CAVB, complete atrioventricular block; AF, atrial fibrillation; AS, aortic stenosis; CMR, cardiac magnetic resonance; ECV, extracellular volume; N-Pro-BNP, N-terminal-pro hormone-brain natriuretic peptide.

Table 1.
Red flags for cardiac amyloidosis.

5.1 Serum biomarkers

5.1.1 ATTR

Witteles et al. propose considering evaluation of ATTR cardiomyopathy in patients older than 65 years (females >75 years) with a diagnosis of heart failure and ≥ 1 clinical finding indicative of ATTR such as suggestive imaging tests results, and/or chronic elevation in biomarkers (troponins, BNP, pro-BNP) [39–41]. Appropriate assessment include evaluation of absence of monoclonal gammopathy using serum free light chains (FLC), serum, and urine immunofixation electrophoresis as serum protein electrophoresis is insensitive leasing to false negative results.

5.1.2 AL cardiac amyloidosis

Pro-BNP concentration is found to be increased in patients with heart failure and in patients with AL amyloidosis before the onset of clinical heart failure. This peptide is considered a marker for cardiac involvement. A report where pro-BNP was measured in patients with AL amyloidosis, found that its concentration was elevated despite the presence of clinical heart failure. Moreover, the diagnostic utility of pro-BNP study in 152 patients identified with amyloidosis where a plasma N-terminal pro-BNP concentration of 152 pmol/L detected cardiac involvement with a sensitivity of 93% and specificity of 90% [42].

5.2 Electrocardiogram (ECG)

Low voltage electrocardiogram QRS (<0.5 mV on limb leads, <1 mV on precordial leads, and Sokolow index defined as the sum of amplitudes of the S-wave in V1 and the R-wave in $V_{5\text{-}6}$ < 1.5 mV) has always been thought to be pathognomonic of cardiac amyloidosis (**Figure 2**). Nevertheless, this finding has been shown to have low sensitivity and its prevalence varies markedly according to the etiology of cardiomyopathy. Low voltage QRS is found in around 60% of AL-type amyloidosis and in close to 20% of ATTR type amyloidosis [43]. However, when present it has been associated with poor survival regardless the type of cardiac amyloidosis [43]. Moreover, a Sokolow index <1.5 mV was shown to be predictive of a combined outcome of time to hospitalization, heart transplant, or death in both AL and ATTR cardiomyopathies [44]. On the other hand, some studies have suggested that an increase in LV mass to EKG voltage relationship (mass-voltage ratio) might be more specific to CA than low voltage alone perse [45, 46]. Left ventricular hypertrophy changes have been described in precordial leads in small group of patients with very uncommon hypertrophy changes noted in limb leads [43].

Other electrocardiographic evaluation using signal-averaged ECG (SAECG) shows that late potentials were significantly more frequents on patients with echocardiographic evidence of cardiac amyloidosis (31% vs. 9% in those with normal echocardiograms) and was independently predictive of an increased risk of sudden cardiac death [47].

5.3 Transthoracic echocardiography

Transthoracic echocardiography is cornerstone in the diagnostic evaluation of patients with heart disease and is considered the standard of care in cases in

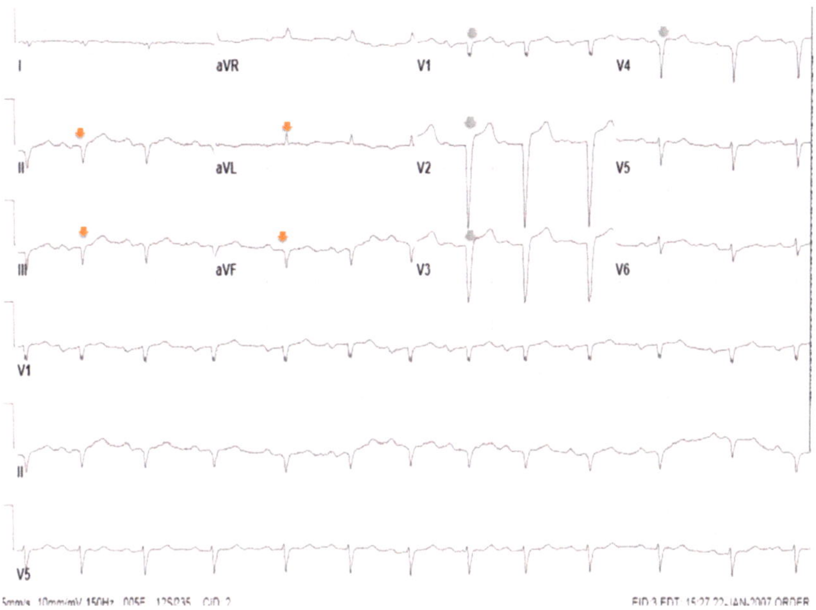

Figure 2.
Low voltage ECG 12-lead electrocardiography depicting the typical changes observed in cardiac amyloidosis. Low voltage limb leads (orange arrowhead) and poor precordial leads "R" wave progression with pseudo infarct pattern (green arrowhead) secondary to amyloid infiltration at the level of the left ventricular myocardium. Also, there is evidence of sinoatrial and atrioventricular conduction defects in this case there is a 1st degree AV block secondary to amyloid infiltration into the conduction system.

which CA is suspected. Cardiac amyloidosis has very distinctive echocardiographic features such as small LV cavity with associated increased left ventricular thickening (>12 mm) (**Figures 1** and **3**), biatrial enlargement, increased thickness of right ventricle, interatrial septum, and atrioventricular valves (**Figure 3**) with near normal LV systolic performance. The often-described increased echogenicity characterized as granular or sparkling texture pathognomonic of cardiac amyloidosis is not very sensitive and only present in a minority of patients especially when disease is advanced (**Figure 3**) [48, 49]. However, this changes which are often referred to as hypertrophy are inaccurate since it is caused by a progressive infiltrative process rather than myocyte hypertrophy as it occurs in other forms of cardiomyopathy. AL and ATTR have overlapping echocardiographic features, although in general ATTR is characterized by thicker walls, owing to the more insidious nature of deposition and late diagnosis versus the toxic aspect of light chains in AL facilitating apoptosis and earlier recognition. However, asymmetric left ventricular thickness, mimicking hypertrophic cardiomyopathy, has been described in patients with familial amyloidosis [50]. Studies have demonstrated that there is a correlation between severity of LV thickness, a higher frequency of associated echocardiographic abnormalities such as left atrial enlargement or granular sparkling appearance and more common reduced systolic function with a decrease survival (median of 1.1 years) in these patients [51]. RV involvement assessed with TAPSE <14 mm is associated with events such as worsening of heart failure, increased mortality and heart transplant (**Figure 3**) [48, 52]. Diastolic dysfunction to different degrees is common and is present in all patients. In advanced CA, doppler mitral flow evaluation shows restrictive pattern characterized with short deceleration time of E wave with decreased A wave velocity (**Figure 3**).

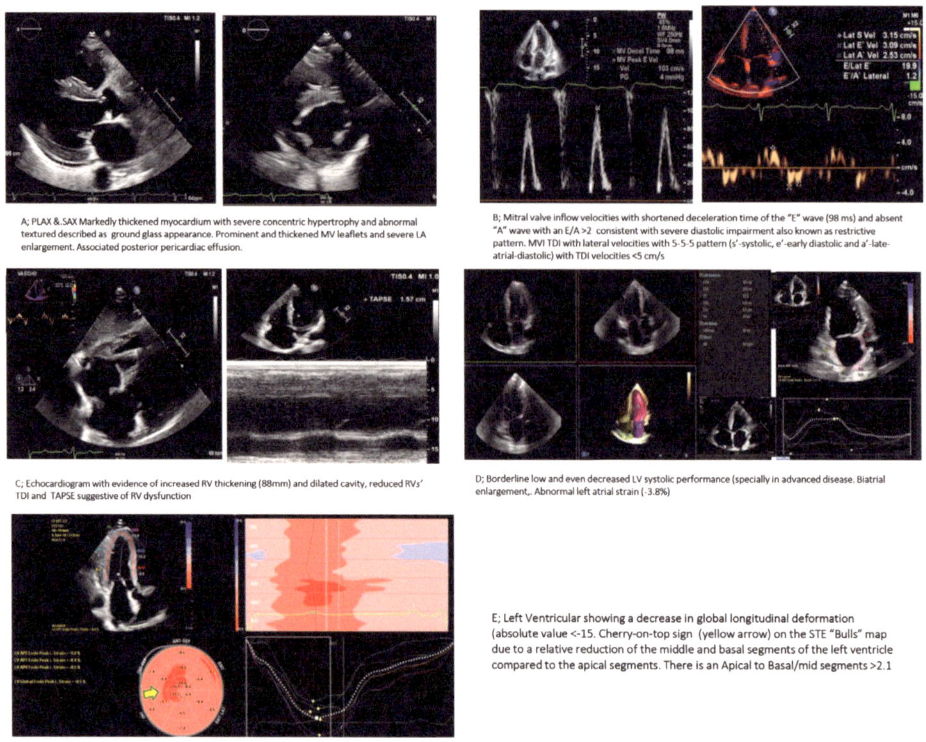

Figure 3.
Transthoracic echocardiogram with characteristic findings of cardiac amyloidosis (A) PLAX & SAX Markedly thickened myocardium with severe concentric hypertrophy and abnormal texture described as ground glass appearance. Prominent and thickened MV leaflets and severe LA enlargement. Associated posterior pericardiac effusion (B) mitral valve inflow velocities with shortened deceleration time of the "E" wave (98 ms) and absent "A" wave with an E/A > 2 consistent with severe diastolic impairment also known as restrictive pattern. MVI TDI with lateral velocities with 5-5-5 pattern (s'—systolic, e'—early diastolic, and a'—late-atrial-diastolic) with TDI velocities <5 cm/s. (C) Echocardiogram with evidence of increased RV thickening (88 mm) and dilated cavity, reduced RVs' TDI and TAPSE suggestive of RV dysfunction. (D) Left ventricular showing a decrease in global longitudinal deformation (absolute value < −15. Cherry-on-top sign (yellow arrow) on the STE "Bulls" map due to a relative reduction of the middle and basal segments of the left ventricle compared to the apical segments. There is an Apical to Basal/mid segments >2.1.

Diminished A wave velocity is due to progression of restrictive disease and intrinsic atrial dysfunction.

Tissue Doppler, strain, and strain rate imaging allows early diagnosis of diastolic dysfunction in patients with cardiac amyloid and helps distinguish cardiac amyloidosis from other restrictive cardiomyopathies etiologies such as constrictive pericarditis. Usually, a mitral annular diastolic velocity (E') <8 cm/s is a good discriminator for restrictive physiology [51, 52]. In patient with more advanced presentation of CA, the "5-5-5" sign with TDI velocities are <5 cm/s (**Figure 3**). Other signs of advanced CA besides tissue velocities include increased isovolumetric contraction time (IVCT) and isovolumetric relaxation time (IVRT) and decreased ejection time. However, regional strain has shown long-axis dysfunction in early cardiac amyloidosis and impairment of longitudinal contraction despite preserved fractional shortening. Reduction in global measures of systolic function, such as left ventricular (LV) ejection fraction, are late manifestations and characteristics of advanced disease. In CA, overall global longitudinal strain (GLS) is < −15 with a characteristically depressed longitudinal strain of the basal and mid-ventricular segment while preserved apical segments, better known as apical sparing or "Cherry-on-top" is common (**Figure 3**). Moreover, reduced GLS have been suggested to be an independent predictor of survival in both AL and ATTR [51]. Left atrial strain analysis by stress echocardiogram (STE) (normal −40%) shows severely decreased LA function with elevated LA volumes and can be helpful for monitoring and prediction of thromboembolic risk (**Figure 3**) [48].

5.4 Cardiac magnetic resonance imaging (MRI)

Cardiac MRI has been used for identification of cardiac amyloidosis in patients with unexplained heart failure and arrhythmias in which echocardiographic findings are suspicious yet inconclusive [52]. It is a highly specific tool for the diagnosis of CA because of its intrinsic capacity to characterized tissue by using late gadolinium enhancement and parametric mapping techniques (T1) and its ability to assess extracellular Volume [ECV]) (**Figure 4**) [53]. In CA, late gadolinium

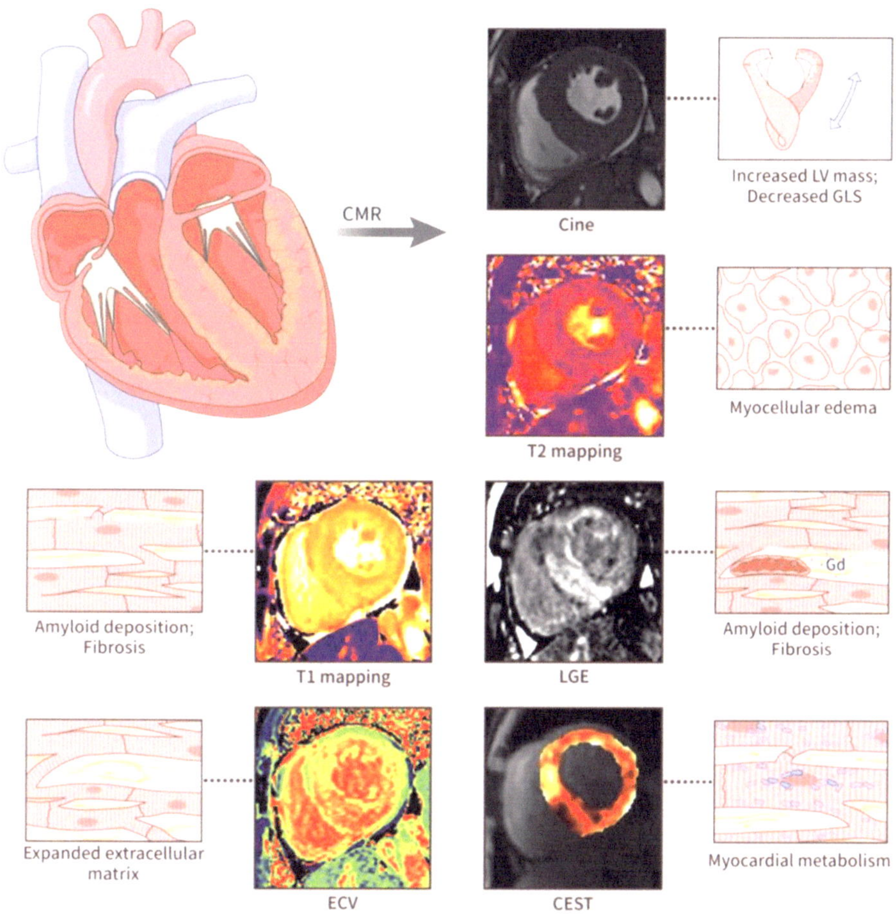

Figure 4.
Common cardiac MRI findings found in cardiac amyloidosis using state-of-the art cardiac MRI approach. The rights of this figure were obtained. Permission for the reproduction of the image was obtained by the authors. Magnetic Resonance Imaging, First published: 30 June 2022, DOI: 10.1002/jmri.28314.

enhancement (LGE) distributes in the extracellular space not following a specific coronary distribution. Different patterns have been observed such as diffuse patterns that can progress from subendocardial to transmural. The circumferential subendocardial LGE has been more frequently seen in patients with AL-CM whereas the diffuse transmural LGE pattern has been more frequently associated with ATTR-CM [54]. The degree and severity of LGE is associated with increased mortality. Native (noncontrast) T1 or T1 time is measured without contrasts and may reflect changes in tissue composition such as in intracellular or extracellular compartments affected by collagen, protein, edema, lipids, and iron content [54]. Whereas postcontrast T1 is used to calculate ECV a which is a surrogate parameter for the extracellular matrix. Both, native T1 and ECV have demonstrated their usefulness as biomarkers for CA diagnosis [54]. A series from National Amyloidosis Centre in the United Kingdom followed hematologic-measured treatment response and correlated them with ECV findings. They concluded that cardiac MRI-detected change in ECV at 6 months to be prognostic for long-term outcomes, even after controlling for the hematologic response. Suggesting that cardiac involvement in AL amyloidosis does not walk so tightly together with hematologic involvement and that serial analysis of the presumed cardiac amyloid burden with cardiac MRI during treatment may be important to comprehensively assess treatment response [55].

5.5 Bone radiotracers

99mTc-PYP/DPD/HMDP cardiac scans have become a chief diagnostic tool used in the diagnosis and differentiation of cardiac amyloidosis. In 1980, it was observed for the first time the uptake of ^{99m}Tc-phosohate in cardiac material from patients undergoing bone scan for evaluation of bone metastasis [56]. Later in 2005, Perugini et al. demonstrated the usefulness of ^{99m}Tc-DPD scintigraphy in diagnosis and successful differentiation of TTR versus AL etiology in patients with documented cardiac amyloidosis [56]. Radiotracer uptake was attributed to possible higher calcium content un ATTR amyloid deposits [57, 58].

There are two approaches for pyrophosphate image interpretation: quantitative vs. semiquantitative evaluation (**Figure 5**). In the quantitative PYP evaluation, a circular target region of interest (ROI) is drawn over the heart on the planar images and are mirrored on the contralateral chest to account for the background of the ribs (H/CL) [52]. Total and absolute counts are measured in each ROI and a ratio of heart-to-contralateral lung determined. When myocardial uptake is visually present in 1 hour, it is considered positive for ATTR if H/CL >1.5. On the other hand, the Perugini grading scale is a semi-quantitative method of scoring cardiac uptake following injection of 99mTc-DPD, 99mTc-Pyrophosphate or 99mTc-HMDP scintigraphy in the investigation of cardiac amyloidosis (particularly ATTR amyloidosis). The grading scale visually compares tracer uptake in the myocardium and ribs and will grade it from 0 to 3 depending on the cardiac uptake compared to the rib with 0 as no cardiac uptake and 3 as cardiac uptake greater than rib uptake. Visual scores greater than 2 on planar ± SPECT/CT imaging without evidence for monoclonal proteins in blood and urine, renders a diagnosis of ATTR cardiac amyloidosis with specificity and positive predictive value >98% (**Figure 5**) [52, 59]. Substantial uptake (Grade 2 or 3) has been reported in more than 20% of patients with AL cardiac amyloidosis.

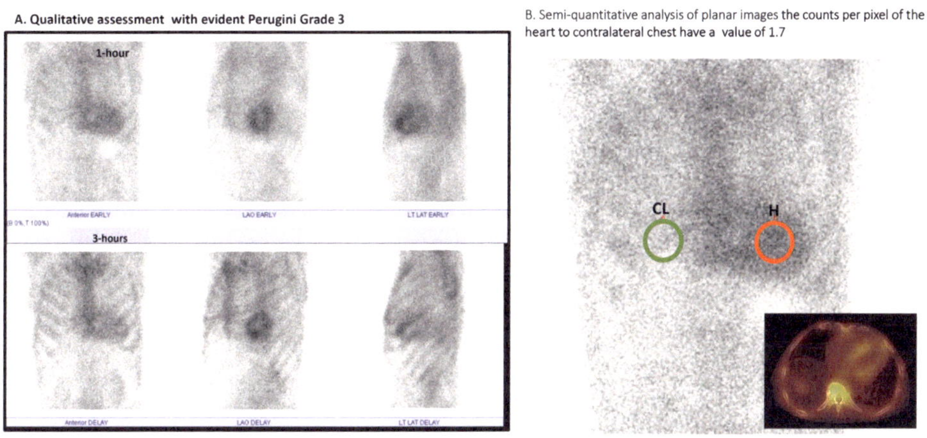

Figure 5.
Cardiac scintigraphy in cardiac amyloidosis. (A) Qualitative assessment with evident Perugini Grade 3. The Perugini visual grading rule as follows: grade 0 = cardiac uptake not visible, grade 1 = mild cardiac uptake visible but inferior to skeletal uptake, grade 2 = moderate cardiac uptake visible equal to or greater than skeletal uptake, and grade 3 = strong cardiac uptake with little or no skeletal uptake. In the (B) semi-quantitative analysis of planar images, the counts per pixel of the heart to contralateral chest have a value of 1.7 (red circle with the H denotes heart or cardiac uptake and green circle with CL denotes contralateral uptake). Semi-quantitative analysis of planar images with both anterior and lateral views planar images are evaluated, by drawing a patient-specific circular ROI on the heart and mirroring it to the contralateral chest to calculate the heart-to-contralateral (H/CL).

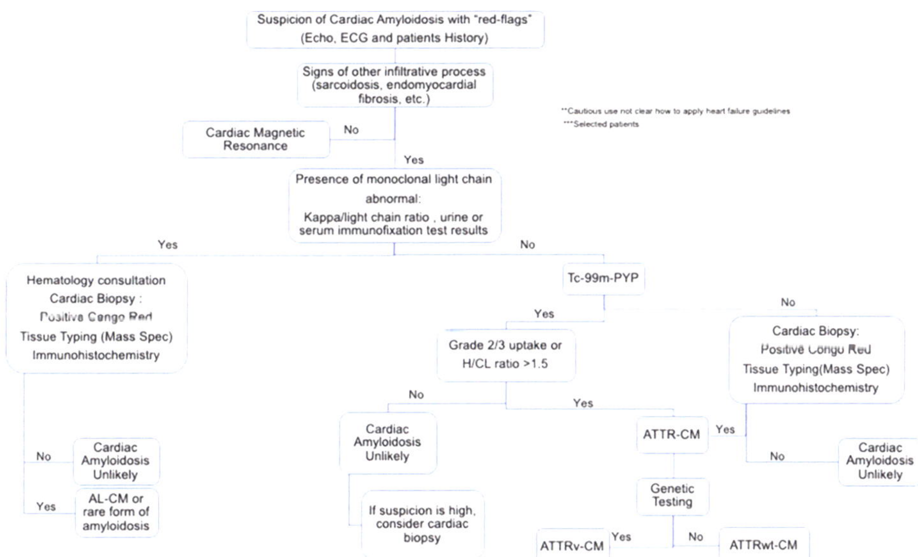

Figure 6.
Cardiac amyloidosis diagnosis flowchart.

5.6 Tissue biopsy

Tissue diagnosis with endomyocardial biopsy remains the goal standard for diagnosis CA. However, since it is invasive, it is usually reserved for those patients in which noninvasive assessment has been equivocal such as in the case of patients where plasma cell dyscrasia cannot be entirely ruled out or those with presence of low-grade uptake [55]. Diagnosis is evident with confirmation of amyloid deposition throughout with evidence of apple-green birefringence using Congo Red staining (**Figure 1**). The type of cardiac amyloidosis can also be determined using mass spectrometry and immunohistochemistry approaches. Another approach that is less invasive is the use of fat pad biopsy, however, its sensitivity is less than that of tissue biopsy (20% vs. 60–80%) [1].

5.7 Genetic testing

All the approaches described above can be used to distinguish between AL amyloidosis and ATTR amyloidosis. However, as it was discussed in Section 3.2 there are two distinct kinds of ATTR, one hereditary and one senile. Therefore, to distinguish between both and to further identify the kind of mutation that exists in the case of ATTRv, genetic testing is granted.

A summarized flowchart for ease and aid of cardiac amyloidosis diagnosis can be found in **Figure 6**.

6. Natural history and prognosis

The overall prognosis of cardiac amyloidosis depends on the type of amyloidogenic protein accumulating in the heart. For instance, AL-CM has the worst prognosis and is considered a hematologic emergency. It has a median survival of 6 months without disease-specific treatment. Therefore, it is imperative to differentiate between AL and ATTR-CM. On the other hand, ATTR is frequently misdiagnosed, leading to delayed diagnosis and treatment. Disease causes significant impairment in physical health, productivity, and lower quality of life. Once ATTR is diagnosed, untreated patients have a median survival of 2–3.5 years. There are multiple staging systems based on clinical as NYHA class, and laboratories such as NT-pro-BNP, troponin, and renal parameters which help delineate treatment strategist (**Table 2**).

7. Treatment options

Management of cardiac amyloidosis consists of treatment and management to stabilize heart failure symptoms while providing medications to stabilize amyloidogenic protein (**Figures** 7 and **8** and **Table 2**). An interdisciplinary treatment approach is paramount in lieu of patients' limited physical capacity and quality of life due to the extensive extracardiac symptom involvement. Diuretics tend to be the first line of management for the control of congestive symptoms. These may be prescribed in combination with mineralocorticoid receptor antagonists. Usually, these patients have higher rate of third spacing with associated right heart failure, thus frequently require diuretics with better bioavailability such as bumetanide and torsemide and addition of mineralocorticoid agents. One of the main challenges patients with CA face is recurrent congestion requiring high dose of diuretics as well as frequent hospitalization. However not all traditional drugs used for the treatment of HF are adequate or have been proven to exert any benefit in patients with cardiac amyloidosis.

On the other hand, neurohormonal antagonists which are typically used in HF treatment are often poorly tolerated and might be counterproductive in some patients.

Transthyretin-CA	AL-CA
Mayo Clinic Model Based on cohort of ATTRwt patients using trop T (>0.05 ng/ml) and NT-pBNP (>3000 levels pg/ml) • Stage I-> No elevated biomarkers. Median survival 66 months • Stage 2-> One elevated biomarker. Median survival 40 months • Stage 3-> Both elevated biomarkers. Median survival 20 months	Revised MAYO (2012) Staging System Incorporated biomarkers with cut off NT- NT-pro-BNP ≥1800 ng/L, cardiac troponin T ≥ 0.025 mcg/L, and the difference between involved and uninvolved serum free light chains (dFLC) ≥18 mg/dL as risk factors. • Stage 1-> No elevation in any of the parameters-> Median Survival 55 months • Stage 2 with elevation of one of the parameters-> Median survival 19 months, • Stage 3 at least two parameters abnormally elevated-> Median survival 12 months • Stage 4 three or more parameters abnormally elevated-> Median survival 5 months
UK Risk Model Based on cohort of wt and hATTR patients with prognostic stages based on renal dysfunction (eGFR threshold <45 ml/min/1.73 m^2 and NT-pBNP (>3000 levels pg/ml) • Stage I-> Both above threshold. Median survival 69.2 months • Stage 2-> One marker above threshold. Median survival 46.7 months • Stage 3-> Both markers above threshold. Median survival 20 months	Mayo Staging Incorporates biomarkers with cut-off of troponin <0.035 mcg/L and NT-pro-BNP <332 ng/L • Stage 1-> No elevation in any of the parameters-> Median Survival 26 months • Stage 2 with elevation of one of the parameters-> Median survival 11 months • Stage 3 at least two parameters abnormally elevated-> Median survival 4 months
Chen et al. incremental value of diuretic dose and NYHA functional to UK and Mayo Clinic Risk Models Based on cohort of wtATTR patients. Addition of NYHA status and diuretic dose to UK model and Mayo Clinic staging • Diuretic dose -> 0 points for 0 mg/kg, 1 point >0–0 5 mg/mg, 2 points >0.5–1 m g/kg, 3 points >1 mg/kg • NYHA functional class -> 1 point NYHA 1, 2 points NYHA 2, 3 points NYHA 3, 4 points NYHA 4	

ATTR, transthyretin amyloidosis; wtATTR, wild type-transthyretin amyloidosis; h or v ATTR, hereditary or variant type-transthyretin amyloidosis; eGFR, estimated glomerular filtration rate; N-Pro-BNP, N-terminal-pro hormone-brain natriuretic peptide; NYHA, New York Heart Association; dFLC, lambda to kappa free light chain ratio difference.

Table 2.
Prognostic staging system for cardiac amyloidosis.

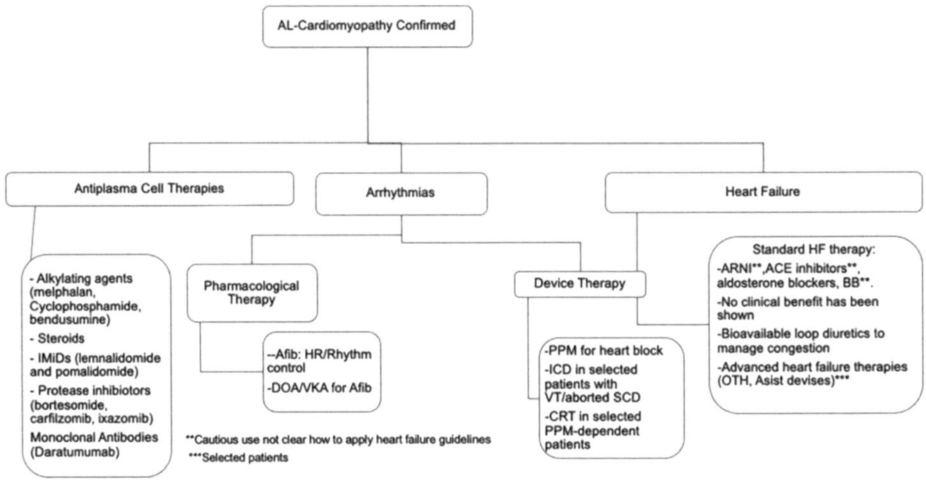

Figure 7.

AL-cardiomyopathy pharmacological therapeutic treatment flowchart. IMiDs, immunomodulator drugs; Afib, atrial fibrillation; DOA, direct oral anticoagulants; VKA, vitamin K antagonist; PPM, permanent pacemaker; ICD, internal cardiac defibrillator; CRT, cardiac resynchronization therapy; VT, ventricular tachycardia; SCD, sudden cardiac death; ARNI, angiotensin receptor-neprilysin inhibitor; ACEI, angiotensin-converting enzyme inhibitor; BB, betablocker; OTH, orthotropic heart transplant.

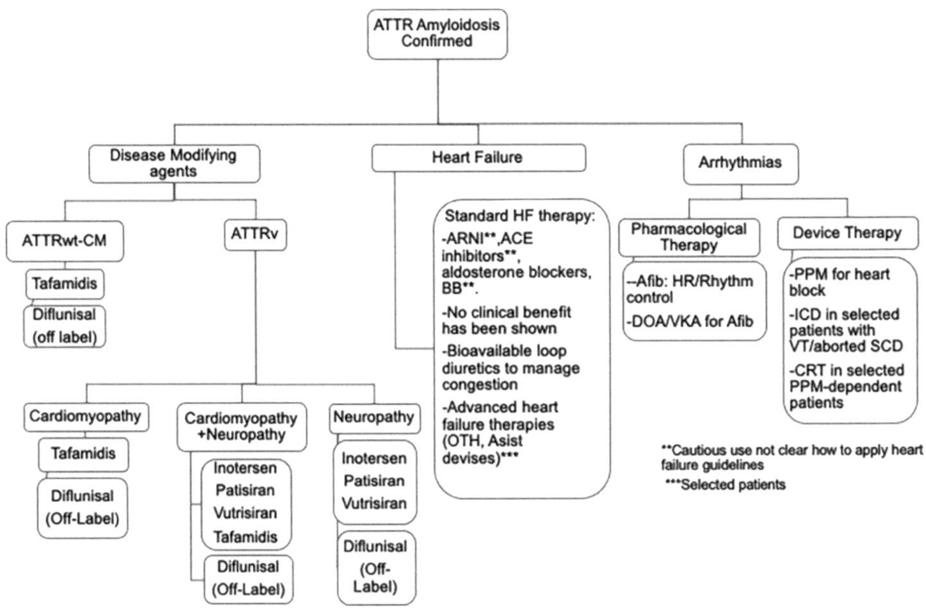

Figure 8.

ATTR-amyloidosis pharmacological therapeutic treatment flowchart. Afib, atrial fibrillation; DOA, direct oral anticoagulants; VKA, vitamin K antagonist; PPM, permanent pacemaker; ICD, internal cardiac defibrillator; CRT, cardiac resynchronization therapy; VT, ventricular tachycardia; SCD, sudden cardiac death; ARNI, angiotensin receptor-neprilysin inhibitor; ACEI, angiotensin-converting enzyme inhibitor; BB, betablocker; OTH, orthotropic heart transplant.

Angiotensin-converting enzyme inhibitors (ACEI), aldosterone receptor blockers (ARB), and aldosterone receptor/Neprilysin inhibitors (ARNI) often lead to hypotension. Moreover, beta-blockers are known to exacerbate bradyarrhythmias in this population. Digoxin binds to amyloid fibrils, leading to potential drug toxicity even when circulating levels are within normal range, and should be avoided unless there is difficulty controlling atrial fibrillation. Similarly, calcium blockers should be avoided as well since they tend to bind irreversibly to amyloid fibers, thus causing bradycardia.

Orthostatic hypotension is a common debilitating symptom in patients with cardiac amyloidosis, often leading to significant deterioration and poor quality of life. Its management include pharmacological interventions such as the use of sympathomimetic agents such as midodrine, droxidopa, the acetylcholinesterase inhibitor pyridostigmine, or the norepinephrine transporter inhibitor atomoxetine along with use of compressions stockings. A retrospective study of patients with AL-CM showed droxidopa is an effective treatment of orthostatic hypotension refractory to midodrine. Slow titration may be important to minimize rapid changes in blood pressure [60].

Cardiac arrhythmias are commonly secondary to infiltration of amyloid proteins to cardiac conduction system as well as fibrosis at the sinoatrial node and atrioventricular nodes which disrupts the transmission of electrical impulses along the conduction fibers, additional direct cytotoxic effects of amyloid fibers have been described in AL-CA [61]. Atrial fibrillation (AF) is the most common rhythm disturbance seen among patients, with a prevalence ranging between 10 and 69% [41, 62]. When it comes to treatment and rhythm control options, patients with cardiac amyloidosis have limited strategies due to intolerance to most of the rate control medications, leading to low output states and hemodynamic deterioration. Nevertheless, AF does not significantly affect the overall survival of patients with ATTR cardiomyopathy. Rhythm control strategies including antiarrhythmic treatment, synchronized cardioversion, and AF ablation are more effective when performed earlier during the disease course [63]. Amiodarone can be used to safely restore heart rhythm and can be considered the agent of choice in those patients with beta blocker intolerance requiring both rhythm and rate control. Anticoagulation is highly recommended in these patients because of higher rates if thrombi and thromboembolic events when compared to aged-matched population without the disease [64]. A retrospective study showed no difference on thrombotic events or major bleeding events between both groups [65]. Hence anticoagulation prescription is indicated to all patient with CA and atrial fibrillation unless prohibitive risk of bleeding. In a comparative study in patients who underwent Left atrial appendage devise placement, it was demonstrated that devise reduce the risk of bleeding complications and ischemic cerebrovascular events in a similar fashion than patients without CA [66]. Sinus bradycardia and bifascicular block are common and progression to complete AV block is not infrequent requiring permanent pacemaker implantation [67]. Biventricular pacing is recommended over regular permanent pacemaker due to risk of induced desynchrony by the last one. It has been found that CRT response was associated with lower rates of cardiac events in this population especially in younger patients [68]. Although sudden cardiac death is common in AL amyloidosis, most of the times it has been the result of electromechanical dissociation rather than ventricular arrhythmias. Therefore, defibrillator implantation is recommended in cases in which a sudden death event has been aborted and it is understood that the patient has a survival of ≥12 months.

7.1 Cardiac amyloidosis disease specific treatment

7.1.1 AL-cardiomyopathy

Patients with amyloid cardiomyopathy due to AL amyloidosis need identification and management with chemotherapeutic regimens that will control production of light chain gammopathy and/or autologous cell transplantation (ASCT) [7]. The goal of treatment in patients with cardiac involvement is to achieve complete resolution or normalization of serum kappa and lambda free light chain (FLC) and FLC ratio. Staging is paramount as the risk of treatment-related mortality associated with ASCT in AL amyloidosis restricts the use of this procedure to a small group of selected patients. Multiple prognostic models have been proposed for patients with amyloidosis, most simple staging models incorporate NT-proBNP and cardiac troponin that can be easily used in clinical settings (**Table 2**) [69]. There are several different choices of anti-plasma cell medications (alkylating agents, immunomodulatory drugs (IMiDs) and proteosomes inhibitors) approved for treatment of myeloma multiple and can be used off-label for the treatment of AL amyloidosis. Daratumumab is the first monoclonal Ab that has been demonstrated to be highly effective in the treatment of AL-CA [70]. The intensity and type of therapy chosen is affected by the number and extent of organ involvement. Patients with AL cardiomyopathy with New York Heart Association (NYHA) functional class 3 and above are not considered for autologous stem cell transplant (ASCT). The treatment goal is to achieve a complete hematological response or extremely low levels of serum FLCs. For those patients who are candidates for stem cell transplantation, ASCT involves administration of high-dose melphalan followed by stem cell rescue (**Figure 7**).

7.1.2 Transthyretin cardiomyopathy

ATTR amyloidosis which was previously managed only by treating symptomatology and volume congestion, is now treated with disease modifying therapies targeted at the level of synthesis, stabilization and/or elimination of the TTR protein. Thus, avoiding overproduction of abnormal TTR protein. Strategies for management are divided in transthyretin tetramer stabilizers, synthesis inhibitors and clearance of amyloid deposits (**Figure 8**).

7.1.2.1 Transthyretin stabilizers

Tafamidis is a transthyretin stabilizer which works by binding to the thyroxine site of TTR with high affinity, thus slowing dissociation of TTR tetramers into monomers and preventing aggregation in amyloid fibrils. It is indicated in ATTR-CM and heart failure with functional class 1–3 (NYHA). The Tafamidis in Transthyretin Cardiomyopathy Clinical Trial (ATTR-ACT) enrolled 441 patients allocated in a 2:1:2 to Tafamidis 80 mg, Tafamidis 20 mg, or placebo [71]. Tafamidis improved survival, reduced cardiovascular (CV)-related hospitalizations, as well as measures of functionality and health-related quality of life (HRQoL) in patients with ATTR-CM. The study was not designed to assess the relative efficacy between study drug dosages, but it showed a significant reduction in the increased NT-pro BNP and troponin I over time in patients with the 80 mg dose over the ones using 20 mg, with higher number of patients with stable or reduced NT-proBNP levels at 30-months. This was better analyzed in the ATTR-ACT long term study treated for additional 60 months using the 80 mg dose. Demonstrating a 30% relative risk reduction of death when compared to the 20 mg dose [72].

In a similar fashion, Diflunisal, a nonsteroidal anti-inflammatory, is known to have capability to stabilize TTR protein by increasing its dissociation barrier by binding to the thyroxine site. It could be used off-label for the treatment of ATTR. Diflunisal has been shown to reduce neurologic deterioration in patients with familial amyloid polyneuropathy due to hereditary transthyretin amyloidosis [73–75].

Additionally, in patients with cardiac involvement, diflunisal treatment resulted in measurable differences in cardiac troponins as well as pro-BNP and echocardiographic parameters of cardiac structure and function after only 1 year of administration [73, 74]. Nevertheless, the medication has been associated the usual side effects seen with NSAIDS such as gastric disturbances, nephrotoxicity as well as cardiac toxicity.

There are other medications in development with ATTR stabilization capabilities, Acoramidis (AG10) and mds84. Acoramidis (AG10) appeared to be safe and well tolerated during phase 2 clinical trial and completely stabilized TTR [76]. The ATTRibute-CM Study is an undergoing phase 3 study with main aim to demonstrate Acoramidis usefulness in improvement of exercise capacity, survival, and secondary end point of improvement of health-related quality of life, all-cause mortality, and rate of cardiovascular-related hospital events when compared to placebo [73]. Lastly, mds84 is bivalent ligand TTR that can bind to the binding groove as well as central protein channel pockets. In vitro studies have demonstrated higher potency capabilities when compared to other TTR stabilizers [73, 74]. So far, there is no evidence of undergoing available clinical trials.

7.1.2.2 Transthyretin gene silencers

Patisiran is a double-stranded small interfering RNA which decreases the production of abnormal TTR by binding to the RNA-induced silencing complex mediating cleavage of the protein's mRNA to prevent TTR synthesis by the liver. It has FDA approval for treatment of ATTRv polyneuropathy. The APOLLO trial demonstrated improvement in the biomarker NT-proBNP as well as echocardiographic parameters such as LV-wall thickness, end-diastolic volume, cardiac output, and global longitudinal strain in those patients with cardiac involvement. Further sub analysis demonstrated improvement in functional capacity, decreased hospitalizations and mortality when compared to placebo [77]. These findings provided off-label alternative use for hereditary (variant) ATTR-CM.

The APOLLO-B, a randomized placebo control trial for treating both types of ATTR-CM designed to determine usefulness of siRNA to improve functional capacity and decrease hospital admissions and MACE. Inotersen, an antisense oligonucleoside inhibitor that causes degradation of TRR mRNA through binding to the TTR mRNA produced by the liver. The medication is administered by subcutaneous injection weekly. Similarly, to Patisiran, it is indicated for treatment of ATTRv polyneuropathy. Dasgupta et al., presented data from a single center which demonstrated long-term treatment in ATTR CM was safe and effective at inhibiting progression and potentially reverting amyloid burden accompanied by increased exercise tolerance and decrease in mean LV mass measured by CMR [78].

There are two ongoing investigational drugs that target gene silencing of TTR undergoing evaluation with phase 3 trials. Eplontersen CARDIO-TTRansform and Vutrisiran (HELIOS-A and HELIOS-B) [73]. In the HELIOS-A, Vutrisiran, preliminary results showed improvement on the exploratory cardiac biomarkers, NT-pro-BNP endpoints when compared to placebo ($P < 0.05$).

7.1.2.3 Transthyretin degraders

Doxycycline is a tetracycline derivative which poses anti-amyloidogenic properties, disrupting pre-formed TTR fibrils in vitro [79, 80]. Tauroursodeoxycholic acid

(TUDCA), a biliary acid has similar effect in reducing non−/pre-fibrillary TTR deposits. This was demonstrated in transgenic mice where the combination of both drugs had a synergistic effect and have shown disease stabilization, good tolerability, and low toxicity profile with 1-year of treatment [80].

Monoclonal anti-serum amyloid protein is an antibody targeting normal non fibrillar glycoprotein SAP promoting a giant cell reaction that will remove visceral amyloid deposits. Medication is administered intravenously. This drug is still undergoing evaluation and a clear utility in amyloid cardiomyopathy has not been demonstrated [73, 74].

7.2 Advanced heart failure therapies

Cardiac amyloidosis is a progressive disease with significant risk of progression of heart failure and mortality associated to a restrictive physiology along with characteristically small, hypertrophied LV ventricle. This leads to a significant anatomic concern as a small LV cavity could lead to suction events by obstructing the inflow cannula thereby predisposing the patient to low flow, hypotension, pump thrombosis as well as arrhythmias and worsening RV dysfunction. Furthermore, this population has frequent RV involvement with associated pulmonary hypertension and right heart failure which would further limit ventricular assistant devise use feasibility. There are only a few small studies with overall conflicting results to draw conclusions. Hence consideration of treatment should be done on a patient-to-patient basis. One small study suggest left ventricular assist device (LVAD) implantation is technically feasible for patients with severe heart failure due to advanced cardiac amyloidosis [81]. Another single-center case series highlighted the feasibility of supporting highly selected CA patients with continuous flow-left ventricular assist devise (CF-LVAD) as bridge to transplant (BTT) or destination therapy (DT including the HeartMate 3 pump) with reasonable outcomes, principally for those with a reduced LVEF and an absence of significant pre-implant RV dysfunction or pulmonary artery pulsatile index (PAPI) ≤ 1.5 [81, 82].

Improvement in treatment options in patients with cardiac amyloidosis has opened the possibility for heart transplant in carefully selected patients with advanced heart failure including those that require combined heart-liver or heart-kidney. Barrette et al. analyzed 31 patients who underwent heart transplants for cardiac amyloidosis (13 with light chain amyloidosis and 18 with transthyretin [ATTR] amyloidosis) that were carefully selected for the procedure. His findings disclosed there was no significant difference in mortality between patients who underwent heart transplantation for amyloid cardiomyopathy and patients who underwent heart transplantation for all other indications [83].

7.3 Transthyretin cardiomyopathy in aortic stenosis

Aortic stenosis (AS) is the most prevalent valvular disease seen in over 4% of octogenarian patients. Multiple studies have described a prevalence of cardiac amyloidosis in patients with aortic stenosis which range from 4% up to 29% [84]. Hence, AS-CA frequently coexists in this population. Aortic stenosis should be graded according to guidelines but taking into consideration that in these settings the patient will present with low flow/low gradient patterns (i.e., AVA <1.0 cm^2, mean gradients <40 mm Hg and stroke volume index <35 ml/m^2). A multicenter prospective of close to 400 patients referred for aortic valve replacement mostly through transcatheter aortic valve replacement (TAVR) showed that even though dual pathology of severe AS-CA conferred overall worse disease by functional capacity, cardiac remodeling and biomarkers, the patients had improved outcome when procedure was performed. Furthermore, their data confirmed AS-CA was common and affected 1 in 8 patients referred for TAVR [85].

8. Conclusions

Cardiac amyloidosis, previously believed to be a rare condition, is often underdiagnosed. Multisystemic presentations cause delays in diagnosis, which reduces the opportunity of treatment at initial stages. The advent of disease advanced multi-imaging modalities has improved identification and diagnosis of disease, with non-invasive diagnosis becoming cornerstone in treatment decision making process. Patient stratification is key for treatment decision and prognosis. Early diagnosis is key for prognosis, course of action, successful response to therapy, and a better treatment outcome.

Conflicts of interest

The contents of this publication do not represent the views of the VA Caribbean Healthcare System, the Department of Veterans Affairs, or the United States Government. Dr. Sonia I. Vicenty is the Director of The Heart Failure Clinic and Associate Director of the Cardiovascular Disease Fellowship Program at the VA Caribbean HealthCare System, San Juan, PR. She is a sponsored speaker for Pfizer, and investigator for IONIS involved CARDIO-TTRansform trial. Dr. Ingrid Bonilla has no conflict of interest to disclose.

Author details

Sonia Vicenty-Rivera* and Ingrid Bonilla-Mercado
Cardiology Section, VA Caribbean Healthcare System, San Juan, Puerto Rico

*Address all correspondence to: soniavicenty@live.com

References

[1] Siddiqi OK, Ruberg FL. Cardiac amyloidosis: An update on pathophysiology, diagnosis, and treatment. Trends in Cardiovascular Medicine. 2018;**28**(1):10-21. DOI: 10.1016/j.tcm.2017.07.004

[2] Sipe JD, Benson MD, Buxbaum JN, et al. Amyloid fibril proteins and amyloidosis: Chemical identification and clinical classification International Society of Amyloidosis 2016 Nomenclature Guidelines. Amyloid. 2016;**23**:209-213

[3] Magy-Bertrand N, Dupond JL, Mauny F, et al. Incidence of amyloidosis over 3 years: The AMYPRO study. Clinical and Experimental Rheumatology. 2008;**26**:1074-1078

[4] Staron A, Connors LH, Zheng L, Doros G, Sanchorawala V. Race/ethnicity in systemic AL amyloidosis: Perspectives on disease and outcome disparities. Blood Cancer Journal. 2020;**10**(11):118. DOI: 10.1038/s41408-020-00385-0 PMID: 33173025; PMCID: PMC7655813

[5] Castaño A, Narotsky DL, Hamid N, et al. Unveiling transthyretin cardiac amyloidosis and its predictors among elderly patients with severe aortic stenosis undergoing transcatheter aortic valve replacement. European Heart Journal. 2017;**38**(38):2879-2887. DOI: 10.1093/eurheartj/ehx350

[6] Liao R, Jain M, Teller P, Connors LH, Ngoy S, Skinner M, et al. Infusion of light chains from patients with cardiac amyloidosis causes diastolic dysfunction in isolated mouse hearts [published correction appears in Circulation. 2013 Sep 10;128(11): e174]. Circulation. 2001;**104**(14):1594-1597

[7] Ma KK, Ogawa T, de Bold AJ. Selective upregulation of cardiac brain natriuretic peptide at the transcriptional and translational levels by pro-inflammatory cytokines and by conditioned medium derived from mixed lymphocyte reactions via p38 MAP kinase. Journal of Molecular and Cellular Cardiology. 2004;**36**:505-513

[8] Carroll A, Dyck PJ, de Carvalho M, Kennerson M, Reilly MM, Kiernan MC, et al. Novel approaches to diagnosis and management of hereditary transthyretin amyloidosis. Journal of Neurology, Neurosurgery, and Psychiatry. 2022;**93**(6):668-678. DOI: 10.1136/jnnp-2021-327909

[9] Luigetti M, Romano A, Di Paolantonio A, Bisogni G, Sabatelli M. Diagnosis and treatment of hereditary transthyretin amyloidosis (hATTR) polyneuropathy: Current perspectives on improving patient care. Therapeutics and Clinical Risk Management. 2020;**16**:109-123. DOI: 10.2147/TCRM.S219979

[10] Koike H, Katsuno M. Ultrastructure in transthyretin amyloidosis: From pathophysiology to therapeutic insights. Biomedicine. 2019;**7**(1):11. DOI: 10.3390/biomedicines7010011

[11] Quarta CC, Buxbaum JN, Shah AM, Falk RH, Claggett B, Kitzman DW, et al. The amyloidogenic V122I transthyretin variant in elderly Black Americans. The New England Journal of Medicine. 2015;**372**(1):21-29. DOI: 10.1056/NEJMoa1404852

[12] Manganelli F, Fabrizi GM, Luigetti M, Mandich P, Mazzeo A, Pareyson D. Hereditary transthyretin amyloidosis overview. Neurological

Sciences. 2022;**43**(Suppl 2):595-604. DOI: 10.1007/s10072-020-04889-2

[13] González-López E, Gallego-Delgado M, Guzzo-Merello G, de Haro-Del Moral FJ, Cobo-Marcos M, Robles C, et al. Wild-type transthyretin amyloidosis as a cause of heart failure with preserved ejection fraction. European Heart Journal. 2015;**36**(38):2585-2594. DOI: 10.1093/eurheartj/ehv338

[14] AbouEzzeddine OF, Davies DR, Scott CG, Fayyaz AU, Askew JW, McKie PM, et al. Prevalence of transthyretin amyloid cardiomyopathy in heart failure with preserved ejection fraction [published correction appears in JAMA Cardiol. 2021 Oct 6; null]. JAMA Cardiology. 2021;**6**(11):1267-1274. DOI: 10.1001/jamacardio.2021.3070

[15] Quock TP, Yan T, Chang E, Guthrie S, Broder MS. Epidemiology of AL amyloidosis: A real-world study using US claims data. Blood Advances. 2018;**2**(10):1046-1053. DOI: 10.1182/bloodadvances.2018016402

[16] Tahir UA, Doros G, Kim JS, Connors LH, Seldin DC, Sam F. Predictors of mortality in light chain cardiac amyloidosis with heart failure. Scientific Reports. 2019;**9**(1).8552. DOI: 10.1038/s41598-019-44912-x

[17] Falk RH, Alexander KM, Liao R, Dorbala S. AL (light-chain) cardiac amyloidosis: A review of diagnosis and therapy. Journal of the American College of Cardiology. 2016;**68**(12):1323-1341. DOI: 10.1016/j.jacc.2016.06.053

[18] Connors LH, Sam F, Skinner M, Salinaro F, Sun F, Ruberg FL, et al. Heart failure resulting from age-related cardiac amyloid disease associated with wild-type transthyretin: A prospective, observational cohort study. Circulation. 2016;**133**(3):282-290. DOI: 10.1161/CIRCULATIONAHA.115.018852

[19] Lindmark K, Pilebro B, Sundström T, Lindqvist P. Prevalence of wild type transtyrethin cardiac amyloidosis in a heart failure clinic. ESC Heart Failure. 2021;**8**(1):745-749. DOI: 10.1002/ehf2.13110

[20] Mohammed SF, Mirzoyev SA, Edwards WD, Dogan A, Grogan DR, Dunlay SM, et al. Left ventricular amyloid deposition in patients with heart failure and preserved ejection fraction. JACC Heart Failure. 2014;**2**(2):113-122. DOI: 10.1016/j.jchf.2013.11.004

[21] Mohammed SF, Mirzoyev SA, Edwards WD, Dogan A, Grogan DR, Dunlay SM, et al. Carpal tunnel syndrome: A common initial symptom of systemic wild-type ATTR (ATTRwt) amyloidosis. Amyloid. 2016;**23**(1):58-63. DOI: 10.3109/13506129.2015.1135792

[22] Geller HI, Singh A, Alexander KM, Mirto TM, Falk RH. Association between ruptured distal biceps tendon and wild-type transthyretin cardiac amyloidosis. Journal of the American Medical Association. 2017;**318**(10):962-963. DOI: 10.1001/jama.2017.9236

[23] Eldhagen P, Berg S, Lund LH, Sörensson P, Suhr OB, Westermark P. Transthyretin amyloid deposits in lumbar spinal stenosis and assessment of signs of systemic amyloidosis. Journal of Internal Medicine. 2021;**289**(6):895-905. DOI: 10.1111/joim.13222

[24] Rapezzi C, Lorenzini M, Longhi S, et al. Cardiac amyloidosis: The great pretender. Heart Failure Reviews. 2015;**20**(2):117-124. DOI: 10.1007/s10741-015-9480-0

[25] Faravelli G, Mondani V, Mangione PP, et al. Amyloid formation by globular proteins: The need to narrow the gap between in vitro and in vivo mechanisms. Frontiers in Molecular

Biosciences. 2022;**9**:830006. DOI: 10.3389/fmolb.2022.830006

[26] Jacobson DR, Alexander AA, Tagoe C, Buxbaum JN. Prevalence of the amyloidogenic transthyretin (TTR) V122I allele in 14 333 African Americans. Amyloid. 2015;**22**(3):171-174. DOI: 10.3109/13506129.2015.1051219

[27] Obi CA, Mostertz WC, Griffin JM, Judge DP. ATTR epidemiology, genetics, and prognostic factors. Methodist DeBakey Cardiovascular Journal. 2022;**18**(2):17-26. DOI: 10.14797/mdcvj.1066

[28] Spencer-Bonilla G, Njoroge JN, Pearson K, Witteles RM, Aras MA, Alexander KM. Racial and ethnic disparities in transthyretin cardiac amyloidosis. Current Cardiovascular Risk Reports. 2021;**15**(6):8. DOI: 10.1007/s12170-021-00670-y

[29] Lousada I, Comenzo RL, Landau H, Guthrie S, Merlin G. Patient experience with hereditary and senile systemic amyloidoses: A survey from the Amyloidosis Research Consortium. Orphanet Journal of Rare Diseases. 2015;**10**(Suppl. 1):22. https://doi.org/10.1186/1750-1172-10-S1-P22b

[30] Tyberg TI, Goodyer AV, Hurst VW 3rd, Alexander J, Langou RA. Left ventricular filling in differentiating restrictive amyloid cardiomyopathy and constrictive pericarditis. The American Journal of Cardiology. 1981;**47**(4):791-796. DOI: 10.1016/0002-9149(81)90175-2

[31] Berk JL, Keane J, Seldin DC, Sanchorawala V, Koyama J, Dember LM, et al. Persistent pleural effusions in primary systemic amyloidosis: Etiology and prognosis. Chest. 2003;**124**(3):969-977. DOI: 10.1378/chest.124.3.969

[32] Chamarthi B, Dubrey SW, Cha K, Skinner M, Falk RH. Features and prognosis of exertional syncope in light-chain associated AL cardiac amyloidosis. The American Journal of Cardiology. 1997;**80**(9):1242-1245. DOI: 10.1016/s0002-9149(97)00653-x

[33] Modesto KM, Dispenzieri A, Gertz M, Cauduro SA, Khandheria BK, Seward JB, Kyle R, et al. Vascular abnormalities in primary amyloidosis. European Heart Journal. 2007;**28**(8):1019-1024. https://doi.org/10.1093/ eurheartj/ehm066

[34] Mueller PS, Edwards WD, Gertz MA. Symptomatic ischemic heart disease resulting from obstructive intramural coronary amyloidosis. The American Journal of Medicine. 2000;**109**(3):181-188. DOI: 10.1016/s0002-9343(00)00471-x

[35] Zabernigg A, Schranzhofer R, Kreczy A, Gattringer K. Continuously elevated cardiac troponin I in two patients with multiple myeloma and fatal cardiac amyloidosis. Annals of Oncology. 2003;**14**(12):1791. DOI: 10.1093/annonc/mdg487

[36] Dispenzieri A, Kyle RA, Gertz MA, Therneau TM, Miller WL, Chandrasekaran K, et al. Survival in patients with primary systemic amyloidosis and raised serum cardiac troponins. Lancet. 2003;**361**(9371):1787-1789. DOI: 10.1016/S0140-6736(03)13396-X

[37] González-Duarte A, Barroso F, Mundayat R, Shapiro B. Blood pressure and orthostatic hypotension as measures of autonomic dysfunction in patients from the transthyretin amyloidosis outcomes survey (THAOS). Autonomic Neuroscience. 2019;**222**:102590. DOI: 10.1016/j.autneu.2019.102590

[38] Barge-Caballero G, Barge-Caballero E, López-Pérez M,

Bilbao-Quesada R, González-Babarro E, Gómez-Otero I, et al. Syncope in patients with transthyretin amyloid cardiomyopathy: Clinical features and outcomes. Postgraduate Medicine. 2022;**134**(4):420-428. DOI: 10.1080/00325481.2022.2054174

[39] Ruberg FL, Grogan M, Hanna M, Kelly JW, Maurer MS. Transthyretin amyloid cardiomyopathy: JACC state-of-the-art review. Journal of the American College of Cardiology. 2019;**73**(22):2872-2891. DOI: 10.1016/j.jacc.2019.04.003

[40] Yamamoto H, Yokochi T. Transthyretin cardiac amyloidosis: An update on diagnosis and treatment. ESC Heart Failure. 2019;**6**(6):1128-1139. DOI: 10.1002/ehf2.12518

[41] Kittleson MM, Maurer MS, Ambardekar AV, Bullock-Palmer RP, Chang PP, Eisen HJ, et al. Cardiac amyloidosis: Evolving diagnosis and management: A scientific statement from the American Heart Association [published correction appears in Circulation 2021 Jul 6;144(1): e10] [published correction appears in Circulation. 2021 Jul 6;144(1): e11]. Circulation. 2020;**142**(1):e7-e22. DOI: 10.1161/CIR.0000000000000792

[42] Palladini G, Campana C, Klersy C, Balduini A, Vadacca G, Perfetti V, et al. Serum N-terminal pro-brain natriuretic peptide is a sensitive marker of myocardial dysfunction in AL amyloidosis. Circulation. 2003;**107**(19):2440-2445. DOI: 10.1161/01.CIR.0000068314. 02595.B2

[43] Cyrille NB, Goldsmith J, Alvarez J, Maurer MS. Prevalence and prognostic significance of low QRS voltage among the three main types of cardiac amyloidosis. The American Journal of Cardiology. 2014;**114**(7):1089-1093. DOI: 10.1016/j.amjcard.2014.07.026

[44] Slivnick JA, Wallner AL, Vallakati A, Truong VT, Mazur W, Elamin MB, et al. Indexed left ventricular mass to QRS voltage ratio is associated with heart failure hospitalizations in patients with cardiac amyloidosis. The International Journal of Cardiovascular Imaging. 2021;**37**(3):1043-1051. DOI: 10.1007/s10554-020-02059-1

[45] Rahman JE, Helou EF, Gelzer-Bell R, Thompson RE, Kuo C, Rodriguez ER, et al. Noninvasive diagnosis of biopsy-proven cardiac amyloidosis. Journal of the American College of Cardiology. 2004;**43**(3):410-415. DOI: 10.1016/j.jacc.2003.08.043B

[46] Zhongwei C, Lin K, Zhuang T, Weiyun C, Wenjuan G, Jia X, et al. Utility of combined indexes of electrocardiography and echocardiography in the diagnosis of biopsy proven primary cardiac amyloidosis. Annals of Noninvasive Electrocardiology. **16**(1):25-29

[47] Dubrey SW, Bilazarian S, LaValley M, Reisinger J, Skinner M, Falk RH. Signal-averaged electrocardiography in patients with AL (primary) amyloidosis. American Heart Journal. 1997;**134**(6):994-1001. DOI: 10.1016/s0002-8703(97)70017-6

[48] Roxana Cristina Rimbas, Anca Balinisteanu, Stefania Lucia Magna, Simona Ionela Visoiu, Andrea Olivia Cliobanu, Elena Beganu, Alina Ioana Nicula, and Dragos Vinereanu. New advanced imaging parameters and biomarkers – a step forward in the diagnosis and prognosis of ATTR cardiomyoathy, Journal of Clinical Medicine2022, 11, 2360. https://doi.org/10.3390/jcm11092360

[49] Wechalekar AD, Gillmore JD, Hawkins PN. Systemic amyloidosis.

Lancet. 2016;**387**(10038):2641-2654. DOI: 10.1016/S0140-6736(15)01274-X

[50] Mörner S, Hellman U, Suhr OB, Kazzam E, Waldenström A. Amyloid heart disease mimicking hypertrophic cardiomyopathy. Journal of Internal Medicine. 2005;**258**(3):225-230. DOI: 10.1111/j.1365-2796.2005. 01522.x

[51] Cueto-Garcia L, Reeder GS, Kyle RA, Wood DL, Seward JB, Naessens J, et al. Echocardiographic findings in systemic amyloidosis: Spectrum of cardiac involvement and relation to survival. Journal of the American College of Cardiology. 1985;**6**(4):737-743. DOI: 10.1016/s0735-1097(85)80475-7

[52] Dorbala S, Ando Y, Bokhari S, Dispenzieri A, Falk RH, Ferrari VA, et al. ASNC/AHA/ASE/EANM/HFSA/ISA/SCMR/SNMMI expert consensus recommendations for multimodality imaging in cardiac amyloidosis: Part 1 of 2-evidence base and standardized methods of imaging [published correction appears in J Nucl Cardiol. 2021 Aug;28(4):1761-1762]. Journal of Nuclear Cardiology. 2019;**26**(6):2065-2123. DOI: 10.1007/s12350-019-01760-6

[53] Dungu JN, Whelan CJ, Gibbs SD, Pinney JH, Banypersad SM, Venner CP, Lachmann HJ et al. Patterns of late gadolinium enhancement in 94 patients with AL or transthyretin cardiac amyloidosis. Journal of Cardiovascular Magnetic Resonance. 2012;**14**(Suppl. 1):O87. https://doi.org/10.1186/1532-429X-14-S1-O87

[54] Guo Y, Li X, Wang Y. State of the art: Quantitative cardiac MRI in cardiac amyloidosis. Journal of Magnetic Resonance Imaging. 2022;**56**(5):1287-1301. DOI: 10.1002/jmri.28314

[55] Bhatti S, Watts E, Syed F, Vallurupalli S, Pandey T, Jambekar K, et al. Clinical and prognostic utility of cardiovascular magnetic resonance imaging in myeloma patients with suspected cardiac amyloidosis. European Heart Journal Cardiovascular Imaging. 2016;**17**(9):970-977. DOI: 10.1093/ehjci/jew101

[56] Perugini E, Guidalotti PL, Salvi F, Cooke RM, Pettinato C, Riva L, et al. Noninvasive etiologic diagnosis of cardiac amyloidosis using 99mTc-3,3-diphosphono-1,2-propanodicarboxylic acid scintigraphy. Journal of the American College of Cardiology. 2005;**46**(6):1076-1084. DOI: 10.1016/j.jacc.2005.05.073

[57] Gillmore JD, Maurer MS, Falk RH, Merlini G, Damy T, Dispenzieri A, et al. Nonbiopsy diagnosis of cardiac transthyretin amyloidosis. Circulation. 2016;**133**(24):2404-2412. DOI: 10.1161/circulationaha.116.021612

[58] Quigley AM, Petrie A, Ross JC, Page J, Martinez-Naharro A, Wechalekar AD, et al. Prognostic utility of the Perugini grading of 99mTc-DPD scintigraphy in transthyretin (ATTR) amyloidosis and its relationship with skeletal muscle and soft tissue amyloid. European Heart Journal Cardiovascular Imaging. 2017;**18**(12):1344-1350. DOI: 10.1093/ehjci/jew325

[59] Cappelli F, Gallini C, Di Mario C, Costanzo EN, Vaggelli L, Tutino F, et al. Accuracy of 99mTc-hydroxymethylene diphosphonate scintigraphy for diagnosis of transthyretin cardiac amyloidosis. Journal of Nuclear Cardiology. 2019;**26**(2):497-504. DOI: 10.1007/s12350-017-0922-z

[60] Ruiz Lopez N, Mendelson LM, Joshi T, Hughes D, Kaku MC,

Sanchorawala V, et al. Droxidopa for treatment of refractory orthostatic hypotension in patients with AL amyloidosis: A case series. Blood. 2021;**138**(1):4737 SSN 0006-4971, https://doi.org/10.1182/blood-2021-151573

[61] Hartnett J, Jaber W, Maurer M, Sperry B, Hanna M, Collier P, et al. Electrophysiological manifestations of cardiac amyloidosis: JACC: CardioOncology state-of-the-art review. JACC CardioOncology. 2021;**3**(4):506-515. DOI: 10.1016/j.jaccao.2021.07.010C

[62] Rapezzi C, Merlini G, Quarta CC, Riva L, Longhi S, Leone O, et al. Systemic cardiac amyloidoses: Disease profiles and clinical courses of the 3 main types. Circulation. 2009;**120**(13):1203-1212. DOI: 10.1161/circulationaha.108.843334

[63] Donnellan E, Wazni OM, Hanna M, Elshazly MB, Puri R, Saliba W, et al. Atrial fibrillation in transthyretin cardiac amyloidosis: Predictors, prevalence, and efficacy of rhythm control strategies. JACC Clinical Electrophysiology. 2020;**6**(9):1118-1127. DOI: 10.1016/j.jacep.2020.04.019

[64] Feng D, Syed IS, Martinez M, Oh JK, Jaffe AS, Grogan M, et al. Intracardiac thrombosis and anticoagulation therapy in cardiac amyloidosis. Circulation. 2009;**119**(18):2490-2497. DOI: 10.1161/circulationaha.108.785014

[65] Mitrani LR, De Los Santos J, Driggin E, Kogan R, Helmke S, Goldsmith J, et al. Anticoagulation with warfarin compared to novel oral anticoagulants for atrial fibrillation in adults with transthyretin cardiac amyloidosis: Comparison of thromboembolic events and major bleeding. Amyloid. 2021;**28**(1):30-34. DOI: 10.1080/13506129.2020.1810010

[66] Amat-Santos IJ, Delgado-Arana JR, Cruz-González I, Gutiérrez H, García-Bolao I, Millán X, et al. Cardiac amyloidosis and left atrial appendage closure. The CAMYLAAC Study. Revista Española de Cardiología (English Edition). 2022 ISSN 1885-5857, https://doi.org/10.1016/j.rec.2022.08.001. (https://www.sciencedirect.com/science/article/pii/S1885585722002080)

[67] Mathew V, Olson LJ, Gertz MA, Hayes DL. Symptomatic conduction system disease in cardiac amyloidosis. The American Journal of Cardiology. 1997;**80**(11):1491-1492. DOI: 10.1016/s0002-9149(97)82785-3

[68] Fischer K, Lellouche N, Damy T, Martins R, Clementy N, Bisson A, et al. Cardiovascular outcomes after cardiac resynchronization therapy in cardiac amyloidosis. ESC Heart Failure. 2022;**9**(1):740-750. DOI: 10.1002/ehf2.13663

[69] Kumar S, Dispenzieri A, Lacy MQ, Hayman SR, Buadi FK, Colby C, et al. Revised prognostic staging system for light chain amyloidosis incorporating cardiac biomarkers and serum free light chain measurements. Journal of Clinical Oncology. 2012;**30**(9):989-995. DOI: 10.1200/JCO.2011.38.5724

[70] Sun C, Wang X, Zhang R, Linhjie X, Bin W, Jian L. Efficacy and safety of intravenous daratumumab-based treatments for AL amyloidosis: A systematic review and meta-analysis. Cancer Cell International. 2022;**22**:222. DOI: https://doi.org/10.1186/s12935-022-02635-

[71] Maurer MS, Schwartz JH, Gundapaneni B, Elliott PM, Merlini G, Waddington-Cruz M, et al. ATTR-ACT study investigators. Tafamidis treatment for patients with transthyretin amyloid

cardiomyopathy. The New England Journal of Medicine. 2018;**379**(11):1007-1016. DOI: 10.1056/NEJMoa1805689

[72] Damy T, Garcia-Pavia P, Hanna M, Judge DP, Merlini G, Gundapaneni B, et al. Efficacy and safety of tafamidis doses in the tafamidis in transthyretin cardiomyopathy clinical trial (ATTR-ACT) and long-term extension study. European Journal of Heart Failure. 2021;**23**(2):277-285. DOI: 10.1002/ejhf.2027

[73] Tschöpe C, Elsanhoury A. Treatment of transthyretin amyloid cardiomyopathy: The current options, the future, and the challenges. Journal of Clinical Medicine. 2022;**11**(8):2148. DOI: 10.3390/jcm11082148

[74] Müller ML, Butler J, Heidecker B. Emerging therapies in transthyretin amyloidosis – a new wave of hope after years of stagnancy? European Journal of Heart Failure. 2020;**22**(1):39-53. DOI: 10.1002/ejhf.1695

[75] Lohrmann G, Pipilas A, Mussinelli R, Gopal DM, Berk JL, Connors LH, et al. Stabilization of cardiac function with diflunisal in transthyretin (ATTR) cardiac amyloidosis. Journal of Cardiac Failure. 2020;**26**(9):753-759. DOI: 10.1016/j.cardfail.2019.11.024

[76] Fox JC, Hellawell JL, Rao S, O'Reilly T, Lumpkin R, Jernelius J, et al. First-in-human study of AG10, a novel, oral, specific, selective, and potent transthyretin stabilizer for the treatment of transthyretin amyloidosis: A phase 1 safety, tolerability, pharmacokinetic, and pharmacodynamic study in healthy adult volunteers. Clinical Pharmacology in Drug Development. 2020;**9**(1):115-129. DOI: 10.1002/cpdd.700

[77] Adams D, Suhr OB, Dyck PJ, Litchy WJ, Leahy RG, Chen J, et al. Trial design and rationale for APOLLO, a Phase 3, placebo-controlled study of patisiran in patients with hereditary ATTR amyloidosis with polyneuropathy. BMC Neurology. 2017;**17**(1):181. DOI: 10.1186/s12883-017-0948-5

[78] Dasgupta NR, Rissing SM, Smith J, Jung J, Benson MD. Inotersen therapy of transthyretin amyloid cardiomyopathy. Amyloid. 2020;**27**(1):52-58. DOI: 10.1080/13506129.2019.1685487

[79] Cardoso I, Merlini G, Saraiva MJ. 4′-iodo-4′-deoxydoxorubicin and tetracyclines disrupt transthyretin amyloid fibrils in vitro producing noncytotoxic species: Screening for TTR fibril disrupters. The FASEB Journal. 2003;**17**(8):803-809. DOI: 10.1096/fj.02-0764com

[80] Obici L, Cortese A, Lozza A, Lucchetti J, Gobbi M, Palladini G, et al. Doxycycline plus tauroursodeoxycholic acid for transthyretin amyloidosis: A phase II study. Amyloid. 2012;**19**(Suppl. 1):34-36. DOI: 10.3109/13506129.2012.678508

[81] Swiecicki PL, Edwards BS, Kushwaha SS, Dispenzieri A, Park SJ, Gertz MA. Left ventricular device implantation for advanced cardiac amyloidosis. The Journal of Heart and Lung Transplantation. 2013;**32**(5):563-568. DOI: 10.1016/j.healun.2013.01.987

[82] Randhawa VK, Gabrovsek A, Soltesz EG, Tong M, Unai S, Chen L, et al. A case series of cardiac amyloidosis patients supported by continuous flow left ventricular assist device. ESC Heart Failure. 2021;**8**(5):4353-4356. DOI: 10.1002/ehf2.13422

[83] Barrett CD, Alexander KM, Zhao H, Haddad F, Cheng P, Liao R, et al. Outcomes in patients with cardiac amyloidosis undergoing heart

transplantation. JACC Heart Failure. 2020;**8**(6):461-468. DOI: 10.1016/j.jchf

[84] Ternacle J, Krapf L, Mohty D, Magne J, Nguyen A, Galat A, et al. Aortic stenosis and cardiac amyloidosis: JACC review topic of the week. Journal of the American College of Cardiology. 2019;**74**(21):2638-2651. DOI: 10.1016/j.jacc.2019.09.056

[85] Nitsche C, Scully PR, Patel KP, Kammerlander AA, Koschutnik M, Dona C, et al. Prevalence and outcomes of concomitant aortic stenosis and cardiac amyloidosis. Journal of the American College of Cardiology. 2021;**77**(2):128-139. DOI: 10.1016/j.jacc.2020.11.006

Section 5

Pediatric Cardiomyopathy

Chapter 6

Cardiomyopathies in Children: Genetics, Pathomechanisms and Therapeutic Strategies

Diana Cimiotti, Seyyed-Reza Sadat-Ebrahimi, Andreas Mügge and Kornelia Jaquet

Abstract

Despite great advances in cardiovascular medicine, cardiomyopathies in children still are challenging for pediatricians as well as cardiologists. Pediatric cardiomyopathies can manifest in diverse phenotypes but are often life-threatening and have a poor prognosis. However, many therapeutic options available for adult patients do not apply for children, leaving a very limited portfolio to attenuate disease progression to avoid or postpone heart transplantation. Childhood cardiomyopathies can arise from different etiologies, but genetic defects such as mutations, for example, in sarcomeric proteins, which are pivotal for the contractile function, are common. This leads to the demand to identify new variants found by genetic screening as pathogenic and furthermore to allow a prognosis or risk assessment for related carriers, thus increasing the need to uncover molecular pathomechanisms of such mutations. This chapter aims to highlight the unique characteristics of pediatric cardiomyopathies in contrast to adult forms, including etiology, pathophysiology, genetics, as well as molecular mechanisms. We will also tackle currents options, challenges, and perspectives in diagnosis and treatment of pediatric cardiomyopathies.

Keywords: pediatric cardiomyopathy, mutations, sarcomere, molecular mechanism, genotype-phenotype correlation, calcium sensitivity, fibrosis, inflammation

1. Introduction

Cardiomyopathies (CM) in children occur relatively rarely with an incidence of less than 1.3 in 100,000 children below 10 years of age and are still challenging for pediatricians, cardiologists, and cardiac surgeons [1]. Cardiomyopathies, which by definition are diseases of the heart muscle, are very heterogeneous and include a cluster of different diseases that often cannot be clearly separated from each other. Generally, CMs are classified into dilated (DCM), hypertrophic (HCM), restrictive (RCM), left ventricular non-compaction (LVNC), arrhythmogenic (ACM), and mixed phenotypes. They further may be subdivided into primary, that is, inherited, and secondary diseases (e.g., metabolic disorders or other genetic diseases as muscular dystrophy). In children, often the pathology is very severe with rapid progression. In addition, comorbidities such as diabetes, renal and pulmonary diseases, and obesity may affect the outcome [2]. There is still a vast amount of known pediatric CM cases that are idiopathic, that is, of unknown cause, often because of lack of causal diagnosis. In consequence, this increases the inefficiency of treatments [3]. Since often suitable therapies besides heart transplantation for diagnosed CM types are not available or inefficient, prognosis is poor [4]. Here, we will describe common features of pediatric CMs concerning their etiology, pathophysiology, and molecular mechanisms, thereby underlining the challenges for classification, diagnosis, and treatment. Also, unique features will be covered, as well as current options and perspectives in diagnosis and treatment.

2. Classification of pediatric cardiomyopathies and their clinical characteristics

The classification of cardiomyopathies in general still is a challenging and debated topic due to different approaches used by larger population-based studies and guidelines provided by different cardiologic societies [2]. In many cases, CMs were (and still are) classified mainly by the morphofunctional phenotype of the myocardium, although, more and more often, pathogenetic and genotypic criteria were included. The different classifications lead to inconsistencies in terminology between different published systems such as the AHA, ACC, or ESC guidelines, thus adding to the difficulty to finding common pathophysiological patterns and therapeutic approaches in different cardiomyopathy studies, even more so for the relatively rare pediatric CMs. One attempt to integrate the different disease characteristics in a single system is the MOGE(S) classification [5]. It includes the morphofunctional phenotype (M), organ involvement (O, e.g., isolated to the heart vs. systemic/multi-organ), genetic inheritance pattern (G), and etiological or explicit genetic defects (E). Optionally, the functional status (S) can be included. But, these characteristics still can be applied in different hierarchies. Thus, the widely used current ESC approach implies the morphofunctional phenotype as the highest category and the genetic and pathogenetic characteristics as subcategories, as the phenotype provides the basis for diagnosis and therapeutic management in the first place. Still, the pathogenetics are of great importance for genetic counseling of mutation-carrier families in order to provide long-term risk assessment and, if necessary, regular monitoring of (as yet) seemingly unaffected family members by a cardiologist. Hereinafter, the different CM types will be discussed with regard to their most prominent morphofunctional aspects and their general prevalence in children. An overview on pediatric CM types is given in **Figure 1**.

2.1 Dilated cardiomyopathy

Dilated cardiomyopathy (DCM) is by far the most common CM in adults as well as in children (50–70% of all pediatric CM cases), though the prognosis is generally much worse for the latter [6]. In a North American study, 46% of 1426 pediatric DCM patients underwent heart transplantation or died during a 5-year follow-up period [6]. The hallmarks of DCM are dilation of the left ventricle (LV) and systolic dysfunction in absence of a hemodynamic cause (e.g., coronary artery and aorta anomalies, sepsis and ischemia) [7]. In addition to LV dilation, other features such as reduced ventricular wall thickness, mass-to-volume ratio, and mitral regurgitation are

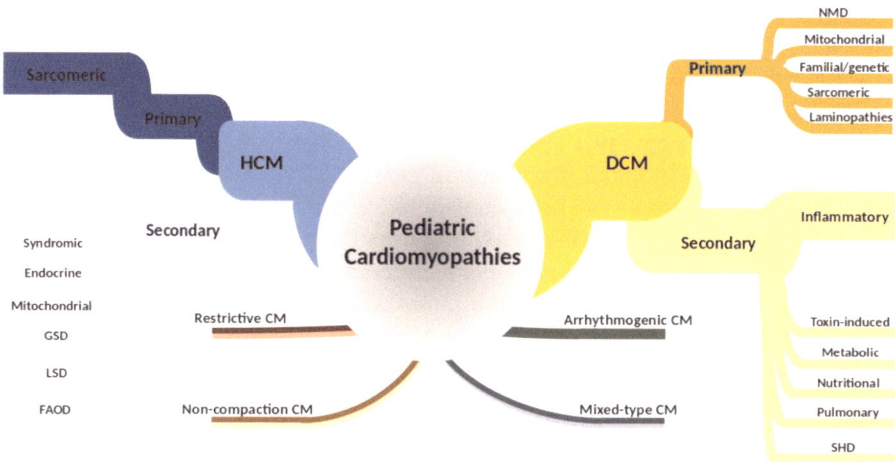

Figure 1.
Overview on pediatric cardiomyopathy (CM) types. The thickness of the branches reflects the relative prevalence in children, except for the rare cardiomyopathies (restrictive, arrhythmogenic, non-compaction, and mixed-type CMs). Here, dual color reflects both primary and secondary etiologies; single-color primary etiology only for arrhythmogenic CM. HCM: Hypertrophic CM; DCM: Dilated CM; NMD: Neuromuscular disorders; GSD: Glycogen storage disorders; LSD: Lysosomal storage disorders; FAOD: Fatty acid oxidation disorders; SHD: Structural heart disease.

observed in the patients. The dilation and decreased contractility can also affect the right ventricle, resulting, for example, in elevated pulmonary pressures and even in pulmonary and peripheral edemas. Again, the phenotype of DCM is highly diverse, ranging from asymptomatic to single or biventricular heart failure, failure to thrive, arrhythmias, and sudden cardiac death [7]. Manifold causes have been described for DCM and encompass primary (genetic and idiopathic) as well as secondary categories [5, 6]. Sometimes, structural heart diseases are associated with DCM, being the end-stage condition of the former, often resulting in the diagnostic "hen and egg" challenge: is the DCM the consequence of the abnormal loading conditions, or are the latter a consequence of an abnormal myocardium? This can often be answered only by successful treatment of the hemodynamic dysfunction (and the subsequent recovery of the myocardium), which is not always possible. The same question applies to DCM associated with pulmonary conditions, which primarily affect the right ventricle.

Primary DCM is difficult to diagnose in absence of identified familial mutations, as all secondary causes have to be excluded first [5]. Thus, patients with de-novo mutations are diagnosed potentially later due to lack of family history. Most cases of idiopathic DCM are considered to have a genetic cause, and there is a growing number of idiopathic DCM cases being reclassified into familial DCM upon further investigation. The estimated occurrence of FDCM is about 30–50% of all DCM cases in children; the 5-year event-free survival rate is 50–60% [6]. The inheritance is autosomal dominant, and the affected genes encompass those encoding for cytoskeletal, sarcomeric, and Z-disk proteins [8]. In addition, DCM is common and a leading cause of mortality in children with neuromuscular disorders (NMDs) such as Duchenne muscular dystrophy, Barth syndrome, myofibrillar myopathies and so on, as well as Emery-Dreyfuss syndrome, caused by a mutation in *LMNA*, the gene encoding for lamin A/C [9, 10]. Primary mitochondrial disorders can also present with a DCM phenotype or develop it over time [11]. Altogether, this underlines the importance of extensive genetic testing of DCM as well as NMD patients.

The distinct feature of secondary DCM (as opposed to primary DCM) is that the underlying causes affect multiple organs and can sometimes be treated, although this is a very broad group of different disorders, accounting for 50–70% of pediatric DCM cases [6]. Also, the phenotype can be very diverse, as well as disease onset and progression. Thus, the common classification criteria here are the dilated morphology and systolic dysfunction in the first place. In case of DCM presentation in very young patients, secondary causes have to be considered in the first place, as primary DCM is expected to be more prevalent in adults. A common type of secondary DCM is the inflammatory DCM, which can be further classified into infectious and non-infectious (e.g., reactions to drugs or toxins, autoimmune diseases etc.) [6]. In children, non-infectious causes are generally rarer than the infectious, with viral myocarditis being the most common cause of inflammatory DCM in children. Especially in cases of viral myocarditis with subsequent DCM, the changes in the morphology of the heart are remarkable, usually starting without significant dilation during the early and acute phase of the infection and remodeling to a dilated phenotype over time. Attributing the myocarditis clearly to a virus can be challenging, though, so that as complete a history and examination as possible should be performed to rule out other causes such as toxin or drug exposure, cancer, metabolic disorders (e.g., thyroid hormone dysregulations, diabetes mellitus), and nutritional disorders/deficiencies [12, 13].

2.2 Hypertrophic cardiomyopathy

The hallmarks of hypertrophic cardiomyopathy (HCM) are a hypertrophied but not dilated ventricle without an underlying hemodynamic cause or physiological hypertrophy and relaxation abnormalities/diastolic dysfunction, whereas the systolic function is usually preserved or even enhanced. Thus, the main diagnostic criterion is the diastolic septal or LV wall thickness, which has to be adjusted for body size in children and is expressed as wall thickness z scores. The wall thickening often presents focally or regionally, so that not the whole ventricle is affected. Nevertheless, the pattern is very diverse, with global biventricular involvement in the most extreme cases. In addition, structural disturbances are common, and mixed phenotypes of HCM with non-compaction and restrictive CM have been described [14, 15]. Similar to other cardiomyopathies, HCM can further be subclassified into primary and secondary forms, with the former being caused by mainly sarcomeric mutations and the latter associated with a multitude of causes, for example, syndromic diseases like Noonan syndrome, lysosomal and glycogen storage diseases (e.g., Anderson-Fabry disease, Pompe and Danon disease), disorders of the fatty acid metabolism, mitochondrial diseases, and hyperinsulinism [2, 16–18]. The latter occurs only in newborn and results from an overproduction of insulin, due to primary causes like pancreatic hyperfunction or to secondary causes like maternal diabetes mellitus. Usually, in these cases, HCM resolves when the underlying hyperinsulinism is treated [2, 14, 19]. In total, HCM accounts for approximately 40% of all pediatric cardiomyopathies and is the second most common CM after DCM in children (**Figure 1**) [20]. The occurrence is ten times higher in children under 1 year of age than in those older than 1 year. In 75% of all HCM cases, idiopathic and genetic/familial HCM are the most common etiologies in children, though it is not clear how many of the idiopathic cases arise from underlying genetic causes that have not been identified yet [21, 22]. Survival in infants with HCM is overall poorer than in older patients, but the prognosis highly depends on etiology and age at diagnosis. For example, inborn errors of metabolism are associated with a very early diagnosis (mean age 6 months) and a 5-year survival rate of only 42%, while for idiopathic non-infantile HCM (age at diagnosis older than 1 year), 94% of children survive 5 years [22]. Thus, early-onset HCM generally has a much worse prognosis, especially in infants with inborn metabolic errors and malformation syndromes, as well as for idiopathic HCM (5-year survival of 82% for early-onset cases vs. 94% for non-infantile cases) [22].

2.3 Restrictive cardiomyopathy

Restrictive cardiomyopathy is in general a rare type of CM, characterized by enhanced ventricular stiffness, abnormal filling patterns, and enlarged atria but absent or very mild hypertrophy or dilation [23]. Thus, the systolic function is nearly normal, while the diastolic function is impaired. The primary diagnostic criterion is the abnormal myocardial stiffness, which is caused by dysfunctions within the myocytes or of the intracellular matrix such as fibrosis, and has to be distinguished from constrictive pericarditis, where the impaired filling results from an abnormal pericardium [24, 25]. As in other cardiomyopathies, the RCM phenotype can vary from asymptomatic to prominent heart failure, pulmonary hypertension, arrhythmias, and sudden death. Causes of RCM can be mutations in sarcomeric and non-sarcomeric genes (primary RCM), as well as infiltration (e.g., amyloidosis), storage disease (e.g., Anderson-Fabry disease), and autoimmune disorders [26]. An important cause of RCM particularly in tropical regions is endomyocardial fibrosis caused by parasitic infections [27]. In children, primary RCM accounts for less than 5% of all CM cases but has the worst outcome [4, 28, 29]. About 66% of the patients present with a pure RCM phenotype and have a 5-year mortality rate of approximately 20% and a 5-year transplantation rate of 58% [28]. In about 50% of children with RCM, pathogenic or likely pathogenic gene variants were found [8].

2.4 Left ventricular non-compaction cardiomyopathy

The most distinctive feature of LVNC is a prominent trabeculation of the left ventricle, as diagnosed by cardiac imaging, which can occur isolated and even without any functional disturbances as well as as part of congenital heart disease or together with skeletal muscle and other systemic abnormalities, for example, Barth syndrome [30]. In addition, it has been associated with atrial and ventricular arrhythmias, atrial fibrillation, and conduction defects. A popular hypothesis suggests that LVNC represents a failure of maturation of the myocardium during embryonic development, although there is also evidence of histological differences of LVNC and normal myocardium even in the embryonic state [31]. The fact that excessive trabeculation does not necessarily lead to functional disturbances also gives rise to controversial views on LVNC as unclassified CM or even just a morphological trait not per se associated with dysfunction [32]. LVNC can occur as mixed phenotype together with, for example, HCM, RCM, or DCM, the latter being the most frequent case in children. Similar to the clinical phenotype, the prognosis in patients with LVNC is highly variable, as the presence of other factors than hypertrabeculation appears to be a major factor [33]. Children with isolated LVNC have a 94% 5-year survival rate, while cases with mixed hypertrophic, restrictive, or dilated phenotypes and/or arrhythmias show significantly poorer outcomes [33]. Barth syndrome is a well-characterized inborn metabolic disease associated with LVNC and DCM. In the United Kingdom and France, about half of the infants diagnosed with Barth syndrome died or received a heart transplant

[34, 35]. Among the transplant-free survivors, cardiac function often stabilized or even recovered after 3 years of age [34, 35].

2.5 Arrhythmogenic cardiomyopathy

Arrhythmogenic cardiomyopathy (ACM) encompasses genetic diseases like AVC (arrhythmogenic ventricular CM), channelopathies, and non-genetic pacing-induced CMs. The clinical and pathological hallmarks of AVC are ventricular arrhythmias, palpitations, syncope in connection to physical exercise, cardiac arrest, impaired ventricular systolic function, and replacement of the myocardium by fibrous and/or fatty tissue. In some cases, patients may also present with ventricular tachycardia and/or heart failure (HF). The formerly used term "arrhythmogenic right ventricular (RV) cardiomyopathy" was established because often the disease affects mainly the right ventricle. But, due to an increasing number of reports of biventricular or even isolated LV involvement, the more general term AVC is now recommended [36, 37]. AVC has an estimated incidence of 1:100 to 1:5000 in the general population and is an important cause of sudden cardiac death (SCD) in children and young adults (11% of all SCD cases and 22% of SCD cases in young athletes), male patients being more often and more severely affected than females [38]. The phenotype is highly diverse though, ranging from nearly normal hearts to severe biventricular dysfunction. The fibrofatty replacement of the muscle tissue is often considered to arise from ischaemic damage of the myocardium, often more prominent in the RV. In contrast, in the LV, often only an isolated fibrofatty scar is observed, leading to a higher risk of severe ventricular arrhythmias and SCD [39]. The diagnosis of AVC is based primarily on cMRI imaging- and/or biopsy-based evidence of fibrofatty replacement in the myocardium and electrocardiographic (ECG) abnormalities. As the disease mostly follows an autosomal-dominant inheritance pattern, family history assessment and genetic screening are also indicated. Common AVC mutations affect desmosomal proteins and proteins involved in cell-cell adhesion. Commercial screening panels are available but do not encompass all genes associated with AVC. For adults, the diagnostic criteria were described in the revised Task Force Criteria of the AHA, but they have only limited validity for pediatric patients, as children often may not exhibit all of the features (e.g., prominent fibrofatty replacement), despite being mutation carriers [40, 41]. Instead, in a larger study, a significantly increased occurrence of SCD and resuscitated SCD was found in pediatric patients compared to adults, while sustained tachycardia was observed significantly less often [42]. Furthermore, athletes were overrepresented among the pediatric patients compared to adults, suggesting an association between endurance exercise during adolescence and pediatric-onset AVC [42].

Channelopathies are inherited arrhythmic diseases typically without structural changes of the heart and myocardium, which is distinctive from, for example, desmosomal, sarcomeric, and cytoskeletal AVC [43]. Channelopathies arise from mutations in genes encoding cardiac ion channels and encompass long- and short-QT syndromes, catecholaminergic polymorphic ventricular tachycardia, Brugada syndrome, and Lenègre disease [43]. Typical phenotypic manifestations are syncopes, cardiac arrest during physical activity, arrhythmias, potentially leading to ventricular fibrillation and SCD. In children, Brugada syndrome has been linked to sudden infant death syndrome [44]. While the heart appears structurally normal, there are prominent changes in the electrocardiographic patterns, which are often characteristic of the specific type of channelopathy, such as prolonged QT intervals in LQTS. Pacing-induced cardiomyopathies arise from ventricular dysfunction caused by tachycardia, arrhythmia, or frequent cardiac ectopy [45]. The phenotype often presents as heart failure symptoms in the presence of tachycardia and ventricular dysfunction or even cardiogenic shock in neonates and infants. Mostly though, the myocardium recovers at least partially after treatment of the underlying arrhythmia [46]. Pacing-induced cardiomyopathy can also occur in children with chronic RV pacing, for example, in cases with atrioventricular block, and develops over time after pacemaker implantation [47]. This type of CM is thought to arise from unwanted abnormal transmission of electric impulses to the LV and can recover after changing to a biventricular pacemaker.

3. Etiology and pathophysiology of pediatric CM

Phenotypes as well as the etiology of pediatric CMs are very heterogeneous. Thus, in inherited CMs, genetic defects may occur in genes encoding proteins of the sarcomere, including the Z-disc proteins, structural proteins (e.g., costameric, desmosomal, cytoskeletal, nucleoskeletal proteins), mitochondrial or Ca^{2+}-handling proteins, signaling proteins such as Ras, or proteins of the Notch signaling pathway, and even mutations in non-coding regions of the genome have been described (see also **Figure 2**). Other causes of pediatric CMs might be inflammation due to viral or bacterial infections and toxins, including chemotherapeutics or neurohormonal or metabolic disorders [48–62]. Inborn errors of metabolism associated with

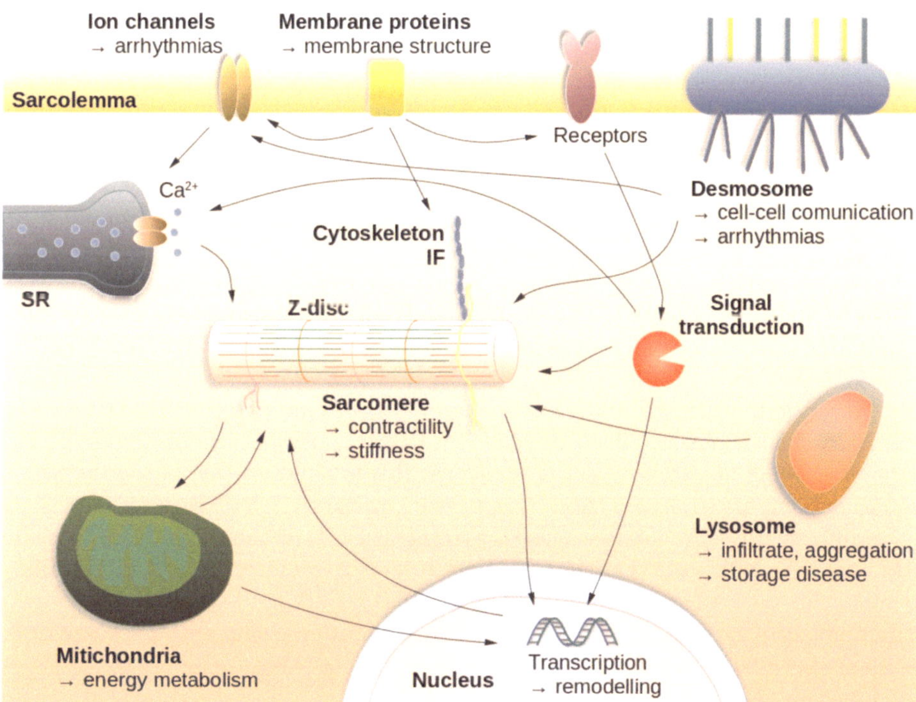

Figure 2.
Cellular compartments affected by genetic mutations causing cardiomyopathy in children. Arrows indicate interactions between different compartments altered in the presence of mutations (e.g., sarcomeric mutations leading to energy depletion and altered transcription). IF: Intermediate filaments.

cardiomyopathies are nicely summarized by [63]. One of these diseases, the Barth syndrome, is associated with CM in early childhood. Characteristically, the Barth syndrome may induce DCM or LNVC, skeletal muscle myopathy, mitochondrial dysfunction, neutropenia, and growth retardation [64]. According to Neuwald [65], a defect in the *TAZ* gene encoding several tafazzins due to alternative splicing might be causative. The taffazin protein family includes acyltransferases involved in phospholipid formation, indicating that the mitochondrial membranes might be defective, leading to an inefficient oxidative phosphorylation and thus to an inefficient energy production for cardiac performance.

LNVC can be caused not only by systemic diseases such as the Barth syndrome but also by gene defects also described in congenital or arrhythmogenic heart disease and restrictive, hypertrophic, or dilated CM. The affected genes identified include those encoding sarcomeric or cytoskeletal proteins as for example *MYH7* (myosin heavy chain 7), *MYL2,3* (myosin light chain 2,3), *MYBPC3* (cardiac myosin binding protein C), *TTN* (titin), *ACTC1* (cardiac alpha actin), *TPM1* (cardiac tropomyosin), *TNNT2* (cardiac troponin T), *TNNI3* (cardiac troponin I), and *ZASP* (LIM binding domain 3), a Z-disc protein [4, 66–71]. Non-sarcomeric gene defects have also been identified, for example, in *HCN4* (hyperpolarisation activated cyclic nucleotide gated potassium channel 4) coding for an ion channel located in pacemaker cells or in genes encoding intermediate filament proteins such as *LMNA* (Lamin A/C), which is involved in heart development, or *DES*, encoding desmin [72, 73]. A list of affected genes in LNVC and their functions can be found in the National Library of Medicine, Medline PLUS. LNVC is mainly due to developmental failure, and it is associated with increased trabeculation, leading to a sponge-like appearance of the heart chambers. Such a remodeling may result in contractile dysfunction, arrhythmia, and sudden cardiac death. The latter is also characteristic of other CMs such as ACM, HCM, or DCM.

DCM, a systolic disorder, is characterized by dilation of the left ventricle or of both ventricles associated with suppressed contractile function. DCM based on genetic defects seems to form the main cause of pediatric DCM, whereby the vast majority of gene mutations is found in sarcomeric proteins, especially in *MYH7*, *TTN*, *TNNT2*, *TPM1*, *MYBPC3*, *MYL2*, *TNNC1* (Troponin C), and *ACTN2*. Others are found in *LMN, DES, VCL* (Vinculin), *TTR* (transthyretin), *BAG3* (associated with apoptosis), *MT-TS2* (encoding a mitochondrial small RNA), or transcription factor encoding PRDM16 [74–78]. In adult and pediatric DCM, the same genes seem to be affected, though unfortunately, most genetic testings have been performed in adults [79]. Besides the genetic causes, inflammation may lead to DCM, the main non-genetic cause in children. Myocarditis is mainly caused by viral infections and is rather challenging for diagnosis and treatment [80]. In most cases, Coxsackieviruses B and adenovirus infections are the causes of myocarditis in children [81]. Recently, SARS-CoV-2 virus has also been described as a possible cause [82]. Besides viral infections, toxins and chemotherapeutics are also emerging as DCM-inducing agents. Especially anthracyclines, which often are used to treat tumors in children as well as in adults, have been linked to the development of heart failure, DCM, or RCM [83]. The onset of cardiomyopathy in cancer patients varies largely; it may develop within a week or less than one year after starting the treatment, depending on various risk factors (e.g., sex, age, dosage, and subtype of the agent) [84].

Most pediatric HCM cases are due to genetic defects mainly in genes encoding sarcomeric proteins, though diagnosis in respect of etiology remains challenging. The HCM mutations often may also cause other CMs such as DCM, RCM, ARVC, or LNVC, even within the same family, indicating additional factors such as further gene mutations, polymorphisms, or comorbidities. Mutations have been identified in genes encoding thick- and thin-filament proteins, whereby most mutations have been identified in *MYBPC3* and *MYH7*. Frequently, mutations have also been described in *TNNT2*, *TNNI3*, and *MYL2* or more seldom in *TPM1* and *ACTN*. HCM in children is even more heterogeneous than in adults. There are also several non-sarcomeric causes recently summarized in [85], which may occur alone or in combination with sarcomeric mutations and then modify the severity and prognosis of the disease [86]. These non-sarcomeric causes of HCM in children include rasopathies, a set of diseases with genetic defects encoding proteins of the Ras signaling cascade, for example, the Noonan syndrome. Others are glycogen storage diseases, including Pompe or Danon disease, characterized by glycogen-filled vacuoles within the cardiomyocytes [87]. In lysosomal storage diseases, for example, mucopolysaccharidoses, partially or undigested macromolecules are accumulated due to dysfunctional lysosomal enzymes [88]. In addition, mitochondrial disorders may occur, which mostly affect oxidative phosphorylation and thus energy production. Thus, HCM is often characterized by an energy deficiency probably due to over-contractility, as might also be the case in RCM.

In contrast to HCM, RCM is characterized by restrictive ventricular filling mostly without an increase in wall thickness. The genetic/familial causes of RCM are mainly due to mutations in genes encoding sarcomeric proteins (listed in [4]). Here, mutations in *TNNI3* occur frequently, but mutations have also been identified in genes of cytoskeletal or nuclear envelope proteins, leading to storage diseases (e.g., Danon disease, Friedrich ataxia, etc.) or infiltrative diseases (cardiac amyloidosis, cardiac sarcoidosis). The latter may also develop due to non-genetic causes.

All CM types are associated with an increased risk of developing severe arrhythmias, but they are most prominent in ACM. ACM is a genetically based disease, whereby most studies have concentrated on adult patients, underlining the need for more studies with children under 18 years of age. Histologically, ACM is characterized by the loss of cardiomyocytes being replaced by fibrofatty tissue [42, 89]. As a consequence of the cardiac remodeling, life-threatening arrhythmia and sudden cardiac death can occur. Causes for this familial disease are mutations in genes encoding desmosomal proteins with a deletion mutation in the junctional plakoglobin gene (*JUP*) being the first identified in ACM [90]. It seems that truncation mutations and splice variants in the *PKP2*, encoding plakophilin 2, are the most frequent causes of ACM, together with mutations in *DSP* (desmoplakin), *DSC2* (desmocollin 2), *DSG2* (desmoglein 2), and *JUP* [91]. Less frequently, mutations in *TMEM43* (Transmembrane Protein 43) and *PLN* (phospholamban) have been described.

4. Molecular mechanisms

Molecular mechanisms of CM development—as far as known to date—often are not specific for a distinct CM type. Generally, contractile function is affected via various mechanisms, and involvement of several cell compartments and cardiac remodeling is common (**Figure 2**).

4.1 Sarcomeric dysfunction

The smallest contractile unit of cross-striated muscles is the sarcomere. It is bordered by the Z-discs from which thin and elastic filaments reach out to the center of the sarcomere (M-Line). The thick filaments emanate bidirectionally from the M-line. Cardiac thin filaments are mainly composed of filamentous cardiac actin, cardiac tropomyosin (cTpm), and the cardiac heterotrimeric troponin complex composed of the tropomyosin-binding subunit (cTnT), the inhibitory subunit (cTnI), and the calcium-binding subunit (cTnC). Cardiac thick filaments are composed of cardiac myosin containing the essential and regulatory myosin light chains (MyLC) and heavy chains (MyHC) and cardiac myosin-binding protein C (cMyBPC), linking thick, thin, and elastic filaments. This implies that MyBPC coordinates the action of the filaments in contraction and relaxation processes. The elastic filament is formed by the giant protein titin. Ca^{2+}-binding to cTnC triggers contraction by enabling actin-myosin interaction and the power stroke (for review, see [92]). In addition, the contraction can be fine-tuned by reversible phosphorylation of many sarcomeric proteins, for example, titin, myosin-binding protein C, myosin light chains, cTnT, cTnI, cTpm, and also Z-disc proteins [93, 94].

CM-inducing mutations may occur in genes encoding filament proteins as well as proteins of the Z-disc. They may lead to single amino acid replacements or loss of a single or several amino acids. As a result, the mutations may alter the very sensitive interplay between the components of the sarcomere and/or protein dynamics and thereby induce contractile dysfunction (for review, see [4]). Furthermore, interactions of sarcomeric proteins with associated proteins might be altered, affecting signaling and thereby protein transcription, metabolism, inflammation, oxidation, cell death, protein degradation, fibrosis, cell–cell communication, Ca^{2+} homeostasis, and so on [95–97].

The intracellular Ca^{2+}- concentration is pivotal for the muscles' contractile function. At submicromolar concentrations, the cardiac muscle is at rest. It contracts upon an up to 100-fold increase in intracellular Ca^{2+}- concentration following a nervous impulse and opening of the voltage-gated L-type Ca-channels, which are located in the T-tubules of cardiomyocytes. The resultant Ca^{2+} inward current triggers the opening of the ryanodine receptors, the Ca^{2+}- channels within the membrane of the sarcoplasmatic reticulum (SR). Thereby, Ca^{2+} is released from the SR Ca^{2+}- stores, which leads to a massive increase in intracellular Ca^{2+}- concentration and to Ca^{2+}-binding to cTnC. This finally enables the power-generating interaction of myosin and actin, leading to contraction. On the other hand, relaxation occurs when Ca^{2+} is dissociated from cTnC. The released Ca^{2+} is then pumped back into the SR via the SR Calcium ATPase (SERCA), into the extracellular space via NCX (Na^{+}-Ca^{2+}-exchanger) and plasma membrane Ca^{2+} ATPases, and into mitochondria [98]. These complex procedure makes clear that alterations in the regulation of intracellular Ca^{2+}-concentrations lead to contractile dysfunction and thus to myocardial diseases. Besides mutations in genes of proteins involved in calcium fluxes (for review, see [99]), mutations in sarcomeric protein genes affect the calcium response of sarcomeric proteins and/or the calcium-binding affinity of the sarcomeres' Ca^{2+}-sensor, cTnC. On a simplified level, it is thought that DCM mutations decrease the calcium sensitivity of the actin-myosin interaction, thereby reducing the contractile capacity, which makes DCM a systolic disorder. Though, in pediatric end-stage DCM, cardiomyocytes exhibit an increased calcium sensitivity [100]. The authors assumed that this is caused by a substantial decrease in cTnI phosphorylation, which however cannot be the main reason, since in adult DCM, cTnI phosphorylation is also reduced (see below). In HCM and RCM, often the Ca^{2+}- sensitivity of the actin-myosin interaction is increased (at least in adults), leading to faster relaxation and re-contraction. Since intracellular Ca^{2+} is increased also due to an increased phosphorylation of Ca^{2+} channels, relaxation is impaired. Increased intracellular Ca^{2+}- concentration leads to hypercontractility, causing energy deficiency and increased production of reactive oxygen species (ROS) due to increased oxidative phosphorylation [101]. Posttranslational modifications and increased ROS might contribute to the development of arrhythmias. ROS induce oxidation of proteins, for example, of the calcium calmodulin kinase (CaMKII), which upon oxidation of methionine residues within the autophosphorylation domain is constantly active, because it cannot be inactivated via dephosphorylation and Ca^{2+}- CaM (calmodulin) dissociation [102, 103]. CaMKII regulates several proteins including those involved in calcium fluxes. Its activation increases intracellular Ca^{2+} levels due to increased open probabilities of Ca^{2+} channels as the L-type Ca^{2+} channel or the Ryanodine receptor. This might contribute to the remodeling of T-tubules further affecting EC coupling and Ca^{2+} homeostasis (for review see [92]).

However, calcium regulation might not only be impaired directly by mutations but also disturb the intermolecular interaction between the components of the sarcomere [104, 105]. Additionally, calcium responses might be affected by cross bridge kinetics or phosphorylation of myosin-binding protein C and cardiac TnI [106]. In pediatric and in adult DCM, cAMP-dependent protein kinase (PKA)-dependent hypophosphorylation of cTnI and MyBPC has been described, leading to a reduced stress response. Furthermore, maximal force and passive force were reduced. Hereby, reduced myofiber densities as proposed by [107] might contribute to the impaired force production. The reduced myofiber density seems not to be caused by an impaired protein quality control system [107]. The underlying mechanism is still unknown.

Most mutations, preferentially truncations leading to adult DCM, have been identified in titin. Controversial study results have been obtained with pediatric DCM. *TTN* and *MYH7* mutations were identified as predominant in a cohort of 106 pediatric patients [74]. In another study analyzing 36 patients, only one *TTN* mutation, a truncation (p.Arg33703*), was identified in a 16-year-old male DCM patient [108]. Mutations occur most frequently in A-band N2Ba/N2B-titin and thus may induce structural and contractile dysfunctions [109]. In A-band titin, interaction sites for myosin and myosin-binding protein C are distributed in a regular pattern [110]. This implies that in the case of A-band titin sequence alterations or truncations, its interaction with myosin and/or myosin-binding protein C might be impaired.

The location of mutations within *MYH7* - another frequent target for pathogenic mutations - seems to determine the DCM type according to Khan et al. [74]. They found that mostly single amino acid replacements in ß-Myosin heavy chain (MYH7) in the range of amino acids 1–600 lead to mixed DCM, a DCM–LNVC phenotype, whereas mutations in the C-terminal part from amino acid 600 lead to pure DCM [74]. The C-terminal rod of myosin heavy chain interacts with other myosin rods, which is essential to build up the thick filament. Myosin consists of 2 heavy chains, with the rod region forming a supercoil. The N-terminal part of each myosin heavy chain consists of a lever arm, a converter region with binding regions for the myosin light chains, and the globular motor domain containing the ATPase domain and actin binding domain. Mutations in the motor domain may affect ATPase activity via altered ATP-binding affinities and/or ATP hydrolysis rate and/or dissociation of the hydrolysis products ADP and P_i. Furthermore, it may impair the interaction of the motor domain with actin. Thus, most DCM mutations seem to weaken the affinity for actin. Furthermore, in contrast to MYH7 HCM mutants, in case of DCM, less force is produced due to a lower occupancy of the force generating state and a reduced ATPase velocity [111]. They predict that less ATP is used to hold a specific force.

Besides MYH7, the gene of cardiac MyBPC is the main target for pediatric and adult cardiomyopathies, whereby mutations in the cardiac MyBPC predominantly lead to HCM and, typically for HCM, are associated with hypercontractility. According to Toepfer et al. [112], mutations in *MYBPC3*, which result in either truncations or single amino acid replacements, affect the dynamics of myosin conformations and the super-relaxed state of myosin. cMyBPC interacts with myosin at several sites (rod, lever arm) and with titin, actin, and troponin and is thought to regulate the number of force-producing myosin motor domains. When phosphorylated, at submaximal Ca^{2+}- levels, it promotes the actin-myosin interaction [113]. Mutations in *MYBPC3* or in genes of interacting proteins might impair the interplay between these proteins and thereby the regulation of contraction. Hereby, an impaired interaction of different proteins with cardiac troponin might also play a role, though the role of the MyBPC-cardiac troponin interaction as well as of its interaction with titin remains to be elucidated [104, 114]. Two fascinating studies revealed that MyBPC regulates sarcomeric contractile oscillations, which might be based on its interplay with all sarcomeric partners [115, 116].

Mutations in the cardiac actin gene are relatively rare and mostly are associated with the development of HCM and DCM. They seem to affect the interaction with myosin heads and/or tropomyosin or troponin [117]. Interactions with MyBPC or actin-associated proteins regulating formation and length of the actin filament have not been considered yet. A nice overview of these proteins and their role is given in the review by Ehler [118]. The first hint that filament formation/structure could be impaired by pathogenic mutations in the cardiac actin gene comes from [119]. They showed that different mutations incorporate differently into the actin filament and destabilize the filaments. A destabilization of actin filaments has also been described by Hassoun et al. [114], and pediatric RCM mutations in *TNNI3* have been demonstrated to largely affect the integrity of reconstituted thin filament structure [104].

Other targets for pathogenic mutations are the genes of the three subunits of the troponin complex: cTnC, cTnI, and cTnT. They are associated mostly with HCM and DCM. However, *TNNI3* mutations frequently result in RCM [4]. They affect Ca^{2+}-sensitivity via impaired intra- and intermolecular interactions as well as via impaired posttranslational modifications. Hypercontractility-induced increase in ROS leads to oxidation of not only lipids, nucleic acids, or protein kinases but also sarcomeric proteins. It has been shown by Budde et al. [120] that oxidation of cardiac troponin I and cardiac MyBPC reduced phosphorylation by PKA and PKC and thereby contributed to the impairment of force production. The effects could be reversed fully by using antioxidants and partly by supplementing PKA. Also, specific oxidations of actin or titin have been associated with development of heart diseases [121, 122].

4.2 Cardiac remodeling

Enhanced ROS production leading to oxidative stress contributes to cardiac remodeling as fibrosis, another hallmark of cardiomyopathies, which leads to further contractile dysfunction via increased stiffness of the ventricular walls and also contributes to arrhythmia. Fibrosis occurs due to the activation of fibroblasts via stimulation of pro-fibrotic factors as TGF-ß, PDGF (platelet-derived growth factor), or cytokines and increased production and deposition of collagen I and III as well as cross-linking of the extracellular matrix (ECM). According to Li et al. [123], TGF-ß increases the expression of SerpinE2/nexin-1, leading to increased collagen deposition. Fibrosis as well as hypertrophic growth have been described to be linked also to ERK1/2, JNK, and p38 pathways. Furthermore, there seems to be an association between fibrosis, oxidative stress, and inflammation (for review see [124]). Even in young children, fibrosis could be observed, though the pathways in children have not been investigated. But there might be differences in signaling between children and adults [125]. Thus, in the case of DCM, a study revealed that children show much less interstitial and perivascular fibrosis than adult patients [126]. Furthermore, it seems that genes leading to an inflammatory response in DCM are expressed in adult but not pediatric patients. Also, differences between young children and adults in receptor physiology have been described. These aberrances will have consequences for the therapy of pediatric heart diseases [127].

Fibrous and/or fibrofatty infiltration leading to life-threatening arrhythmia is a hallmark of ACM, which is caused by genetic defects [128]. Genes modified include those encoding mostly desmosomal proteins (e.g., placophilin 2) and rarely junctional proteins as catenins, cytoskeletal proteins as TMEM43, and so on [129]. The molecular mechanisms of ACM development especially in children are not quite understood. ACM is strongly correlated to cardiomyocyte loss, which might be due to a stimulated apoptosis, since defects in desmosomal or junctional proteins lead to reduced cell adhesion and impaired sarcolemmal structure [130]. Apoptosis might be triggered by stimulated hippo pathways and fibrosis via WNT inhibition and TGF-ß pathways [129]. Fibrosis (together with deposits of protein aggregates, amyloidosis, glycogen storage defects), probably due to an impaired protein control system, might also be the causative for the stiffness observed especially with RCM [4]. Increased myocardial stiffness, however, is also observed in other heart diseases than RCM, as in heart failure with preserved rejection fraction, LNVC, and HCM. Increased myocardial stiffness leads to a reduced filling of the heart chambers with blood. Besides fibrosis and protein aggregates, the microtubular network, that is, microtubule density and its cross-linking with intermediate filaments, also contributes to the myocardial elasticity [131]. In addition, sarcomeric titin is a major player in myocardial stiffness. The ratio of the isoforms N2Ba and N2B is decisive [132]. But posttranslational modifications such as changes in titin phosphorylation also contribute to the alterations in stiffness [132–136].

For HCM and RCM but not ACM, another hallmark is the myocyte disarray, which according to Garcia-Canadilla et al. [137] in case of HCM mutations occurs very early, even before birth, indicating a developmental impairment at least in mice. In addition, cardiomyocyte disarray might contribute to arrhythmia associated with HCM/RCM. Molecular mechanisms leading to myocyte disarray are not known. In [138], a cell-to-cell imbalance in the expression of mutant proteins was described, which might lead to arrhythmias, myocyte disarray, and fibrosis.

Epigenetic modulations play a role in all cardiomyopathies. Thus, in HCM, hypertrophic growth is mediated by stimulating the expression of sarcomeric proteins. Hereby, a reprogramming occurs; fetal instead of adult proteins are expressed in adult HCM patients. In newborn CM patients, there might be a different mechanism, since some cardiac-specific genes such as *TNNI3* are expressed within the first year of life and gradually replace the fetal skeletal muscle isoform. In hypertrophic growth and reprogramming, calicneurin and the transcription factors NFAT, GATA4, NFkappaB, and MEF2 play a central role, nicely summarized by Dirkx et al. [139]. NFAT also regulates the expression of micro RNAs (miRNAs), which regulate mRNAs. In hypertrophy, miR23 is induced by targeting MURF1 and FOXO3a, both involved in cardiac remodeling [140, 141]. Epigenetic studies are largely missing in infant cardiomyopathy patients, and investigations are urgently needed. One of the few studies is [142], investigating miRNA profiles in children with heart failure. They found 17 miRNAs that were either not regulated (miR-130b, miR-204, miR-331-3p, miR-188-5p, miR-1281, miR-572, miR-765, miR-223, miR-125a-3p, and miR-1268) or antithetically regulated (miR-638, miR-7, miR-132, and miR-146a) in adult heart failure. Several of these miRs regulate genes, such as SMAD4, which are involved in the transition of hypertrophy to heart failure. In DCM, altered DNA methylation patterns and histone modifications and altered miR and lncRNA (long noncoding RNA) regulation have been identified in adult CM patients, but again, investigations in children are missing [143].

5. Diagnosis of cardiomyopathy in children

Considering the substantial risk of developmental disorders, disabilities, and mortality of children with cardiomyopathies, early detection, accurate classification, and treatment of cardiomyopathies in children are imperative [144–146]. Nevertheless, there is a gap in knowledge and a lack of consensus in the diagnostic approach, definition, and classification of cardiomyopathies in children [2]. Thus, the American Heart Association, in their latest publication, provided some suggestions in the form of a scientific statement instead of a clinical practice guideline. In this statement, a classification system for cardiomyopathy based on a hierarchy incorporating the required elements of the MOGE(S) classification was suggested. Manifestations of cardiomyopathy in children can range from a sole histopathological variation in cardiac tissue to congestive heart failure or sudden death [147–149]. The clinical presentation of patients with cardiomyopathy can resemble those with heart failure with reduced ejection fraction, including dyspnea on exertion, fluid retention and edema, lethargy, orthopnea, presyncope, syncope, and paroxysmal nocturnal dyspnea [26, 32]. Nevertheless, clinicians should be attentive to the rare types of cardiomyopathies such as LVNC or arrhythmogenic right ventricular (RV) dysplasia [37, 150]. Considering the variety of manifestations of cardiomyopathy, taking a thorough history of the patient and other family members as well as general physical examination concerning not only cardiac disorders but also possible extracardiac abnormalities, that is, Noonan syndrome, are essential for choosing the most relevant diagnostic modalities [2].

5.1 Laboratory parameters and biomarkers

A few biomarkers are used in the routine clinical approach to children with cardiomyopathies, which to some extent is due to the lack of reliable evidence. A high cardiac troponin concentration in serum can support a diagnosis of myocarditis considering that other causes of ischemia (e.g., acute coronary syndrome and acute myocardial strain such as that induced by pulmonary embolism or recreational drug use) are uncommon in children. Given that natriuretic peptides have been reported in a study on adult patients to be markedly higher in patients with RCM, N-terminal pro-B-type natriuretic peptide may offer supportive evidence for RCM versus constrictive pericarditis [151]. However, studies are warranted to verify their applicability in children. Thus, for example, fibrotic pathways seem to vary age-dependently.

According to Woulfe et al. [152], fibrotic pathways in children (<18 years) were less active than in adults, though here again many more studies are needed [126, 153, 154]. A study of Miyamoto et al. [155] showed that the ß1: ß2 adrenoreceptor ratio differed significantly in pediatric HF patients from the one in adult patients. cAMP levels were commonly decreased in both adult and pediatric HF but were significantly higher in HF children than in HF adults. In addition, gene expressions of BNP, Cx43, and PP1ß and PP2A were regulated antithetically, indicating that signaling is differentially regulated in children and adults. However, it is already difficult to determine a normal BNP level since it alters with age of the children probably due to the maturation process of the heart from fetal to adult including alterations in gene expression and metabolism [156]. This development largely takes place within the first year after birth.

Several biological roles of miRNAs have been identified so far in cardiac development and diseases [157]. Accordingly, emerging studies have revealed the potential utility of miRNAs as biomarkers for the detection of DCM, myocarditis, and the evaluation of heart failure in children [158–160]. The study of Jiao et al. [159] reported an area under the curve (AUC) of up to 0.992, suggesting that these circulating miRNAs may be useful for DCM detection and diagnosis in children. Nevertheless, the studies evaluating the diagnostic role of miRNA in cardiomyopathy in children are sparse. Furthermore, the study of Miyamoto et al. [158] emphasized the inapplicability of employing an adult miRNA profile as a circulating biomarker for pediatric patients, highlighting the significance of developing a signature of circulating miRNAs in this population. Moreover, there are not many miRNAs that are consistent among studies. Therefore, further studies are warranted to find common miRNAs to be accepted as validated biomolecules in the diagnostics of cardiomyopathies.

5.2 Genetic testing

Considering that genetic causes play a major role in pediatric cardiomyopathies, genetic tests are indicated in most cases, not only for better classification but also for determining the cause and screening other family members. Autosomal-dominant inheritance is the most common mode of inheritance in familial isolated cardiomyopathy diagnosed in childhood, but X-linked inheritance and autosomal-recessive inheritance are also reported less frequently [18, 20]. Children with HCM and those with an affected first-degree relative have the highest likelihood of inheritance of a disease-causing mutation among those with isolated cardiomyopathy. Furthermore, HCM that develops in childhood is more likely to be caused by multiple disease-causing mutations compared with HCM that emerges in adulthood [161]. Therefore, it is advised to take into account a broad panel rather than targeted genetic testing when HCM manifests throughout childhood [161]. Thus, whole exome or even whole genome screening should be the gold standard to detect pathogenic or likely pathogenic mutations [162, 163]. Moreover, because the signs of syndromes may be missed at the initial presentation, particularly in infants or critically ill children, a comprehensive genetic examination is helpful. Nevertheless, comprehensive genetic counseling and a thorough family pedigree are essential for understanding the scope and implications of genetic testing. When a child with cardiomyopathy is confirmed to have a pathogenic mutation known to be related to cardiomyopathy, cascade genetic testing of family members is typically advised [2]. Notably, there are various limitations of genetic testing in children. A negative or nondiagnostic test result does not rule out the diagnosis of cardiomyopathy or the possibility that the cardiomyopathy may have a hereditary etiology. Moreover, adult data is the only source of information for commercial panels that may not be applicable to children [2].

5.3 Functional and structural assessment

Assessment of myocardial structural, valvular or coronary artery abnormalities, and cardiac functions by means of proper imaging techniques is considered the cornerstone for the diagnosis and classification of cardiomyopathies.

Electrocardiography and electrophysiology are essential in the diagnosis of some types of pediatric cardiomyopathies, such as ACM. Slow intraventricular conduction in electrophysiology examinations is typically detected in ACM, and most often, right bundle-branch block with right precordial repolarization variations can be detected in electrocardiography. Scar or delayed conduction can be evaluated in 3D using an emerging approach for the diagnosis of ACM called electroanatomic mapping [164–166].

Echocardiography, which is often the initial imaging modality in cardiomyopathy evaluation, provides an overview of structural parameters including chamber dimensions, volumes, wall dimensions, assessment of cardiac functional features such as Doppler traces of ventricular contractility (dP/dt), systolic-to-diastolic ratio, as well as tissue Doppler imaging and extents of myocardial deformation (strain and strain rate) [167]. Notably, no absolute values are attainable as the cutoff point for morphological parameters obtained from echocardiography in children, such as LV end-systolic dimension (LVESD), LV end-diastolic volume, and LV end-diastolic dimension (LVEDD), and they all should be interpreted regarding the z scores adjusted for patient size [168–170]. These parameters are essential to the classification of morphological types. A high LVEDD or LV end-diastolic volume, besides low LV functional parameters, is marker of a dilated, hypokinetic type. Increased wall thickness proposes HCM. Measuring the thickness-to-dimension ratio can aid in distinguishing between idiopathic DCM and myocarditis [2]. However, it is not easy to determine deviations from normal LV morphology, as somatic growth has to be taken into account while monitoring the progression, for example, of HCM or DCM [171]. Thus, performing an accurate assessment by echocardiography in children can be difficult. Specifically, evaluation of diastolic function in children has low interobserver consistency, and the results are not properly associated with invasive haemodynamic investigations; thus, it may not be able to accurately discriminate between cardiomyopathy phenotypes [172, 173].

Cardiac magnetic resonance imaging (cMRI) offers great advantages over echocardiography for the diagnosis and assessment of cardiomyopathies and transcends some limitations of echocardiography in children. Determination of structural features including chamber dimensions, wall thicknesses, and ventricular mass as well as functional parameters including flow rates, shunts, and regional wall motion abnormalities using cMRI can aid in the diagnosis and accurate classification of the cardiomyopathy [174, 175]. Furthermore, assessment of the presence and pattern of fibrosis in tissue with late gadolinium enhancement and also the determination of edema and hyperemia in cMRI are some exceptional properties of cMRI that aid in the noninvasive investigation of patients with cardiomyopathy (e.g., to distinguish the different types of HCM or to discriminate DCM versus myocarditis) [176]. The information acquired from cMRI can also help determine the possible causes of cardiomyopathies (e.g., cardiomyopathies secondary to iron overload). Strain parameters and RV morphology and physiology, which are important in diagnosing and classifying cardiomyopathies, can be evaluated more accurately with cMRI than with echocardiography.

Cardiac computed tomography (CT) and cardiac catheterization are rarely considered for the diagnosis and evaluation of pediatric cardiomyopathies. Cardiac catheterization can be helpful for haemodynamic assessment, performing endomyocardial biopsy, and surgical interventions in patients with amenable lesions [177]. In general, morphological evaluation of the heart in children and infants by imaging techniques as well as cardiac catheterization can be challenging due to the requirement of specialized training and equipment. The availability of both specialized medical professionals as well as equipment still is a major obstacle worldwide to improve the quality of care for patients with pediatric cardiomyopathies.

6. Treatment of pediatric cardiomyopathy

Pediatric cardiomyopathy is treated according to the distinct symptoms that each patient presents [15]. Various factors, including the specific type of cardiomyopathy, the disease's progression at the time of diagnosis, the patient's age, any coexisting medical conditions, the patient's tolerance for particular medications, and other factors, may affect the specific therapeutic procedures and interventions [15]. The therapeutic approach for pediatric cardiomyopathy options may include staged therapy for heart failure, lifestyle modifications, nutrition and strenuous physical activity restrictions, patient and parent education, implanted cardioverter-defibrillator installation, and, in refractory situations, consideration of heart transplantation [178, 179]. A multidisciplinary team of healthcare professionals, including pediatricians, pediatric cardiologists, hematologists, surgeons who specialize in pediatric cardiothoracic surgery, physical therapists, occupational therapists, and/or other healthcare professionals, may be needed to provide this type of treatment [179]. It is crucial to consider that medications and surgical methods for treating cardiomyopathy have mostly been tried and evaluated in adults. Thus, as also stated in a review by Loss et al. [180], pediatric management in general follows the guidelines for adult HF treatment. This is due to the lack of clinical trials with children, which are especially challenging due to difficulties in recruiting an adequate number of probands, high costs, and so on.

6.1 Noninvasive treatment

The usefulness of drugs developed mainly for adults in treating pediatric cardiomyopathy is only dimly documented. There are some studies showing that utilization of medicals as well as signaling differ in children and in adult heart failure patients. In the study of Pan et al. [156], diastolic diseases in children were treated with ACE-inhibitors (angiotensin-converting enzyme), ß-blockers, digitalis, calcium channel blockers, dopamine, and diuretics. In children with diastolic diseases but not CM, the medical treatment was largely successful and improved cardiac function. However, children with CM did not improve. Though, in this study, only few children with CM were included. However, the results underline the observation that medical treatments prescribed for adult patients with CM may not be proper for children with CM. For review on possible medical treatments in pediatric RCM, see [29]. Another nice review on HF drug therapies highlighting the gaps for pediatric HF management is by Das et al. [181].

Thus, to ascertain the long-term safety and efficacy of such medicines in the pediatric population, more studies are required. Some ongoing studies evaluate emerging methods for treatment of pediatric cardiomyopathies such as reducing mitochondrial oxidative stress by MitoQ (mitoquinol mesylate) for DCM, oral Ifetroban for Duchenne muscular dystrophy cardiomyopathy and DCM, or gene therapy for male patients with Danon disease [182–184]. Nonetheless, more investigations are required to determine the optimal therapy approaches for cardiomyopathies in children.

6.2 Minimally invasive and invasive treatments

Altarabsheh et al. evaluated the early and late results of children (<21 years) who underwent transaortic septal myectomy for obstructive HCM [185]. Although the results of this study supported the safety and efficiency of this approach, technical challenges are reported to be augmented in children due to limited exposure during the procedure and subsequently increased risk of suboptimal removal of obstructive muscle, iatrogenic injuries to aortic/mitral valves or papillary muscles, and aneurysm formation in ventricular apex due to excessive muscular resection. Some alternative approaches are also introduced in adult patients such as radiofrequency catheter ablation (RFCA) and alcohol septal ablation, but limited or no data are available for children with HCM [186–188]. There are also ongoing studies evaluating novel methods like intracoronary transplantation of stem cells in pediatric CM [189, 190]. Additionally, surgery in adults is also considered in cases with complex LV morphologic abnormalities, such as papillary muscle anomalies, aberrant intraventricular muscle bundles, intrinsic mitral valve disease (requiring repair or replacement), and associated CAD that necessitates bypass grafting [191].

Cardiac resynchronization therapy (with or without implantable cardioverter-defibrillator) is also available as another option for pediatric and adult patients with DCM with ventricular conduction delay. The goal of this treatment is to enhance heart function by reducing the delay in activation of the left ventricular free wall, which is frequently observed in patients with left ventricular systolic dysfunction. The treatment has been demonstrated to enhance survival in this group, restore coordination and relaxation of the heart chambers, and cause favorable cardiac remodeling. However, using the current suggested criteria, up to a third of patients do not see any therapeutic improvement [192]. Furthermore, recommendations about electrical device therapies for children with DCM are mainly adopted from those for adults but based on considerably less evidence [193].

Despite these promising approaches, often heart transplantation remains as the only treatment option for pediatric CM. The main problem is that waiting for a suitable heart often takes a long time, which the children do not have to survive. The mortality of children while on transplant wait-list might be as high as 17–30% and even higher for infants, due to the general shortage of donor hearts and the high refusal rate due to poor quality (80%) [194, 195]. Also here, a lack of consensus between different centers and listing programs leads to prominent differences in the potential outcomes. Thus, the waiting time has to be bridged by a mechanical circulatory support or total artificial heart, which is suboptimal especially for newborns and infants, due to the limited availability of suitable devices and the adverse effects on the following heart transplantation due to, for example, adhesions. Alternatively, an allograft transplantation can be tried, although here the same problems as the donor heart availability and utilization apply [196]. After transplantation, the problem of immunosuppression arises, bearing the risk of infections or developing cancer. Thus, at Duke University hospital, recently a newborn who in addition to heart failure had a T-cell deficiency has been successfully transplanted a heart together with thymus for the first time in spring 2022. In general, the posttransplant survival rates in children are highly variable and largely depend on comorbidities, general clinical status, the use of mechanical support devices, and, as a major factor, disease progression due to wait-list time.

7. Conclusion and future perspectives

Although pediatric cardiomyopathies share many aspects with CMs in adults, there is rising evidence of unique features that have implications for diagnosis and treatment. First of all, a standard guideline for the classification of CM by the scientific society is desperately needed, as a mutual approach is required for developing protocols and reporting the findings. Age-based scales for diagnostic parameters for distinguishing between normal and abnormal conditions have to be established and adjusted for children.

Furthermore, we need to increase awareness of the medical community to avoid using the same CM therapeutic protocols of adults for children when their experimental evidence did not include children or excluded them. In the future, besides genetic testing (whole exome or whole genome), family analysis and analysis of specific biomarkers and investigation of molecular mechanisms in children will further support diagnosis and treatment design. In addition, large well-conceived trials are needed to increase the efficacy of medical treatments in children. Not only physical/mental effects but also developmental effects of therapeutic practices have to be investigated in long-term cohort studies.

Specifically optimized, mechanical circulatory supports for small children have to be developed that will reduce the deaths while awaiting heart transplantation. The assessment of donor heart suitability needs to be improved and standardized to reduce transplantation wait-list time. Also, increased allograft utilization may contribute to improved survival rates until transplantation, together with modified postoperative care and monitoring optimized for pediatric patients.

An interesting, though controversial, topic in the future might be xenotransplantation, considering the increasing demands for pediatric heart transplantation and advances in tissue engineering and genetic modification of, for example, animal donors. Though ethically highly debated, a survey of congenital heart surgeons revealed a generally high acceptance (80–88%) of xenotransplantation [197].

Acknowledgements

Part of this work was kindly supported by the Boehringer Ingelheim Fonds (S.-R. Sadat-Ebrahimi).

Conflict of interest

The authors declare no conflict of interest.

Author details

Diana Cimiotti[1*†], Seyyed-Reza Sadat-Ebrahimi[2†], Andreas Mügge[2†] and Kornelia Jaquet[2,3†]

1 Institute of Clinical Pharmacology, Ruhr-University Bochum, Bochum, Germany

2 Department of Cardiology, St. Josef Hospital and BG Bergmannsheil, Clinics of the Ruhr-University Bochum, Bochum, Germany

3 Experimental and Molecular Cardiology, St. Josef Hospital, Clinic of the Ruhr-University Bochum, Bochum, Germany

*Address all correspondence to: diana.cimiotti@rub.de

† These authors contributed equally.

References

[1] Yuan SM. Cardiomyopathy in the pediatric patients. Pediatrics and Neonatology. 2018;**4**(59):120-128

[2] Lipshultz SE, Law YM, Asante-Korang A, Austin ED, Dipchand AI, Everitt MD, et al. Cardiomyopathy in children: Classification and diagnosis: A scientific statement from the American Heart Association. Circulation. 2019; **7**(140):E9-E68. DOI: 10.1161/CIR.0000000000000682

[3] Harmon WG, Sleeper LA, Cuniberti L, Messere J, Colan SD, Orav EJ, et al. Treating children with idiopathic dilated cardiomyopathy (from the pediatric cardiomyopathy registry). The American Journal of Cardiology. 2009;**7**(104):281-286

[4] Cimiotti D, Budde H, Hassoun R, Jaquet K. Genetic restrictive cardiomyopathy: Causes and consequences—An integrative approach. International Journal of Molecular Sciences. 2021;**1**(22):558

[5] Arbustini E, Narula N, Dec GW, Reddy KS, Greenberg B, Kushwaha S, et al. The MOGE(S) classification for a phenotype-genotype nomenclature of cardiomyopathy: Endorsed by the world heart federation. Journal of the American College of Cardiology. 2013;**12**(62): 2046-2072

[6] Towbin JA, Lowe AM, Colan SD, Sleeper LA, Orav EJ, Clunie S, et al. Incidence, causes, and outcomes of dilated cardiomyopathy in children. Journal of the American Medical Association. 2006;**10**(296):1867. DOI: 10.1001/jama.296.15.1867

[7] Kirk R, Dipchand AI, Rosenthal DN, Addonizio L, Burch M, Chrisant M, et al. The International Society for Heart and Lung Transplantation guidelines for the management of pediatric heart failure: Executive summary [corrected]. The journal of heart and lung transplantation: The official publication of the International Society for Heart. Transplantation. 2014;**9**(33):888-909

[8] Ware SM. Genetics of paediatric cardiomyopathies. Current Opinion in Pediatrics. 2017;**10**(29):534-540

[9] Feingold B, Mahle WT, Auerbach S, Clemens P, Domenighetti AA, Jefferies JL, et al. Management of Cardiac Involvement Associated with Neuromuscular Diseases: A scientific statement from the American Heart Association. Circulation. 2017;**9**(136): e200-e231. DOI: 10.1161/CIR.0000000000000526

[10] Bonne G, Barletta MRD, Varnous S, Bécane HM, Hammouda EH, Merlini L, et al. Mutations in the gene encoding Lamin A/C cause autosomal dominant Emery-Dreifuss muscular dystrophy. Nature Genetics. 1999;**3**(21):285-288

[11] El-Hattab AW, Scaglia F. Mitochondrial cardiomyopathies. Frontiers in Cardiovascular Medicine. 2016,**7**(3):25

[12] Kühl U, Schultheiss HP. Myocarditis in children. Heart Failure Clinics. 2010; **10**(6):483-496 viii-ix

[13] Baughman KL. Diagnosis of myocarditis: Death of Dallas criteria. Circulation. 2006;**1**(113):593-595

[14] Wang S, Zhu C. Hypertrophic cardiomyopathy in children. Asian Cardiovascular and Thoracic Annals. 2022;**1**(30):92-97

[15] Lipshultz SE, Cochran TR, Briston DA, Brown SR, Sambatakos PJ,

Miller TL, et al. Pediatric cardiomyopathies: Causes, epidemiology, clinical course, preventive strategies and therapies. Future Cardiology. 2013;**11**(9):817-848. DOI: 10.2217/fca.13.66

[16] Kimura A, Harada H, Park JE, Nishi H, Satoh M, Takahashi M, et al. Mutations in the cardiac troponin I gene associated with hypertrophic cardiomyopathy. Nature Genetics. 1997; **8**(16):379-382

[17] Teekakirikul P, Zhu W, Huang HC, Fung E. Hypertrophic cardiomyopathy: An overview of genetics and management. Biomolecules. 2019;**12**(9): 878

[18] Kaski JP, Syrris P, Esteban MTT, Jenkins S, Pantazis A, Deanfield JE, et al. Prevalence of sarcomere protein gene mutations in preadolescent children with hypertrophic cardiomyopathy. Circulation: Cardiovascular. Genetics. 2009;**10**(2):436-441. DOI: 10.1161/CIRCGENETICS.108.821314

[19] Huang T, Kelly A, Becker SA, Cohen MS, Stanley CA. Hypertrophic cardiomyopathy in neonates with congenital hyperinsulinism. Archives of Disease in Childhood - Fetal and Neonatal Edition. 2013;7(98):F351-F354. DOI: 10.1136/archdischild-2012-302546

[20] Lipshultz SE, Sleeper LA, Towbin JA, Lowe AM, Orav EJ, Cox GF, et al. The incidence of pediatric cardiomyopathy in two regions of the United States. New England Journal of Medicine. 2003;**4**(348):1647-1655. DOI: 10.1056/NEJMoa021715

[21] Nugent AW, Daubeney PEF, Chondros P, Carlin JB, Colan SD, Cheung M, et al. Clinical features and outcomes of childhood hypertrophic cardiomyopathy. Circulation. 2005; **8**(112):1332-1338. DOI: 10.1161/CIRCULATIONAHA.104.530303

[22] Colan SD, Lipshultz SE, Lowe AM, Sleeper LA, Messere J, Cox GF, et al. Epidemiology and cause-specific outcome of hypertrophic cardiomyopathy in children: Findings from the pediatric cardiomyopathy registry. Circulation. 2007;**2**(115): 773-781

[23] Tariq M. Importance of genetic evaluation and testing in pediatric cardiomyopathy. World Journal of Cardiology. 2014;**6**:1156

[24] Talreja DR, Edwards WD, Danielson GK, Schaff HV, Tajik AJ, Tazelaar HD, et al. Constrictive pericarditis in 26 patients with histologically Normal pericardial thickness. Circulation. 2003;**10**(108): 1852-1857. DOI: 10.1161/01.CIR.0000087606.18453.FD

[25] Garcia MJ. Constrictive pericarditis versus restrictive cardiomyopathy? Journal of the American College of Cardiology. 2016;**5**(67):2061-2076

[26] Muchtar E, Blauwet LA, Gertz MA. Restrictive cardiomyopathy. Circulation Research. 2017;**9**(121): 819-837. DOI: 10.1161/CIRCRESAHA.117.310982

[27] Bloomfield GS, Barasa FA, Doll JA, Velazquez EJ. Heart failure in sub-Saharan Africa. Current Cardiology Reviews. 2013;**5**(9):157-173

[28] Webber SA, Lipshultz SE, Sleeper LA, Lu M, Wilkinson JD, Addonizio LJ, et al. Outcomes of restrictive cardiomyopathy in childhood and the influence of phenotype. Circulation. 2012;**9**(126):1237-1244. DOI: 10.1161/CIRCULATIONAHA.112.104638

[29] Ditaranto R, Caponetti AG, Ferrara V, Parisi V, Minnucci M, Chiti C, et al. Pediatric restrictive cardiomyopathies. Frontiers in Pediatrics. 2022;**1**(9):1684

[30] Maron BJ, Towbin JA, Thiene G, Antzelevitch C, Corrado D, Arnett D, et al. Contemporary definitions and classification of the cardiomyopathies. Circulation. 2006;**4**(113):1807-1816. DOI: 10.1161/CIRCULATIONAHA.106.174287

[31] Jensen B, van der Wal AC, Moorman AFM, Christoffels VM. Excessive trabeculations in noncompaction do not have the embryonic identity. International Journal of Cardiology. 2017;**1**(227):325-330

[32] Elliott P, Andersson B, Arbustini E, Bilinska Z, Cecchi F, Charron P, et al. Classification of the cardiomyopathies: A position statement from the european society of cardiology working group on myocardial and pericardial diseases. European Heart Journal. 2007;**12**(29):270-276. DOI: 10.1093/eurheartj/ehm342

[33] Jefferies JL, Wilkinson JD, Sleeper LA, Colan SD, Lu M, Pahl E, et al. Cardiomyopathy phenotypes and outcomes for children with left ventricular myocardial noncompaction: Results from the pediatric cardiomyopathy registry. Journal of Cardiac Failure. 2015;**11**(21):877-884

[34] Kang SL, Forsey J, Dudley D, Steward CG, Tsai-Goodman B. Clinical characteristics and outcomes of cardiomyopathy in Barth syndrome: The UK experience. Pediatric Cardiology. 2016;**1**(37):167-176

[35] Rigaud C, Lebre AS, Touraine R, Beaupain B, Ottolenghi C, Chabli A, et al. Natural history of Barth syndrome: A national cohort study of 22 patients. Orphanet Journal of Rare Diseases. 2013;**5**(8):1-13. DOI: 10.1186/1750-1172-8-70

[36] Beffagna G, Zorzi A, Pilichou K, Marra MP, Rigato I, Corrado D, et al. Arrhythmogenic cardiomyopathy. European Heart Journal. 2020;**12**(41):4457-4462

[37] Corrado D, Basso C, Judge DP. Arrhythmogenic cardiomyopathy. Circulation Research. 2017;**9**(121):784-802. DOI: 10.1161/CIRCRESAHA.117.309345

[38] Tabib A, Loire R, Chalabreysse L, Meyronnet D, Miras A, Malicier D, et al. Circumstances of death and gross and microscopic observations in a series of 200 cases of sudden death associated with Arrhythmogenic right ventricular cardiomyopathy and/or dysplasia. Circulation. 2003;**12**(108):3000-3005. DOI: 10.1161/01.CIR.0000108396.65446.21

[39] Sen-Chowdhry S, Syrris P, Prasad SK, Hughes SE, Merrifield R, Ward D, et al. Left-dominant arrhythmogenic cardiomyopathy: An under-recognized clinical entity. Journal of the American College of Cardiology. 2008;**12**(52):2175-2187

[40] Marcus FI, McKenna WJ, Sherrill D, Basso C, Bauce B, Bluemke DA, et al. Diagnosis of arrhythmogenic right ventricular cardiomyopathy/dysplasia: Proposed modification of the task force criteria. European Heart Journal. 2010;**4**(31):806-814. DOI: 10.1093/eurheartj/ehq025

[41] Etoom Y, Govindapillai S, Hamilton R, Manlhiot C, Yoo SJ, Farhan M, et al. Importance of CMR within the task force criteria for the diagnosis of ARVC in children and adolescents. Journal of the American

College of Cardiology. 2015;**3**(65): 987-995

[42] te Riele ASJM, James CA, Sawant AC, Bhonsale A, Groeneweg JA, Mast TP, et al. Arrhythmogenic right ventricular dysplasia/cardiomyopathy in the pediatric population. JACC: Clinical Electrophysiology. 2015;**12**(1):551-560

[43] Corrado D, Basso C, Thiene G. Is it time to include ion channel diseases among cardiomyopathies? Journal of Electrocardiology. 2005;**10**(38):81-87

[44] Dettmeyer RB, Kandolf R. Cardiomyopathies—Misdiagnosed as sudden infant death syndrome (SIDS). Forensic Science International. 2010; **1**(194):e21-e24

[45] Gopinathannair R, Etheridge SP, Marchlinski FE, Spinale FG, Lakkireddy D, Olshansky B. Arrhythmia-induced cardiomyopathies: Mechanisms, recognition, and management. Journal of the American College of Cardiology. 2015;**10**(66): 1714-1728

[46] Moore JP, Patel PA, Shannon KM, Albers EL, Salerno JC, Stein MA, et al. Predictors of myocardial recovery in pediatric tachycardia-induced cardiomyopathy. Heart Rhythm. 2014; **7**(11):1163-1169

[47] Kim JJ, Friedman RA, Eidem BW, Cannon BC, Arora G, Smith EO, et al. Ventricular function and Long-term pacing in children with congenital complete atrioventricular block. Journal of Cardiovascular Electrophysiology. 2007;**4**(18):373-377. DOI: 10.1111/j.1540-8167.2006.00741.x

[48] Morimoto S. Sarcomeric proteins and inherited cardiomyopathies. Cardiovascular Research. 2007;**12**(77): 659-666. DOI: 10.1093/cvr/cvm084

[49] Watkins H, Ashrafian H, Redwood C. Inherited cardiomyopathies. New England Journal of Medicine. 2011; **4**(364):1643-1656. DOI: 10.1056/NEJMra0902923

[50] Towbin JA. Inherited cardiomyopathies. Circulation Journal. 2014;**78**:2347-2356

[51] Bates MGD, Bourke JP, Giordano C, d'Amati G, Turnbull DM, Taylor RW. Cardiac involvement in mitochondrial DNA disease: Clinical spectrum, diagnosis, and management. European Heart Journal. 2012;**12**(33):3023-3033. DOI: 10.1093/eurheartj/ehs275

[52] Taylor MRG, Slavov D, Ku L, Lenarda AD, Sinagra G, Carniel E, et al. Prevalence of Desmin mutations in dilated cardiomyopathy. Circulation. 2007;**3**(115):1244-1251. DOI: 10.1161/CIRCULATIONAHA.106.646778

[53] Kindel SJ, Miller EM, Gupta R, Cripe LH, Hinton RB, Spicer RL, et al. Pediatric cardiomyopathy: Importance of genetic and metabolic evaluation. Journal of Cardiac Failure. 2012;**5**(18): 396-403

[54] Fiorillo C, Astrea G, Savarese M, Cassandrini D, Brisca G, Trucco F, et al. MYH7-related myopathies: Clinical, histopathological and imaging findings in a cohort of Italian patients. Orphanet Journal of Rare Diseases. 2016;**7**(11): 1-14. DOI: 10.1186/s13023-016-0476-1

[55] Jhang WK, Choi JH, Lee BH, Kim GH, Yoo HW. Cardiac manifestations and associations with gene mutations in patients diagnosed with RASopathies. Pediatric Cardiology. 2016;**12**(37):1539-1547. DOI: 10.1007/s00246-016-1468-6

[56] Kaski JP, Syrris P, Burch M, Tome-Esteban MT, Fenton M, Christiansen M,

et al. Idiopathic restrictive cardiomyopathy in children is caused by mutations in cardiac sarcomere protein genes. Heart. 2008;7(94): 1478-1484. DOI: 10.1136/hrt.2007.134684

[57] Choudhry S, Puri K, Denfield SW. An update on pediatric cardiomyopathy. Current Treatment Options in Cardiovascular Medicine. 2019;**8**(21):36. DOI: 10.1007/s11936-019-0739-y

[58] Salman OF, El-Rayess HM, Khalil CA, Nemer G, Refaat MM. Inherited cardiomyopathies and the role of mutations in non-coding regions of the genome. Frontiers in Cardiovascular Medicine. 2018;**6**(5):77. DOI: 10.3389/fcvm.2018.00077/full

[59] Purevjav E, Towbin JA. The Z-Disk Final Common Pathway in Cardiomyopathies. IntechOpen Book: Cardiomyopathy - Disease of the Heart Muscle; 2021

[60] McNally EM, Golbus JR, Puckelwartz MJ. Genetic mutations and mechanisms in dilated cardiomyopathy. Journal of Clinical Investigation. 2013; **1**(123):19-26

[61] Florczyk-Soluch U, Polak K, Dulak J. The multifaceted view of heart problem in Duchenne muscular dystrophy. Cellular and Molecular Life Sciences: CMLS. 2021;**7**(78):5447-5468

[62] Jui E, Singampalli KL, Shani K, Ning Y, Connell JP, Birla RK, et al. The immune and inflammatory basis of acquired pediatric cardiac disease. Frontiers in Cardiovascular Medicine. 2021;7(8):812. DOI: 10.3389/fcvm.2021.701224/full

[63] Norrish G, Elliott PM. Cardiomyopathies in children: Mitochondrial and storage disease. Progress in Pediatric Cardiology. 2018; **12**(51):16-23

[64] Sabbah HN. Barth syndrome cardiomyopathy: Targeting the mitochondria with elamipretide. Heart Failure Reviews. 2021;**3**(26):237-253. DOI: 10.1007/s10741-020-10031-3

[65] Neuwald AF. Barth syndrome may be due to an acyltransferase deficiency. Current Biology: CB. 1997;**8**(7):R462-R466

[66] Probst S, Oechslin E, Schuler P, Greutmann M, Boyé P, Knirsch W, et al. Sarcomere gene mutations in isolated left ventricular noncompaction cardiomyopathy do not predict clinical phenotype. Circulation: Cardiovascular. Genetics. 2011;**8**(4):367-374. DOI: 10.1161/CIRCGENETICS.110.959270

[67] Miller EM, Hinton RB, Czosek R, Lorts A, Parrott A, Shikany AR, et al. Genetic testing in pediatric left ventricular noncompaction. Circulation: Cardiovascular. Genetics. 2017;**12**:10. DOI: 10.1161/CIRCGENETICS.117.001735

[68] Postma AV, van Engelen K, van de Meerakker J, Rahman T, Probst S, Baars MJH, et al. Mutations in the sarcomere gene ¡i¿MYH7¡/i¿ in Ebstein anomaly. Circulation: Cardiovascular. Genetics. 2011;**2**(4):43-50. DOI: 10.1161/CIRCGENETICS.110.957985

[69] Arndt AK, Schafer S, Drenckhahn JD, Sabeh MK, Plovie E, Caliebe A, et al. Fine mapping of the 1p36 deletion syndrome identifies mutation of PRDM16 as a cause of cardiomyopathy. The American Journal of Human Genetics. 2013;**7**(93):67-77

[70] Klaassen S, Kühnisch J, Schultze-Berndt A, Seidel F. Left ventricular

noncompaction in children: The role of genetics, morphology, and function for outcome. Journal of Cardiovascular Development and Disease. 2022;**6**(9):206

[71] Vatta M, Mohapatra B, Jimenez S, Sanchez X, Faulkner G, Perles Z, et al. Mutations in cypher/ZASPin patients with dilated cardiomyopathy and left ventricular non-compaction. Journal of the American College of Cardiology. 2003;**12**(42):2014-2027

[72] Camozzi D, Capanni C, Cenni V, Mattioli E, Columbaro M, Squarzoni S, et al. Diverse Lamin-dependent mechanisms interact to control chromatin dynamics. Nucleus. 2014; **9**(5):427-440. DOI: 10.4161/nucl.36289

[73] Kulikova O, Brodehl A, Kiseleva A, Myasnikov R, Meshkov A, Stanasiuk C, et al. The Desmin (DES) mutation p. A337P is associated with left-ventricular non-compaction cardiomyopathy. Genes. 2021;**1**(12):121

[74] Khan RS, Pahl E, Dellefave-Castillo L, Rychlik K, Ing A, Yap KL, et al. Genotype and cardiac outcomes in pediatric dilated cardiomyopathy. Journal of the American Heart Association. 2022;**1**(11):22854. DOI: 10.1161/JAHA.121.022854

[75] Hawley MH, Almontashiri N, Biesecker LG, Berger N, Chung WK, Garcia J, et al. An assessment of the role of vinculin loss of function variants in inherited cardiomyopathy. Human Mutation. 2020;**9**(41):1577-1587. DOI: 10.1002/humu.24061

[76] Toro R, Pérez-Serra A, Campuzano O, Moncayo-Arlandi J, Allegue C, Iglesias A, et al. Familial dilated cardiomyopathy caused by a novel frameshift in the BAG3 gene. PLoS One. 2016;**7**(11):e0158730. DOI: 10.1371/journal.pone.0158730

[77] Ware SM, Wilkinson JD, Tariq M, Schubert JA, Sridhar A, Colan SD, et al. Genetic causes of cardiomyopathy in children: First results from the pediatric cardiomyopathy genes study. Journal of the American Heart Association. 2021; **5**(10):17731. DOI: 10.1161/JAHA.120.017731

[78] Wu T, Liang Z, Zhang Z, Liu C, Zhang L, Gu Y, et al. PRDM16 is a compact myocardium-enriched transcription factor required to maintain compact myocardial Cardiomyocyte identity in left ventricle. Circulation. 2022;**2**(145):586-602. DOI: 10.1161/CIRCULATIONAHA.121.056666

[79] Sarohi V, Srivastava S, Basak T. A comprehensive outlook on dilated cardiomyopathy (DCM): State-of-the-art developments with special emphasis on OMICS-based approaches. Journal of Cardiovascular Development and Disease. 2022;**6**(9):174

[80] Pomiato E, Perrone MA, Palmieri R, Gagliardi MG. Pediatric myocarditis: What have we learnt so far? Journal of Cardiovascular Development and Disease. 2022;**5**(9):143

[81] Bowles NE, Ni J, Kearney DL, Pauschinger M, Schultheiss HP, McCarthy R, et al. Detection of viruses in myocardial tissues by polymerase chain reaction. Journal of the American College of Cardiology. 2003;**8**(42): 466-472

[82] Sanna G, Serrau G, Bassareo PP, Neroni P, Fanos V, Marcialis MA. Children's heart and COVID-19: Up-to-date evidence in the form of a systematic review. European Journal of Pediatrics. 2020;**7**(179):1079-1087. DOI: 10.1007/s00431-020-03699-0

[83] Lipshultz SE, Alvarez JA, Scully RE. Anthracycline associated cardiotoxicity

in survivors of childhood cancer. Heart. 2007;**10**(94):525-533. DOI: 10.1136/hrt.2007.136093

[84] Tunuguntla HP, Puri K, Denfield SW. Management of Advanced Heart Failure in children with cancer therapy-related cardiac dysfunction. Children. 2021;**9**(8):872

[85] Monda E, Rubino M, Lioncino M, Fraia FD, Pacileo R, Verrillo F, et al. Hypertrophic cardiomyopathy in children: Pathophysiology, diagnosis, and treatment of non-sarcomeric causes. Frontiers in Pediatrics. 2021;**2**(9):94

[86] Nguyen MB, Mital S, Mertens L, Jeewa A, Friedberg MK, Aguet J, et al. Pediatric hypertrophic cardiomyopathy: Exploring the genotype-phenotype association. Journal of the American Heart Association. 2022;**3**(11):24220. DOI: 10.1161/JAHA.121.024220

[87] Charron P. Danon's disease as a cause of hypertrophic cardiomyopathy: A systematic survey. Heart. 2004;**8**(90): 842-846. DOI: 10.1136/hrt.2003.029504

[88] Muenzer J. Overview of the mucopolysaccharidoses. Rheumatology. 2011;**12**(50):v4-v12

[89] Cohen MI, Atkins MB. Arrhythmogenic right ventricular cardiomyopathy in the pediatric population. Current Opinion in Cardiology. 2022;**1**(37):99-108. DOI: 10.1097/HCO.0000000000000937

[90] McKoy G, Protonotarios N, Crosby A, Tsatsopoulou A, Anastasakis A, Coonar A, et al. Identification of a deletion in plakoglobin in arrhythmogenic right ventricular cardiomyopathy with palmoplantar keratoderma and woolly hair (Naxos disease). The Lancet. 2000; **6**(355):2119-2124

[91] van Lint FHM, Murray B, Tichnell C, Zwart R, Amat N, Deprez RHL, et al. Arrhythmogenic right ventricular cardiomyopathy-associated Desmosomal variants are rarely De novo. Circulation: Genomic and Precision Medicine. 2019; **8**(12):e002467. DOI: 10.1161/CIRCGEN.119.002467

[92] Crocini C, Gotthardt M. Cardiac sarcomere mechanics in health and disease. Biophysical Reviews. 2021; **10**(13):637-652. DOI: 10.1007/s12551-021-00840-7

[93] Westfall MV. Contribution of post-translational phosphorylation to sarcomere-linked cardiomyopathy phenotypes. Frontiers in Physiology. 2016;**9**(7):407

[94] Solaro RJ. Multiplex kinase signaling modifies cardiac function at the level of Sarcomeric proteins. Journal of Biological Chemistry. 2008;**10**(283): 26829-26833

[95] Ladha FA, Thakar K, Pettinato AM, Legere N, Cohn R, Romano R, et al. Identifying cardiac actinin interactomes reveals sarcomere crosstalk with RNA-binding proteins. bioRxiv. 2020;**5**. DOI: 10.1101/2020.03.18.994004. Available from: https://www.biorxiv.org/content/early/2020/05/05/2020.03.18.994004. Eprint: https://www.biorxiv.org/content/early/2020/05/05/2020.03.18.994004.full.pdf

[96] Martin TG, Kirk JA. Under construction: The dynamic assembly, maintenance, and degradation of the cardiac sarcomere. Journal of Molecular and Cellular Cardiology. 2020;**11**(148): 89-102

[97] Kötter S, Krüger M. Protein quality control at the sarcomere: Titin protection and turnover and implications for

disease development. Frontiers in Physiology. 2022;**6**(13):1315

[98] Bers DM. Cardiac excitation–contraction coupling. Nature. 2002; **1**(415):198-205

[99] Schartner V, Laporte J, Böhm J. Abnormal excitation-contraction coupling and calcium homeostasis in myopathies and cardiomyopathies. Journal of Neuromuscular Diseases. 2019;**9**(6):289-305

[100] Nakano SJ, Walker JS, Walker LA, Li X, Du Y, Miyamoto SD, et al. Increased myocyte calcium sensitivity in end-stage pediatric dilated cardiomyopathy. American Journal of Physiology-Heart and Circulatory Physiology. 2019;**12**(317):H1221-H1230. DOI: 10.1152/ajpheart.00409.2019

[101] Ashrafian H, Redwood C, Blair E, Watkins H. Hypertrophic cardiomyopathy:A paradigm for myocardial energy depletion. Trends in Genetics. 2003;**5**(19):263-268

[102] Erickson JR, He BJ, Grumbach IM, Anderson ME. CaMKII in the cardiovascular system: Sensing redox states. Physiological Reviews. 2011; **7**(91):889-915

[103] Hudmon A, Schulman H. Structure-function of the multifunctional Ca2 +/calmodulin-dependent protein kinase II. The Biochemical Journal. 2002; **6**(364):593-611

[104] Cimiotti D, Fujita-Becker S, Möhner D, Smolina N, Budde H, Wies A, et al. Infantile restrictive cardiomyopathy: cTnI-R170G/W impair the interplay of sarcomeric proteins and the integrity of thin filaments. PLoS One. 2020;**3**(15):e0229227. DOI: 10.1371/journal.pone.0229227

[105] Cheng Y, Regnier M. Cardiac troponin structure-function and the influence of hypertrophic cardiomyopathy associated mutations on modulation of contractility. Archives of Biochemistry and Biophysics. 2016; **7**(601):11-21

[106] Solís C, Solaro RJ. Novel insights into sarcomere regulatory systems control of cardiac thin filament activation. Journal of General Physiology. 2021;**7**:153

[107] Bollen IAE, van der Meulen M, de Goede K, Kuster DWD, Dalinghaus M, van der Velden J. Cardiomyocyte hypocontractility and reduced myofibril density in end-stage pediatric cardiomyopathy. Frontiers in Physiology. 2017;**12**(8):1103

[108] Zaklyazminskaya E, Mikhailov V, Bukaeva A, Kotlukova N, Povolotskaya I, Kaimonov V, et al. Low mutation rate in the TTN gene in paediatric patients with dilated cardiomyopathy – A pilot study. Scientific Reports. 2019;**12**(9): 16409

[109] Herman DS, Lam L, Taylor MRG, Wang L, Teekakirikul P, Christodoulou D, et al. Truncations of Titin causing dilated cardiomyopathy. New England Journal of Medicine. 2012; **2**(366):619-628. DOI: 10.1056/nejmoa1110186

[110] LeWinter MM, Granzier H. Cardiac Titin. Circulation. 2010;**5**(121): 2137-2145. DOI: 10.1161/CIRCULATIONAHA.109.860171

[111] Ujfalusi Z, Vera CD, Mijailovich SM, Svicevic M, Yu EC, Kawana M, et al. Dilated cardiomyopathy myosin mutants have reduced force-generating capacity. Journal of Biological Chemistry. 2018; **6**(293):9017-9029

[112] Toepfer CN, Wakimoto H, Garfinkel AC, McDonough B, Liao D, Jiang J, et al. Hypertrophic cardiomyopathy mutations in ¡i¿MYBPC3¡/i¿ dysregulate myosin. Science Translational Medicine. 2019;**1**: 11. DOI: 10.1126/scitranslmed.aat1199

[113] Kensler RW, Shaffer JF, Harris SP. Binding of the N-terminal fragment C0–C2 of cardiac MyBP-C to cardiac F-actin. Journal of Structural Biology. 2011; **4**(174):44-51

[114] Hassoun R, Budde H, Mannherz HG, Lódi M, Fujita-Becker S, Laser KT, et al. De novo missense mutations in TNNC1 and TNNI3 causing severe infantile cardiomyopathy affect myofilament structure and function and are modulated by troponin targeting agents. International Journal of Molecular Sciences. 2021;**9**(22):9625

[115] Napierski NC, Granger K, Langlais PR, Moran HR, Strom J, Touma K, et al. A Novel "Cut and Paste" Method for In Situ Replacement of cMyBP-C Reveals a New Role for cMyBP-C in the Regulation of Contractile Oscillations. Circulation Research. 2020 3;126:737-749. doi: 10.1161/CIRCRESAHA.119.315760.

[116] Harris SP. Making waves: A proposed new role for myosin-binding protein C in regulating oscillatory contractions in vertebrate striated muscle. Journal of General Physiology. 2021;**3**:153

[117] Despond EA, Dawson JF. Classifying cardiac actin mutations associated with hypertrophic cardiomyopathy. Frontiers in Physiology. 2018;**4**(9):405

[118] Ehler E. Actin-associated proteins and cardiomyopathy - the 'unknown' beyond troponin and tropomyosin. Biophysical Reviews. 2018;**8**(10): 1121-1128. DOI: 10.1007/s12551-018-0428-1

[119] Erdmann C, Hassoun R, Schmitt S, Kikuti C, Houdusse A, Mazur AJ, et al. Integration of cardiac actin mutants causing hypertrophic (p.A295S) and dilated cardiomyopathy (p.R312H and p. E361G) into cellular structures. Antioxidants. 2021;**7**(10):1082

[120] Budde H, Hassoun R, Tangos M, Zhazykbayeva S, Herwig M, Varatnitskaya M, et al. The interplay between s-glutathionylation and phosphorylation of cardiac troponin i and myosin binding protein c in end-stage human failing hearts. Antioxidants. 2021;**7**(10):1134

[121] Rouyère C, Serrano T, Frémont S, Echard A. Oxidation and reduction of actin: Origin, impact in vitro and functional consequences in vivo. European Journal of Cell Biology. 2022; **6**(101):151249

[122] Loescher CM, Breitkreuz M, Li Y, Nickel A, Unger A, Dietl A, et al. Regulation of titin-based cardiac stiffness by unfolded domain oxidation (UnDOx). Proceedings of the National Academy of Sciences of the United States of America. 2020;**9**(117): 24545-24556. DOI: 10.1073/pnas.2004900117

[123] Li X, Zhao D, Guo Z, Li T, Qili M, Xu B, et al. Overexpression of SerpinE2/protease nexin-1 contribute to pathological cardiac fibrosis via increasing collagen deposition. Scientific Reports. 2016;**12**(6):37635

[124] Schirone L, Forte M, Palmerio S, Yee D, Nocella C, Angelini F, et al. A review of the molecular mechanisms underlying the development and progression of cardiac remodeling.

Oxidative Medicine and Cellular Longevity. 2017;**2017**:1-16

[125] Tian J, An X, Niu L. Myocardial fibrosis in congenital and pediatric heart disease. Experimental and Therapeutic Medicine. 2017;**5**(13):1660-1664. DOI: 10.3892/etm.2017.4224

[126] Patel MD, Mohan J, Schneider C, Bajpai G, Purevjav E, Canter CE, et al. Pediatric and adult dilated cardiomyopathy represent distinct pathological entities. JCI Insight. 2017;7:2

[127] Recla S, Schmidt D, Logeswaran T, Esmaeili A, Schranz D. Pediatric heart failure therapy: Why β1-receptor blocker, tissue ACE-I and mineralocorticoid-receptor-blocker? Translational Pediatrics. 2019;**4**(8): 127-127

[128] Cicenia M, Drago F. Arrhythmogenic cardiomyopathy: Diagnosis, evolution, risk stratification and pediatric population—Where are we? Journal of Cardiovascular Development and Disease. 2022;**3**(9):98

[129] Austin KM, Trembley MA, Chandler SF, Sanders SP, Saffitz JE, Abrams DJ, et al. Molecular mechanisms of arrhythmogenic cardiomyopathy. Nature Reviews Cardiology. 2019;**9**(16): 519-537

[130] Li D, Liu Y, Maruyama M, Zhu W, Chen H, Zhang W, et al. Restrictive loss of plakoglobin in cardiomyocytes leads to arrhythmogenic cardiomyopathy. Human Molecular Genetics. 2011;**12**(20): 4582-4596. DOI: 10.1093/hmg/ddr392

[131] Ward M, Iskratsch T. Mix and (mis-)match – The mechanosensing machinery in the changing environment of the developing, healthy adult and diseased heart. Biochimica et Biophysica Acta (BBA) - molecular Cell Research. 2020:**3**;1867:118436

[132] Wu Y, Cazorla O, Labeit D, Labeit S, Granzier H. Changes in Titin and collagen underlie diastolic stiffness diversity of cardiac muscle. Journal of Molecular and Cellular Cardiology. 2000;**12**(32):2151-2161

[133] Hamdani N, Herwig M, Linke WA. Tampering with springs: Phosphorylation of titin affecting the mechanical function of cardiomyocytes. Biophysical Reviews. 2017;**6**(9):225-237. DOI: 10.1007/s12551-017-0263-9

[134] Hamdani N, Paulus WJ. Myocardial Titin and collagen in cardiac diastolic dysfunction. Circulation. 2013;7(128): 5-8. DOI: 10.1161/CIRCULATIONAHA. 113.003437

[135] Bhupathi SS, Chalasani S, Rokey R. Stiff heart syndrome. Clinical Medicine & Research. 2011;**6**(9):92-99. DOI: 10.3121/cmr.2010.899

[136] Chung CS, Hutchinson KR, Methawasin M, Saripalli C, Smith JE, Hidalgo CG, et al. Shortening of the elastic tandem immunoglobulin segment of Titin leads to diastolic dysfunction. Circulation. 2013;7(128):19-28. DOI: 10.1161/ CIRCULATIONAHA.112.001268

[137] Garcia-Canadilla P, Cook AC, Mohun TJ, Oji O, Schlossarek S, Carrier L, et al. Myoarchitectural disarray of hypertrophic cardiomyopathy begins pre-birth. Journal of Anatomy. 2019;**11**(235): 962-976. DOI: 10.1111/joa.13058

[138] Kraft T, Montag J. Altered force generation and cell-to-cell contractile imbalance in hypertrophic cardiomyopathy. Pflügers Archiv - European Journal of Physiology. 2019;

5(471):719-733. DOI: 10.1007/s00424-019-02260-9

[139] Dirkx E, da Costa Martins PA, Windt LJD. Regulation of fetal gene expression in heart failure. Biochimica et Biophysica Acta (BBA) - Molecular Basis of Disease. 1832;**2013**(12):2414-2424

[140] Wang K, Lin ZQ, Long B, Li JH, Zhou J, Li PF. Cardiac hypertrophy is positively regulated by MicroRNA miR-23a. Journal of Biological Chemistry. 2012;**1**(287):589-599

[141] Lin Z, Murtaza I, Wang K, Jiao J, Gao J, Li PF. miR-23a functions downstream of NFATc3 to regulate cardiac hypertrophy. Proceedings of the National Academy of Sciences. 2009; **7**(106):12103-12108. DOI: 10.1073/pnas.0811371106

[142] Stauffer BL, Russell G, Nunley K, Miyamoto SD, Sucharov CC. miRNA expression in pediatric failing human heart. Journal of Molecular and Cellular Cardiology. 2013;**4**(57):43-46

[143] Yu J, Zeng C, Wang Y. Epigenetics in dilated cardiomyopathy. Current Opinion in Cardiology. 2019;**5**(34):260-269

[144] Marino BS, Lipkin PH, Newburger JW, Peacock G, Gerdes M, Gaynor JW, et al. Neurodevelopmental outcomes in children with congenital heart disease: Evaluation and management. Circulation. 2012;**8**(126): 1143-1172. DOI: 10.1161/CIR.0b013e318265ee8a

[145] Burstein DS, Shamszad P, Dai D, Almond CS, Price JF, Lin KY, et al. Significant mortality, morbidity and resource utilization associated with advanced heart failure in congenital heart disease in children and young adults. American Heart Journal. 2019; **3**(209):9-19

[146] Dipchand AI. Current state of pediatric cardiac transplantation. Annals of Cardiothoracic Surgery. 2018;**1**(7):31-55

[147] Bagnall RD, Weintraub RG, Ingles J, Duflou J, Yeates L, Lam L, et al. A prospective study of sudden cardiac death among children and young adults. New England Journal of Medicine. 2016; **6**(374):2441-2452. DOI: 10.1056/NEJMoa1510687

[148] Jortveit J, Eskedal L, Hirth A, Fomina T, Døhlen G, Hagemo P, et al. Sudden unexpected death in children with congenital heart defects. European Heart Journal. 2016;**2**(37):621-626. DOI: 10.1093/eurheartj/ehv478

[149] Imanaka-Yoshida K. Inflammation in myocardial disease: From myocarditis to dilated cardiomyopathy. Pathology International. 2020;**1**(70):1-11. DOI: 10.1111/pin.12868

[150] Towbin JA, Ballweg J, Johnson J. Left Ventricular Noncompaction Cardiomyopathy. In: Jefferies JL, Chang AC, Rossano JW, Shaddy RE, Towbin JA, editors. Heart Failure in the Child and Young Adult. Boston: Academic Press: Elsevier; 2018. pp. 269-290. Available from: https://www.sciencedirect.com/science/article/pii/B978012802393800020X. ISBN: 978-0-12-802393-8. DOI: 10.1016/B978-0-12-802393-8.00020-X

[151] Leya FS, Arab D, Joyal D, Shioura KM, Lewis BE, Steen LH, et al. The efficacy of brain natriuretic peptide levels in differentiating constrictive pericarditis from restrictive cardiomyopathy. Journal of the American College of Cardiology. 2005; **6**(45):1900-1902

[152] Woulfe KC, Siomos AK, Nguyen H, SooHoo M, Galambos C, Stauffer BL, et al. Fibrosis and fibrotic gene expression in pediatric and adult patients

with idiopathic dilated cardiomyopathy. Journal of Cardiac Failure. 2017;**4**(23): 314-324

[153] Wittnich C, Belanger MP, Bandali KS. Newborn hearts are at greater 'metabolic risk' during global ischemia – Advantages of continuous coronary washout. Canadian Journal of Cardiology. 2007;**3**(23):195-200

[154] Lai L, Leone TC, Keller MP, Martin OJ, Broman AT, Nigro J, et al. Energy metabolic reprogramming in the hypertrophied and early stage failing heart. Circulation. Heart Failure. 2014; **11**(7):1022-1031. DOI: 10.1161/CIRCHEARTFAILURE.114.001469

[155] Miyamoto SD, Stauffer BL, Nakano S, Sobus R, Nunley K, Nelson P, et al. Beta-adrenergic adaptation in paediatric idiopathic dilated cardiomyopathy. European Heart Journal. 2014;**1**(35):33-41. DOI: 10.1093/eurheartj/ehs229

[156] Pan B, Hu D, Sun H, Lv T, Xu W, Tian J. Pediatric diastolic heart failure: Clinical features description of 421 cases. Frontiers in Pediatrics. 2022; **5**(10):656

[157] Sadat-Ebrahimi SR, Aslanabadi N. Role of MicroRNAs in diagnosis, prognosis, and treatment of acute heart failure: Ambassadors from intracellular zone. Galen Medical Journal. 2020;**6**(9): e1818

[158] Miyamoto SD, Karimpour-Fard A, Peterson V, Auerbach SR, Stenmark KR, Stauffer BL, et al. Circulating microRNA as a biomarker for recovery in pediatric dilated cardiomyopathy. The Journal of Heart and Lung Transplantation. 2015; **5**(34):724-733

[159] Jiao M, You HZ, Yang XY, Yuan H, Li YL, Liu WX, et al. Circulating microRNA signature for the diagnosis of childhood dilated cardiomyopathy. Scientific Reports. 2018;**12**(8):724

[160] Oh JH, Kim GB, Seok H. Implication of microRNA as a potential biomarker of myocarditis. Clinical and Experimental Pediatrics. 2022;**5**(65): 230-238

[161] Bales ND, Johnson NM, Judge DP, Murphy AM. Comprehensive versus targeted genetic testing in children with hypertrophic cardiomyopathy. Pediatric Cardiology. 2016;**6**(37):845-851. DOI: 10.1007/s00246-016-1358-y

[162] Lee TM, Hsu DT, Kantor P, Towbin JA, Ware SM, Colan SD, et al. Pediatric cardiomyopathies. Circulation Research. 2017;**9**(121):855-873. DOI: 10.1161/CIRCRESAHA.116.309386

[163] Al-Hassnan ZN, Almesned A, Tulbah S, Alakhfash A, Alhadeq F, Alruwaili N, et al. Categorized genetic analysis in childhood-onset cardiomyopathy. Circulation: Genomic and Precision Medicine. 2020;**10**(13): 504-514. DOI: 10.1161/CIRCGEN.120.002969

[164] Haanschoten DM, Adiyaman A, 't Hart NA, Jager PL, Elvan A. Value of 3D mapping-guided endomyocardial biopsy in cardiac sarcoidosis. European Journal of Clinical Investigation. 2021;**4**(51): e13497. DOI: 10.1111/eci.13497

[165] Esposito A, Palmisano A, Antunes S, Maccabelli G, Colantoni C, Rancoita PMV, et al. Cardiac CT with delayed enhancement in the characterization of ventricular tachycardia structural substrate. JACC: Cardiovascular Imaging. 2016;7(9):822-832

[166] Zeppenfeld K. Ventricular Tachycardia Ablation in Nonischemic

Cardiomyopathy. JACC: Clinical Electrophysiology. 2018 9;4:1123-1140.

[167] Kim KH, Park JC, Yoon HJ, Yoon NS, Hong YJ, Park HW, et al. Usefulness of aortic strain analysis by velocity vector imaging as a new echocardiographic measure of arterial stiffness. Journal of the American Society of Echocardiography. 2009; **12**(22):1382-1388

[168] Lang RM, Bierig M, Devereux RB, Flachskampf FA, Foster E, Pellikka PA, et al. Recommendations for chamber quantification: A report from the American Society of Echocardiography's guidelines and standards committee and the chamber quantification writing group, developed in conjunction with the European Association of Echocardiography, a branch of the European Society of Cardiology. Journal of the American Society of Echocardiography. 2005;**12**(18): 1440-1463

[169] Lee CK, Margossian R, Sleeper LA, Canter CE, Chen S, Tani LY, et al. Variability of M-mode versus two-dimensional echocardiography measurements in children with dilated cardiomyopathy. Pediatric Cardiology. 2014;**4**(35):658-667. DOI: 10.1007/s00246-013-0835-9

[170] Pettersen MD, Du W, Skeens ME, Humes RA. Regression equations for calculation of Z scores of cardiac structures in a large cohort of healthy infants, children, and adolescents: An echocardiographic study. Journal of the American Society of Echocardiography. 2008;**8**(21):922-934

[171] Khoury PR, Mitsnefes M, Daniels SR, Kimball TR. Age-specific reference intervals for indexed left ventricular mass in children. Journal of the American Society of Echocardiography. 2009;**6**(22):709-714

[172] Dragulescu A, Mertens L, Friedberg MK. Interpretation of left ventricular diastolic dysfunction in children with cardiomyopathy by echocardiography: Problems and limitations. Circulation Cardiovascular Imaging. 2013;**3**(6):254-261

[173] Ezon DS, Maskatia SA, Sexson-Tejtel K, Dreyer WJ, Jeewa A, Denfield SW. Tissue Doppler imaging measures correlate poorly with left ventricular filling pressures in pediatric cardiomyopathy. Congenital Heart Disease. 2015;**9**(10):E203-E209. DOI: 10.1111/chd.12267

[174] Mozaffarian D, Benjamin EJ, Go AS, Arnett DK, Blaha MJ, Cushman M, et al. Heart disease and stroke statistics—2016 update. Circulation. 2016;**1**(133):e38-e48. DOI: 10.1161/CIR.0000000000000350

[175] Buechel EV, Kaiser T, Jackson C, Schmitz A, Kellenberger CJ. Normal right- and left ventricular volumes and myocardial mass in children measured by steady state free precession cardiovascular magnetic resonance. Journal of Cardiovascular Magnetic Resonance. 2009;**12**(11):19. DOI: 10.1186/1532-429X-11-19

[176] Ziółkowska L, Petryka J, Boruc A, Kawalec W. Comparison of echocardiography with tissue Doppler imaging and magnetic resonance imaging with delayed enhancement in the assessment of children with hypertrophic cardiomyopathy. Archives of Medical Science. 2017;**2**:328-336. DOI: 10.5114/aoms.2016.60404

[177] Ryan TD, Madueme PC, Jefferies JL, Michelfelder EC, Towbin JA, Woo JG, et al. Utility of echocardiography in the

assessment of left ventricular diastolic function and restrictive physiology in children and young adults with restrictive cardiomyopathy: A comparative echocardiography-catheterization study. Pediatric Cardiology. 2017;**2**(38):381-389. DOI: 10.1007/s00246-016-1526-0

[178] Masarone D, Valente F, Rubino M, Vastarella R, Gravino R, Rea A, et al. Pediatric heart failure: A practical guide to diagnosis and management. Pediatrics & Neonatology. 2017;**8**(58):303-312

[179] Colan SD. Pediatric Cardiomyopathy - NORD (National Organization for Rare Disorders); 2019. Available from: https://rarediseases.org/rare-diseases/pediatric-cardiomyopathy/?filter=complete-report [Accessed: 24-11-2022]

[180] Loss KL, Shaddy RE, Kantor PF. Recent and upcoming drug therapies for pediatric heart failure. Frontiers in Pediatrics. 2021;**11**(9):1192

[181] Das BB, Moskowitz WB, Butler J. Current and future drug and device therapies for pediatric heart failure patients: Potential lessons from adult trials. Children. 2021;**4**(8):322

[182] Halliday B. Examining the Effects of Mitochondrial Oxidative Stress in DCM - Full Text View. 2022. Available from: ClinicalTrials.gov.

[183] Renno M. Oral Ifetroban in Subjects with Duchenne Muscular Dystrophy - Full Text View. 2017. Available from: ClinicalTrials.gov.

[184] Rossano J, Taylor M, Greenberg B. Gene Therapy for Male Patients with Danon Disease (DD) Using RP-A501; AAV9.LAMP2B - Full Text View. 2019. Available from: ClinicalTrials.gov.

[185] Altarabsheh SE, Dearani JA, Burkhart HM, Schaff HV, Deo SV, Eidem BW, et al. Outcome of septal Myectomy for obstructive hypertrophic cardiomyopathy in children and young adults. The Annals of Thoracic Surgery. 2013;**2**(95): 663-669

[186] Sreeram N, Emmel M, Giovanni JVD. Percutaneous radiofrequency septal reduction for hypertrophic obstructive cardiomyopathy in children. Journal of the American College of Cardiology. 2011; **12**(58):2501-2510

[187] Emmel M, Sreeram N, deGiovanni JV, Brockmeier K. Radiofrequency catheter septal ablation for hypertrophic obstructive cardiomyopathy in childhood. Zeitschrift für Kardiologie. 2005;**10**(94):699-703. DOI: 10.1007/s00392-005-0282-6

[188] Liebregts M, Steggerda RC, Vriesendorp PA, van Velzen H, Schinkel AFL, Willems R, et al. Long-term outcome of alcohol septal ablation for obstructive hypertrophic cardiomyopathy in the young and the elderly. JACC: Cardiovascular Interventions. 2016;**3**(9):463-469

[189] Aghdami N. Intracoronary Transplantation of Bone Marrow Derived Mononuclear Cells in Pediatric Cardiomyopathy - Full Text View. 2017. Available from: Clinical Trials.gov.

[190] Srour S. New Horizons for the Treatment of Cardiomyopathy in Children - Full Text View. 2021. Available from: ClinicalTrials.gov.

[191] Maron BJ, Ommen SR, Semsarian C, Spirito P, Olivotto I, Maron MS. Hypertrophic cardiomyopathy. Journal of the American College of Cardiology. 2014; **7**(64):83-99

[192] Jefferies JL, Towbin JA. Dilated cardiomyopathy. The Lancet. 2010; **2**(375):752-762

[193] Weintraub RG, Semsarian C, Macdonald P. Dilated cardiomyopathy. The Lancet. 2017;**7**(390):400-414

[194] Deshpande S, Sparks JD, Alsoufi B. Pediatric heart transplantation: Year in review 2020. The Journal of Thoracic and Cardiovascular Surgery. 2021; **8**(162):418-421

[195] Giafaglione J, Morrison A, Gowda C, Gajarski R, Nandi D. Pediatric donor heart allocation in the United States, 2006-2017: Current patterns and potential for improvement. Pediatric Transplantation. 2020;**9**(24):e13743. DOI: 10.1111/petr.13743

[196] Khan AM, Green RS, Lytrivi ID, Sahulee R. Donor predictors of allograft utilization for pediatric heart transplantation. Transplant International. 2016;**12**(29):1269-1275. DOI: 10.1111/tri.12835

[197] Padilla LA, Rhodes L, Sorabella RA, Hurst DJ, Cleveland DC, Dabal RJ, et al. Attitudes toward xenotransplantation: A survey of parents and pediatric cardiac providers. Pediatric Transplantation. 2021;**3**:25. DOI: 10.1111/petr.13851

Section 6

Miscellaneous Cardiomyopathy

Chapter 7

Takotsubo Cardiomyopathy

Shivangi Patel, Mario Madruga and Neelima Katukuri

Abstract

Takotsubo cardiomyopathy Takotsubo cardiomyopathy occurs worldwide. The condition is thought to be responsible for 2% of all acute coronary syndromes' cases presenting to hospitals. Although it has generally been considered a self-limiting disease, spontaneously resolving over the course of days to weeks, a subset of patients may present with symptoms arising from its complications, e.g., heart failure, pulmonary oedema, stroke, cardiogenic shock, or cardiac arrest. It occurs more commonly in postmenopausal women.

Keywords: cardiomyopathy, cardiac imaging, cardiac MRI, Takotsubo, familial cardiomyopathy

1. Introduction

Takotsubo syndrome (TTS), also known as stress cardiomyopathy or 'broken heart syndrome', has been described for the first time in Japan in 1990. It is an acute cardiac condition characterized by systolic and diastolic left ventricular (LV) dysfunction with apical hypokinesis that is typically transient. Approximately 90% of patients are postmenopausal women with a mean presentation between 62 and 75 years of age. It has been described in medical literature across the globe, spanning virtually every major ethnic group. Historic evidence suggests that patients with TTS have less traditional risk factors for coronary artery disease [1].

2. Pathophysiology

Despite increasing diagnosis and awareness of TTS, the exact mechanism remains unknown. The most accepted etiologic theory of Takotsubo syndrome is one of excess catecholaminergic-induced myocardial stunning. The association between stressful emotional states and development of TTS has been well-documented. Studies have measured the plasma concentration of catecholamines (dopamine, epinephrine, norepinephrine) present in patients with TTS, finding them higher (two to threefold) than both the general population and patients with ACS [2]. The mechanism by which supraphysiologic catecholaminergic state causes myocardial injury is a continued debate. Multivessel coronary artery spasm, cardiac microvascular dysfunction, and direct cardiomyocyte injury are proposed mechanisms [3].

Direct myocyte injury is thought to occur via beta-2 inhibitory effects of G-protein [guanine nucleotide-binding protein] coupled receptors resulting in negative inotropy with resultant LV dysfunction. Normal circulating levels of catecholamines bind to Beta-2 adrenergic receptors of ventricular cardiomyocytes resulting in stimulation of Gs protein-adenylyl cyclase-protein kinase A pathway and thus a positive inotropic effect. The inhibitory effect happens with *supra*physiologic levels of catecholamines, though to take place to protect myocytes from apoptosis occurring with strong stimulation of Gs, a phenomenon known as 'stimulus trafficking' [4].

The gender disparity in disease presentation remains a point of ambiguity. Men have higher basal levels of sympathetic hormone than women, they produce higher amounts of catecholamines when presented with stressors and have a higher degree of catecholamine-mediated vasoconstriction. Yet, women seem to have a higher susceptibility to adrenergic myocardial stunning as exampled in LV dysfunction after subarachnoid hemorrhage. The cardioprotective effects of estrogen including protection against atherosclerosis and endothelial dysfunction is well known. There is the additional proposed benefit that estrogen downregulates beta-adrenergic receptors. Studies performed on ovariectomized rats subjected to stress demonstrated a higher deleterious cardiovascular response compared to groups provided with estrogen supplementation [5]. The overwhelming majority of patients with TTS are post-menopausal, further correlating that estrogen deficiency may predispose women to developing TTS. This may be the rationale behind the higher mortality of TTS seen in men. Men with TTS have an approximate mortality rate of 4.4%, comparable to the mortality rate of men with ST elevation myocardial infarction treated with primary percutaneous coronary intervention [6].

A hallmark feature of TTS is underlying inflammatory injury and edema of myocardial cells. In TTS, edema is generally diffuse and transmural in nature but worsened in areas with regional wall motion abnormalities and not limited to a vascular territory. Endomyocardial biopsies show mononuclear infiltrates, contraction-band necrosis, and myocardial inflammation-mediated edema.

Recent studies have demonstrated that elevated neutrophil/lymphocyte ratios, inflammatory markers, and even elevated neoplastic markers as a surrogate for systemic inflammation are independent risk factors for increased in-hospital complications, long-term adverse events, and death [7].

3. Diagnosis

The Mayo Clinic diagnostic criteria for stress cardiomyopathy must include all four of the following for diagnosis:

1. Transient LV systolic dysfunction with wall motion abnormalities extending beyond a single epicardial coronary artery distribution. (Excepts include rare focal and global subtypes).

2. Absence of obstructive coronary artery disease (CAD) or angiographic evidence of acute plaque rupture. If CAD is found, diagnosis of stress cardiomyopathy can still be made if the wall motion abnormalities are not in the distribution of the coronary artery.

3. New electrocardiographic abnormalities (ST elevation, ST depression, T wave inversions) or moderate elevation in cardiac troponin.

4. Absence of pheochromocytoma or myocarditis [8]

Presentation often mimics acute coronary syndrome (ACS): chest pain, ST elevations on electrocardiography, and elevated cardiac biomarkers. Diagnostic coronary angiography is typically performed revealing normal or nonobstructive coronary artery disease in the vast majority of patients. It is estimated that approximately 2% of all patients undergoing emergent coronary angiography for presumed ACS have TTS [3]. Though ACS and TTS may share similar features, theorized pathogenesis, management, and prognosis of TTS is unique.

4. Diagnostic modalities

Traditionally, transthoracic echocardiography is one of the first non-invasive diagnostic tools utilized in patients with suspected Takotsubo syndrome. Transthoracic echocardiography depicts LV geometry, LV function and anatomic variants. In recent years, assessing global longitudinal strain (GLS) using speckle-tracking echocardiography, has become a sensitive marker for myocardial dysfunction with increasing prognostic utility (**Figure 1**). GLS is a simple parameter that expresses longitudinal shortening as a percentage (change in length as a proportion to baseline length) [7]. Not only does strain pattern help differentiate acute TTS from ACS, but it can help identify persistent LV dysfunction even after recovery of ejection fraction (EF) [9]. There is an increasing population of patients that have continued abnormal GLS even after complete LVEF recovery. The clinical implications of persistently abnormal GLS with association to recurrence of TTS has yet to be investigated.

Cardiac Magnetic Resonance (CMR) has become an increasingly utilized imaging tool in patients with TTS. Like echocardiography, CMR can visualize wall motion abnormalities and identify areas of LV dysfunction. More significantly, CMR can identify the presence of reversible (edema) and irreversible myocardial damage (scarring). CMR can also identify potential complications of TTS, such as LV outflow tract (LVOT) obstruction, valve disease, pericardial effusion, and LV thrombus. In TTS, the hallmark features of inflammatory injury and edema are visualized on CMR as signal hyperintensity in the T2- weighted sequences. Not only can the extent of edema

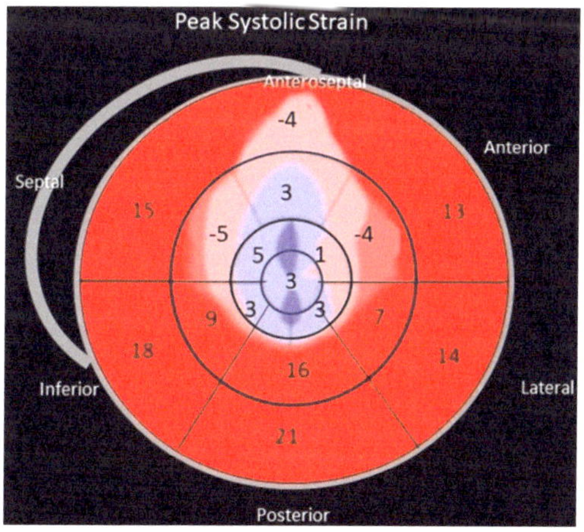

Figure 1.
Global longitudinal strain plot on transthoracic echocardiography with 'evil eye' pattern seen in Takotsubo syndrome.

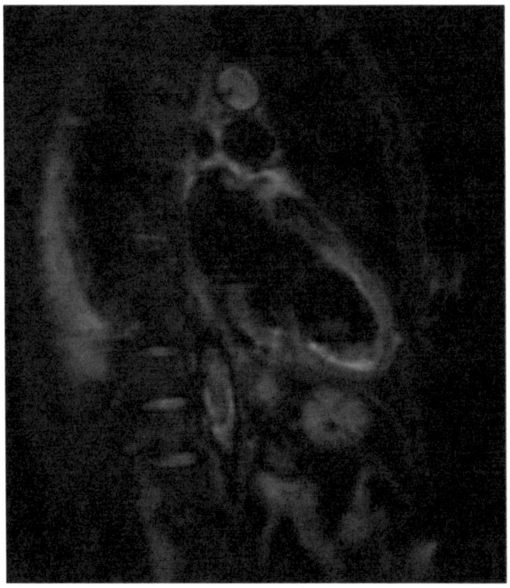

Figure 2.
Late gadolinium enhancement of apical and lateral wall segments in apical-type Takotsubo syndrome.

be quantified with more diagnostic accuracy, CMR has the capability to identify potential areas of irreversibility. To assess for the presence/absence of scarring tissue, short and long axis acquisitions are performed after contrast injection using an inversion-recovery gradient echo sequence to help identify late gadolinium enhancement (LGE) (**Figure 2**). Though not common in TTS, LGE can identify areas of contraction-band necrosis often seen in endomyocardial biopsies in TTS patients [10].

Cardiac imaging advances not only assist in monitoring recovery and identifying persistent injury; they can also aid in elucidating pathogenesis of Takotsubo syndrome. Microcirculatory dysfunction as a pathologic mechanism of TTS has been previously underrecognized due to lack of imaging modalities. New studies involving single-photon emission computed tomography perfusion have shown a decrease in tracer uptake during the acute phase of TTS and a return to normal at follow-up, suggesting a role for coronary microvascular dysfunction as a trigger of myocardial ischemia in this condition. Additionally, perfusion CMR has corroborated disruptions in coronary microcirculation in the absence of obstructive epicardial disease in patients with TTS.

5. Treatment

The treatment for Takotsubo syndrome is largely empiric and supportive. Angiotensin-converting enzyme inhibitors (ACE-i), angiotensin II receptor blockers (ARB), and/or beta-blockers are often utilized in stable patients. Beta-blockade initiated in the acute phase of TTS has been associated with a statistically significant higher long-term survival with a greater benefit seen in hypertensive patients or those who developed cardiogenic shock [11]. Neither beta-blockers nor ACE-i/ARB were shown to reduce the recurrence of TTS [12]. There exists a plethora of evidence regarding optimized medical treatment for patients with reduced LV function due to other etiologies. Again, few data exist regarding optimum regimen for patients with TTS.

6. Outcomes

Historically, Takotsubo syndrome was often thought to portend a more benign course with favorable outcomes compared to ACS. More recent, larger-scale analyses are revealing that up to 50% of patients suffer from acute complications and acute mortality rates similar to ACS. In most patients, recovery of LV function can be seen within 1–6 months. The risk factors that influence rate of LV recovery process are unknown. Concerningly, factors that lead to delayed resolution of wall motion abnormalities also remain unknown. The nebulous nature of this disease course has significant clinical implications. Patients without early LV recovery have higher prevalence of in-hospital complications and higher mortality and should be monitored closely. Patients with persistent wall motion abnormalities also require close monitoring with repeat cardiac imaging. Recurrence rates of TTS average between 2 and 10% [12]. A variable TTS pattern at recurrence is common in up to 20% of recurrence cases (see **Figure 3** for variant patterns of TTS). Despite these findings, few data exist regarding treatment, long-term prognosis, and risk stratification.

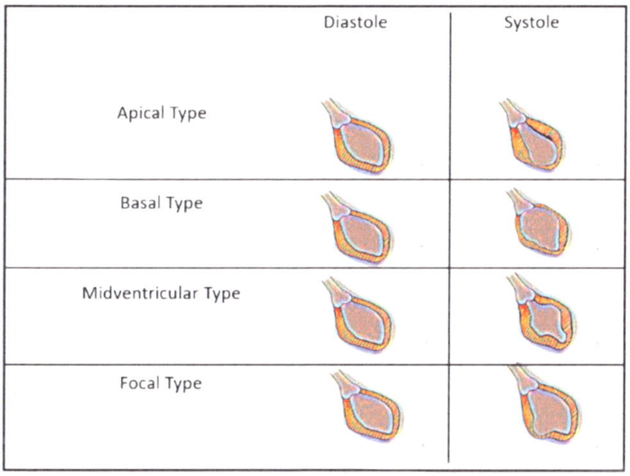

Figure 3.
Variants of Takotsubo cardiomyopathy.

7. Future implications

Though Takotsubo syndrome remains an enigma in many aspects, new capabilities of cardiac imaging are emerging that can assist with clarifying pathogenesis, tracking injury patterns, and preventing recurrence. With the utilization of global longitudinal strain on transthoracic echocardiography, persistent LV dysfunction can be detected even when ejection fraction has recovered, a feature that can potentially be used to identify which patients are at a higher risk of recurrence. CMR affords clinicians the opportunity to identify pathogenic features not previously recognized as large contributors to TTS etiology, ultimately enhancing treatment options. Further studies are being conducted investigating both genetic predispositions and biomarkers to better assess disease course. It is our hope that with each new discovery, we become closer to deciphering the complexities of Takotsubo syndrome.

Conflict of interest

The authors declare no conflict of interest.

Abbreviations

TTS	Takotsubo syndrome
LV	left ventricular
CAD	coronary artery disease
ACS	acute coronary syndrome
ACE-i	Angiotensin-converting enzyme inhibitors
ARB	angiotensin II receptor blockers

Author details

Shivangi Patel[1], Mario Madruga[1] and Neelima Katukuri[2*]

1 Orlando Heart and Vascular Institute, USA

2 Orlando VA Medical Center, USA

*Address all correspondence to: pneelu@gmail.com

References

[1] Khalid N et al. Takotsubo cardiomyopathy and myopericarditis: Unraveling the inflammatory hypothesis. International Journal of Cardiology. 2015;**196**(1):168-169. DOI: 10.1016/j.ijcard.2015.05.175

[2] Pelliccia F et al. Pathophysiology of Takotsubo syndrome. Circulation. 2017;**135**(24):2426-2441. DOI: 10.1161/circulationaha.116.027121

[3] Merchant EE et al. Takotsubo cardiomyopathy: A case series and review of the literature. Western Journal of Emergency Medicine. 2008;**9**(2):104

[4] Ueyama T et al. Chronic Estrogen supplementation following Ovariectomy improves the emotional stress-induced cardiovascular responses by indirect action on the nervous system and by direct action on the heart. Circulation Journal. 2007;**71**(4):565-573. Available from: www.jstage.jst.go.jp/article/circj/71/4/71_4_565/_article. DOI: 10.1253/circj.71.565

[5] Pascual I et al. Observed and expected survival in men and women after suffering a STEMI. Journal of Clinical Medicine. 2020. Available from: www.ncbi.nlm.nih.gov/pmc/articles/PMC7230566/;**9**(4). DOI: 10.3390/jcm9041174

[6] Wittstein IS et al. Neurohumoral features of myocardial stunning due to sudden emotional stress. New England Journal of Medicine. 2005;**352**(6):539-548. DOI: 10.1056/nejmoa043046

[7] Komamura K. Takotsubo cardiomyopathy: Pathophysiology, diagnosis and treatment. World Journal of Cardiology. 2014;**6**(7):602. DOI: 10.4330/wjc.v6.i7.602

[8] Scantlebury DC, Prasad A. Diagnosis of Takotsubo cardiomyopathy. Circulation Journal. 2014;**78**(9):2129-2139. DOI: 10.1253/circj.cj-14-0859

[9] Santoro F et al. Prognostic role of neoplastic markers in Takotsubo syndrome. Scientific Reports. 2021;**11**(1). DOI: 10.1038/s41598-021-95990-9

[10] Silverio A et al. Beta-blockers are associated with better long-term survival in patients with Takotsubo syndrome. Heart. 2022;**108**(17):1369-1376. DOI: 10.1136/heartjnl-2021-320543

[11] Santoro F et al. Lack of efficacy of drug therapy in preventing Takotsubo cardiomyopathy recurrence: A meta-analysis. Clinical Cardiology. 2014;**37**(7):434-439. DOI: 10.1002/clc.22280

[12] Angelini P. Recurrent Takotsubo cardiomyopathy: An opportunity to clarify causation and prognosis. Texas Heart Institute Journal. 2018;**45**(4):252-253. DOI: 10.14503/thij-18-6778

Chapter 8

Long-Term Beta-Blocker Therapy Outcomes in Acute and Chronic Stimulant Abuse

Jessica Bugbee

Abstract

Fear of BBT (beta-blocker therapy) has initiated after a small amount of evidence proposing beta-blockers given during acute stimulant toxicity may create an unopposed alpha-receptor stimulation leading to worse medical outcomes. The objective is to investigate how long-term BBT (both selective and non-selective) affect cardiovascular outcomes compared to no BBT regarding prevention of stimulant-induced-cardiomyopathy. Method is review of most current medical literature. The use of either selective or non-selective beta-blockers to treat the acute effects of cocaine or methamphetamine toxicity demonstrates safety and efficacy. Long-term BBT either selective or non-selective shows success in the prevention of cardiomyopathy in cocaine users by demonstrating a lower rate of death, MI, hospital readmission and improvement of LVEF and NYHA functional class compared to no BBT use. Both selective and non-selective long-term BBT prevent the progression of cardiomyopathy in active cocaine users but not methamphetamine.

Keywords: acute coronary syndrome, cocaine, amphetamines, beta-blockers, HFrEF, mortality, alpha-receptor stimulation

1. Introduction

As many medical providers can attest first-hand, the devastation due to the methamphetamine problem does not spare a single person. Methamphetamine abuse is on the rise and recognition of its devastating cardiovascular risks are more important than ever. Similarly, cocaine use does not have benign effects on the heart. In the United States, heart failure (HF) is accountable for more than 1 million hospitalizations and $32 billion in costs annually [1, 2]. Long-term stimulant abuse is a known cause of cardiomyopathy. Beta-blockers have shown improvement of systolic heart failure but use regarding prevention of stimulant-induced-cardiomyopathy is not well investigated. One of the proposed mechanisms of myocardial injury is thought due to catecholamine excess causing increased workload on the heart, which may benefit from BBT. However, BBT has been controversial in this patient population due to reported cases of worsening vasoconstriction due to unopposed alpha-receptor stimulation; and it has been suggested to avoid them altogether in this population with heart failure [1–4].

IntechOpen

If BBT can decrease the extent and progression of stimulant-induced cardiomyopathy then patients might have a greater chance of regaining cardiac function if they one day decide to quite stimulant abuse. Patients may also have improvement in cardiac function and symptoms leading to less heart failure-related hospital admissions; which in turn could decrease the current financial burden placed on healthcare.

There is a lack of quality studies investigating the use of long-term BBT in active cocaine users and almost no data investigating this same issue in regards to methamphetamine. Recent research has suggested that the phenomenon of excessive alpha-stimulation might not be related to beta-blocker use [1, 2, 4]. Therefore, in patients who actively engage in stimulant drug abuse, how does long-term BBT (both selective and non-selective) affect cardiovascular outcomes compared to no BBT regarding prevention of stimulant-induced-cardiomyopathy?

2. Beta-blocker therapy in acute stimulant toxicity

Current literature recommends against the use of beta-blockers in the setting of cocaine-induced-chest-pain. Small catheter-based-human-studies and case reports have suggested they might exacerbate coronary vasospasm and the toxic effects of cocaine by inducing "unopposed" alpha-adrenergic stimulation [1–3]. Two high quality systematic clinical reviews have demonstrated lack of evidence preventing the use of BBT in both acute methamphetamine and cocaine intoxication. Findings show the superiority of beta-blockers in the management of both stimulant-induced HTN and tachycardia when compared to first-line treatment choices calcium-channel blockers and nitrates; which were shown to only attenuate HTN and not tachycardia [1, 2].

The most recent 2012 ACCF/AHA guidelines endorse the use of labetalol (non-selective with alpha-properties) in acute stimulant toxicity given certain vital sign parameters and only after a vasodilator is given prior. These guidelines also endorse there is a lack of literature investigating these effects in methamphetamine users; and currently recommend that treatment for acute methamphetamine toxicity the same as cocaine toxicity pending future investigation [5].

Current evidence shows that providers have been using BBT during acute stimulant toxicity without causing any adverse cardiac events [1, 2, 6]. For instance, a retrospective study examined 376 patients presenting to the emergency department (ED) with acute coronary syndrome (ACS) and self-reported cocaine use within 24-hours in the presence of positive urine drug screen (UDS) for cocaine. Beta-blockers given were metoprolol (45%), carvedilol (26%), labetalol (27%), or atenolol (2%). No differences were found between selective, non-selective beta-blockers, rate of death, stroke or arrhythmia compared to those not receiving BBT [6]. These findings demonstrate that it is safe to implement BBT during the management of patients presenting with ACS secondary to acute cocaine intoxication.

A systematic review and meta-analysis of five studies were performed involving 1794 patients presenting with cocaine-associated-chest-pain (CACP). The authors found no increased risk of non-fatal MI or all-cause mortality in patients given BBT versus no BBT [7]. This evidence supports the idea that BBT is safe in patients experiencing concomitant stimulant toxicity. This same idea can be applied to the use of long-term BBT. If BBT is safe in acute toxicity then it should demonstrate safety in patients who are prescribed beta-blockers daily who also abuse cocaine or methamphetamine.

3. Beta-blocker therapy after hospital discharge

BBT has shown safety in patients experiencing acute stimulant intoxication. Safety has also been demonstrated in patients discharged on BBT immediately after hospitalization for cocaine-related-chest-pain. It has been demonstrated that taking either selective or nonselective BBT following hospital discharge has a 70% reduction in the rate of death over a median follow-up of 972 days compared to no BBT. The authors of this same study admit that patients with CACP have been shown to exhibit a high mortality rate, and outpatient BBT may help protect against cardiovascular death [8].

A prospective single-center study examined outcomes in 57 patients ≤50 years of age admitted with ACS and urine drug screen (UDS) positive for cocaine. Patients discharged on BBT showed a 12.5% increase in 90-day survival. Discharge on BBT also had 14.7% less chance of death and 2.6% less chance of hospital admission secondary to MI compared to discharge without BBT [4]. Overall, the authors of this study support the use of long term BBT in this patient population.

A retrospective cohort study examined 60 patients with positive UDS for cocaine. Of these patients, 40 (66%) received selective beta-blockers (propranolol, metoprolol, atenolol), 13 patients (21%) received nonselective beta-blockers (carvedilol, labetalol), and 8 patients (13%) received both. Results showed proportionately fewer cases of death and myocardial infarction (MI) during hospital admission and during 5-year follow-up in patients that received BBT (6.1%) compared to none (25.9%) [9].

BBT has been shown to improve outcomes after MI in non-stimulant users [8]. Evidence from the previously mentioned studies suggests the safety of discharge on BBT after cocaine-related ACS by demonstrating a decreased rate of death and cardiac-related complications during the time period following hospital discharge.

4. Long-term beta-blocker therapy in active methamphetamine use

Beta-blockers use regarding prevention of methamphetamine-induced cardiomyopathy has been minimally investigated [1]. Investigators performed a study based out of 2 medical centers in Germany in order to describe clinical characteristics and histological changes in the myocardium of 24 subjects with methamphetamine-associated-cardiomyopathy (MACM). Of patients receiving BBT, 20 patients stopped using methamphetamine while 4 patients continued methamphetamine abuse. Mean age was 30-years and echocardiograms showed severe systolic dysfunction and left ventricular chamber dilatation. The majority had regurgitant valve lesions, ventricular thrombi, and pleural or pericardial effusions. All patients were treated with standard heart failure therapy including the use of BBT. Follow-up averaged 12 months later and improvement in symptoms and ventricular function were only identified in the patients who discontinued methamphetamine abuse [10].

No benefit of BBT was identified during ongoing methamphetamine use, however, the study only involved 4 patients using BBT yielding results of low statistical value. Further limitations of this study include an inability to confirm outpatient adherence to BBT therapy and that methamphetamines were not the sole drugs of abuse. Most patients profiled used other substances such as alcohol, heroin, and cocaine which are all known to have cardiotoxic effects. Since most methamphetamine users often simultaneously abuse alcohol and other drugs [10]. It is difficult to say whether or not BBT could counteract the cardiotoxic effects of multiple substances used simultaneously.

This study suggests that only cessation of methamphetamine abuse is associated with improvement in cardiac function and symptoms; whereas continued methamphetamine abuse leads to ongoing heart failure and worse outcome despite concurrent long-term BBT. Given the limitations of the study, randomized controlled experimental studies are needed to investigate these findings further.

5. Long-term beta-blocker therapy in active cocaine use

It has been suggested that long-term BBT is ineffective in reducing cardiomyopathy in active methamphetamine users according to a single experimental study. The use of long-term BBT in the prevention of cocaine-induced cardiomyopathy has been investigated on a larger scale. A meta-analysis studied outcomes of BBT among 90-systolic heart failure (HF) patients who actively abuse cocaine compared to 177 patients with non-ischemic systolic HF without cocaine use. The authors found no differences in HF readmissions, major adverse cardiovascular events or death when comparing the two groups over a 4000-day interval. Within HF patients with active cocaine use, mortality rates were not different between nonselective BBT versus selective BBT [11].

Findings of this study suggest that BBT produces the same outcomes in systolic HF patients whether or not they abuse cocaine. Findings demonstrate the safety of long-term BBT with cocaine use and suggest that this population should not be precluded from its' benefits. Limitations of this study include a sample size of mostly males and significant differences between cocaine positive and cocaine-negative groups involving age, BMI, co-morbidities, and ACE-I use. Another limitation is that this study does not include outcomes of cocaine use without BBT.

Fortunately, a single-center retrospective cohort study decided to investigate outcomes with and without BBT in active cocaine users. The study investigates 268 adult patients with heart failure with reduced ejection fraction (HFrEF) who tested positive for cocaine on UDS. Of the patients involved, 86% were placed on long-term BBT while 14% were not. Results show that 30-day readmission rates related to either all-cause or HF were 21% less with BBT compared to none. No differences were found between these same groups after 1-year [12].

Limitations of this study include the significantly larger number of patients placed on long-term BBT compared to none, thereby lowering the statistical significance of findings. Another limitation involves significant variation in intervals of follow-up echocardiograms. The authors were unable to evaluate the effects of BBT on LVEF in cocaine users and instead could only measure the incidence of all-cause mortality. The authors' inability to assess LVEF in this study is unfortunate since the use of BBT in this population is meant to reduce the instance of cardiomyopathy.

A case-series of four patients investigated long-term BBT outcomes by measuring changes in the instance of cardiomyopathy. Results found clinical and echocardiographic (ECHO) recovery with carvedilol therapy in severe systolic HF with ongoing cocaine use. None of the patients were prescribed beta-blockers on admission, after 2.5 months each patient was being treated with carvedilol 25 mg twice daily. At mean follow up of 9.25 months, New York Heart Association functional class (NYHA) on average improved by 1.5 and left ventricular ejection fraction (LVEF) improved by 36.5% at follow-up [13].

None of the patients required hospitalization 1-year after enrollment. Furthermore, each had almost full recovery of LVEF during ongoing treatment with carvedilol and concomitant cocaine use during a 2-year follow-up. The authors concluded that patients with severe cocaine-induced-cardiomyopathy are capable of achieving full clinical and echocardiographic recovery with maximum dose of carvedilol [13].

Limitations of this study include case series design and lack of comparison without BBT use. Unfortunately, this limits the significance of the study's findings. Strengths include actual measurement of LVEF to determine the success of long-term BBT. Findings from the study are promising and prompt need for future large randomized studies.

Most recently, a retrospective analysis was performed on 72 beta-blocker-naive active cocaine users affected by HFrEF <40%. After 12-months, 38 patients receiving BBT were more likely to have an improvement in their NYHA class and left ventricular ejection fraction (LVEF). Results also included lower rates of cardiovascular events and HF hospitalizations compared to 34 patients not receiving BBT. When comparing 23 patients receiving carvedilol against 15 patients receiving metoprolol succinate no difference was found in LVEF improvement while NYHA class showed larger improvement with carvedilol [3]. Overall, this study provides evidence supporting the equal success of long-term therapy with both selective and non-selective beta-blockers in regards to reducing cardiomyopathy in active cocaine users compared to no BBT.

The majority of patients in the study were able to achieve full or almost full recovery of their LVEF after one year of long-term BBT. Limitations include failure to fully investigate the pathological substrate of HF since coronary angiography was performed in the majority (72%) but not all patients. Also, a cardiovascular magnetic resonance was not performed in order to investigate the extent of myocardial fibrosis and edema. Therefore, large experimental studies involving coronary imaging are strongly needed to explore the findings of this study further.

6. Discussion

6.1 Strengths

Common strengths of the previously mentioned studies include the fact that patients given BBT were reported to be at higher risk for cardiovascular events compared to those not given BBT [6, 8, 9]. Patients were older, had higher presenting systolic BPs, and more often had a history of hypertension. They were also more likely to be taking outpatient angiotensin-converting enzyme inhibitors (ACEIs) or angiotensin receptor blockers (ARBs), statins, and aspirin. Those who received BBT in the ED showed a statistically larger decrease in systolic blood pressure compared to those receiving BBT in the hospital ward only [8].

Patients had increased risk of systolic dysfunction compared to patients not given BBT [6, 8, 9]. Even though the most common limitation between the studies involves the use of UDS to determine illicit drug toxicity, most emergency departments determine cocaine and other illicit drug ingestion through utilization of UDS [9]. Further strengths include the recency of the studies used [3, 4, 7, 10–12].

6.2 Limitations

Common limitations of the studies used include retrospective cohort study design [3, 4, 6, 8, 9, 12] and the inclusion of a case series [13]. There was an inability to determine the timing of cocaine ingestion with use of UDS since cocaine can be present in urine 48–72 hours after last ingestion [4, 6–9]. Lack of data regarding cocaine serum levels and knowledge on time of cocaine ingestion could be problematic. Acute cocaine toxicity may have different effects compared to cocaine toxicity determined by positive UDS [9].

Further limitations include several studies failed to provide data on selectivity, route, and type of BBT used [4, 7, 10, 12]. Authors were unable to assess interim behaviors and treatments after discharge and relied only on data obtained from the index hospitalization and the National Death Index to determine long-term mortality [8]. Also, there was a lack of quantitative data measuring the frequency of cocaine use [3, 8, 10–13] including compliance with BBT during follow-up [3, 4, 8, 10–12].

7. Conclusion

The use of either selective or non-selective beta-blockers to treat the acute effects of cocaine or methamphetamine toxicity demonstrates safety and efficacy. Avoidance of using BBT in this population is secondary to the fear of causing adverse cardiac events during acute toxicity. Since safety has been demonstrated in recent literature, then the use of long-term BBT in patients that regularly use these drugs should demonstrate safety as well. Long-term BBT either selective or non-selective shows success in the prevention of cardiomyopathy in cocaine users by demonstrating a lower rate of death, MI, hospital readmission and improvement of LVEF and NYHA functional class compared to no BBT use. Therefore, both selective and non-selective long-term BBT prevents the progression of cardiomyopathy in active cocaine users but not methamphetamine. Since a single study has attempted to investigate this topic in methamphetamine users' additional experimental studies are strongly needed in order to determine if long-term BBT can decrease cardiomyopathy in this population.

Funding

The author received no financial support for the research, author-ship, and/or publication of this chapter.

Disclosures

The author reports no relationships that could be construed as a conflict of interest.

Author details

Jessica Bugbee
University of the Pacific Master of Physician Assistant – Certified,
Sacramento, California, USA

*Address all correspondence to: jessica.bugbee1@gmail.com

References

[1] Richards JR, Albertson TE, Derlet RW, Lange RA, Olson KR, Horowitz BZ. Treatment of toxicity from amphetamines, related derivatives, and analogues: A systematic clinical review. Drug and Alcohol Dependence. 2015;**150**:1-13

[2] Richards JR, Garber D, Laurin EG, Albertson TE, Derlet RW, Amsterdam EA, et al. Treatment of cocaine cardiovascular toxicity: a systematic review. Clinical Toxicology. 2016;**54**(5):345-364

[3] Lopez PD, Akinlonu A, Mene-Afejuku TO, Dumancas C, Saeed M, Cativo EH, et al. Clinical outcomes of B-blocker therapy in cocaine-associated heart failure. International Journal of Cardiology. 2019;**277**:153-158

[4] Cediel G, Carrillo X, García-García C, Rueda F, Oliveras T, Labata C, et al. β-Blocker treatment and prognosis in acute coronary syndrome associated with cocaine consumption: The RUTI-Cocaine Study. International Journal of Cardiology. 2018;**260**:7-10

[5] Anderson JL, Adams CD, Antman EM, Bridges CR, Califf RM, Casey DE, et al. 2012 ACCF/AHA focused update incorporated into the ACCF/AHA 2007 guidelines for the management of patients with unstable angina/non–ST-elevation myocardial infarction: A report of the American College of Cardiology Foundation/American Heart Association Task Force on Practice Guidelines. Journal of the American College of Cardiology. 2013;**61**(23):e179-e347

[6] Fanari Z, Kennedy KK, Lim MJ, Laddu AA, Stolker JM. Comparison of in-hospital outcomes for beta-blocker use versus non–beta blocker use in patients presenting with cocaine-associated chest pain. The American Journal of Cardiology. 2014;**113**(11):1802-1806

[7] Pham D, Addison D, Kayani W, Misra A, Jneid H, Resar J, et al. Outcomes of beta-blocker use in cocaine-associated chest pain: A meta-analysis. Emergency Medical Journal. 2018;**35**(9):559-563

[8] Rangel C, Shu RG, Lazar LD, Vittinghoff E, Hsue PY, Marcus GM. β-Blockers for chest pain associated with recent cocaine use. Archives of Internal Medicine. 2010;**170**(10):874-879

[9] Dattilo PB, Hailpern SM, Fearon K, Sohal D, Nordin C. B-blockers are associated with reduced risk of myocardial infarction after cocaine use. Annals of Emergency Medicine. 2008;**51**(2):117-125

[10] Schürer S, Klingel K, Sandri M, Majunke N, Besler C, Kandolf R, et al. Clinical characteristics, histopathological features, and clinical outcome of methamphetamine-associated cardiomyopathy. JACC: Heart Failure. 2017;**5**(6):435-445

[11] Nguyen P, Kamran H, Nasir S, Chan W, Shah T, Deswal A, et al. Comparison of frequency of cardiovascular events and mortality in patients with heart failure using versus not using cocaine. The American Journal of Cardiology. 2017;**119**(12):2030-2034

[12] Egbuche OE, Ekechukwu IR, Maduabum N, Obinwa U, Ukpaka KL, Maihemuti A, et al. Effect of beta-blocker therapy on hospital readmission and mortality in heart failure patients

with ongoing cocaine use. Journal of Cardiac Failure. 2017;**23**(8):S61

[13] Littmann L, Narveson SY, Fesel NM, Marconi SL. Beta blocker treatment of heart failure patients with ongoing cocaine use. International Journal of Cardiology. 2013;**168**(3):2919-2920

Chapter 9

Emerging Hallmarks of Mitochondrial Biochemistry in Cardiac Trabecular Morphogenesis and Left Ventricular Noncompaction (LVNC)

Gowthami Mahendran and Margaret A. Schwarz

Abstract

Functioning as a pivotal platform for energy production and transduction, mitochondria generate ATP to meet the dynamic demands of embryonic development. Consequently, disruption or alteration in mitochondrial activity influences not only cellular status, but also can impact organ formation. Disrupted mitochondrial performance not only impairs cardiovascular function but can also disrupt cardiac maturation through prevention of the myocardium's transition between the trabeculation to the compaction phase. During embryonic development, proliferating cardiomyocytes create a trabecular mesh network. Gradual compaction of this network transforms the intra-trabecular spaces into the capillaries of the coronary circulation. Achievement of functional compaction and ultimately normal cardiac function is dependent in part on mitochondrial well-being with failure to complete remodeling of the inner trabecular layer contributing to disrupted endocardial vasculature and fibrosis, left ventricular noncompaction (LVNC). LVNC, commonly associated with mitochondrial genetic alterations, is speculated to occur due to an interruption during the process of compaction at the early developmental stages of the left ventricle (LV). Mitochondrial mutations, remain the common etiology of LVNC with a wide spectrum of these genes associated with other cardiomyopathies related to LVNC. Understanding the impact that mitochondrial genetic alterations have on the evolution of cardiac noncompaction could provide new treatment opportunities.

Keywords: trabeculation, mitochondria, LVNC, mutations, cardiomyopathy

1. Introduction

Cardiac development consists of four stages including embryonic cardiac chamber maturation [Carnegie stage (CS) 11 in humans and embryonic day (E) 8.5 in mice], trabeculation (at CS 12 in humans and E9.5 in mice), compaction (CS 22 in humans and E14.5 in mice) and cardiomyocyte proliferation (E11-E17.5 in mice). Originating from embryonic mesodermal germ layer cells that differentiate into mesothelium, endothelium, and myocardium followed by gastrulation, the exterior lining of the heart is made up of mesothelial pericardium. Whereas the interior lining of the heart, lymphatic, and blood vessels, arise from endothelium. During cardiac development, the atrial septation (primary atrial septum formation) begins at E10.5 to E13.5 in mice, which is comparable to Carnegie stages (CS 14 to 18) in humans or estimated gestational age (EGA) of 6 6/7–8 weeks. The ventricular septation proceeds from E11.5 to E13.5 in mice and EGA 8–9 1/7 weeks (CS 18–22) in human fetuses. Outflow septation, the transformation of a right ventricle (RV) single outflow tract into pulmonary and aortic arteries originating from the right and left ventricles, starts at E11.5–E13.5 in the mouse and EGA 7 3/7–8 weeks (CS 16–18) in humans [1]. While the separation of atrioventricular (AV) valves from endocardial cushions at the center of cardiac loop occurs at 9 1/7 weeks (CS 22). By the end of 9 1/7 weeks (CS22), all of the major structures of the heart are formed, with the average spanning period of EGA 6 4/7–9 3/7 weeks [2–4].

During cardiac development, trabeculation followed by a compaction step (CS 12 to CS 22), is vital in the developmental stages of humans (**Figure 1**). Emerging from the developing ventricular wall and stretching into the ventricular lumen, trabeculae projections consist of cardiomyocytes lined by an endothelial layer of the endocardium and are an important element of ordered ventricular formation. Any defects during trabeculation, compaction of remodeling junctions, or cardiac chamber maturation, could lead to the inhibition of well compacted myocardium with persisting trabeculations resulting in the condition left ventricular noncompaction (LVNC).

The trabeculation process is further defined by three sequential steps resulting in fusion with myocardium layer that is compacted and progression into a mature thickened ventricular wall. Initially, the trabecular ridges start to emerge while the myocardial projections progress into the lumen. This is followed by the expansion of trabeculae projections, creating a trabeculae network. In the final remodeling step of trabeculae formation, trabeculae growth ceases and they compact together contributing to ventricular radial thickening [6, 7]. Importantly, the LV of a healthy heart has three distinct trabeculation types (hypertrophic, fibrotic or both) [8] and is less trabeculated than RV [9]. Upon stimulation of ventricular trabeculations during the compaction phase of embryonic development, the growth of trabecula ceases and the ends of the trabecula thicken, with the spaces in between the trabecular buds developing into capillaries [10, 11]. The persistence of a trabecular mesh caused by myocardial noncompaction can occur due to irregularities arising in the maturation process of the cardiac chamber. However, the step of remodeling ventricular trabeculae for compaction is believed to be correlated with congenital or acquired mutations of genes associated with cardiomyocytes and the powerhouse of the cell, mitochondria. Unfortunately, complications arising from disruption in the compaction process, referred to as noncompaction, can result in heart failure and neonatal death [12].

In normal human embryo development, the compaction of myocardium begins after the 5th week of embryonic life. To form a well-developed compacted epicardial and a well-compacted endocardial layer, vascular endothelial growth factor (VEGF) and angiopoietin [13] triggers these loosely interwoven muscle fibers of the myocardium to condense, thus removing the large flattened trabeculae spongy mesh from early embryonic development prior to resolving the intertrabecular recesses into capillaries. This gradual progression of trabeculae compaction occurs faster in the LV than in the RV. However, the etiology of LVNC is poorly understood and occurs as a spectrum of pathological conditions, ranging from asymptomatic to the risk of RV failure and fetal heart failure [14]. Due to its relatively low prevalence in combination

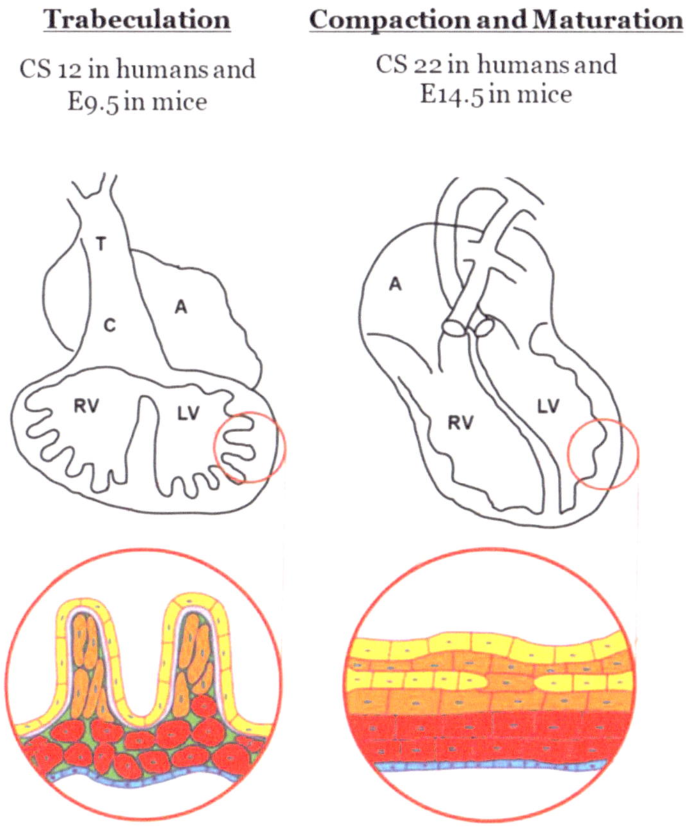

Figure 1.
Progression of left ventricular trabeculation to compaction: Trabeculation and compaction of endocardial cells (yellow), cardiomyocytes (orange in left image, red in right image), cardiac jelly (purple), epicardial cells (blue) of a LV followed by the maturation step in mouse and human are shown (figure adapted and modified from Zhang et al. [5]).

with less sensitive detection techniques for noncompaction, less is known regarding its etiology and therapy compared to other cardiomyopathies. While the occurrence of LVNC is independent of sex or age, the prevalence varies among different ethnic groups: with a greater occurrence within black populations. Lastly, the pathophysiological impact of LV noncompaction is poorly understood, though it is expected to a have an association with altered ventricular systolic and diastolic function [15, 16].

2. Cardiac energy metabolism: role of the mitochondria

Cardiac energy metabolism relies on regular mitochondrial function and energy production. Thus, inborn errors of metabolism impacting the mitochondrial dysfunction are a common pathological factor of LVNC. Mitochondrial cardiomyopathy is a myocardial condition defined by an aberrant heart-muscle structure or function, that involves mitochondrial respiratory chain pathways. Failure in the regulation of these metabolic pathway mechanisms can lead to cardiac dysfunction associated with noncompaction [17]. Thus, the proper functioning of mitochondrial enzyme complexes is crucial for the normal progression of cardiac morphogenesis. This review focuses specifically on the mitochondrial influence on trabecula morphogenesis and its influence on the compaction of LV myocardium. Moreover, we describe the mechanisms contributing to LVNC and explore the current diagnostic and therapeutic strategies available for this type of mitochondrial myopathy [18, 19].

A double membrane-bound organelle, mitochondria have their own genome and exhibit maternal inheritance patterns. The mitochondrial genome is composed of 22 tRNAs, 2 rRNAs, and 37 genes encoding 13 different proteins that form subunits of enzyme complexes within the oxidative phosphorylation system (OXPHOS). Although comparatively smaller than the nuclear genome, the human mitochondrial genome possesses thousands of mitochondria, each encoding dozens of copies of the mitochondrial genome. Unlike the nuclear genome, mitochondria have higher mutation rates (100 fold higher) due to the absence of a mismatch base repairing mechanism [20]. Notably, deficiencies in NADH-coenzyme Q (CoQ) reductase (complex I) and cytochrome-c oxidase (complex IV) have been commonly studied in many mitochondrial disorders [20, 21]. OXPHOS pathway involves around 80 different proteins to make five electron transport complexes (complex I–V) [22]. Many of the mutations and defects in genes involved in OXPHOS impacts the mitochondrial energy production. As such they are the primary source of reactive oxygen species (ROS) generation. Hence, the overproduction of ROS causes mitochondrial damage through a range of pathologies that affects the rest of the cell (**Figure 2**). In addition to oxidative phosphorylation system, mitochondria also control apoptosis and cytosol calcium concentrations. Importantly within the cardiac muscle, calcium signaling propagated within the cytosol, is trafficked through the mitochondrial membrane via the voltage dependent anion channel (VDAC) and an inner membrane located calcium uniporter or a Na^{+}/Ca^{2+} exchanger. Thus, a vital feature of cellular life any alterations in mitochondrial Ca^{2+} homeostasis can cause profound effects in the mitochondrial function with defects contributing to cell death [23].

Mitochondrial energy production is influenced by maternally inherited mitochondrial DNA (mtDNA) and nuclear DNA [24] with mitochondrial gene mutations causing irregular function. Energy released upon electrons transfer between the 5 enzyme complexes of the mitochondrial electron transport chain (ETC) within the inner mitochondrial membrane, acts as a proton pump across the mitochondrial membrane. This electrochemical gradient is important for cellular energetic homeostasis [25]. Defects in the five enzyme complexes of mitochondrial ETC, some of which are encoded by mitochondrial DNA, can reduce ATP energy generation resulting in an energy insufficiency. Additionally, cardiac mitochondrial function is also coupled with ROS production from oxidative damage during the OXPHOS cycle. Elevated free iron levels and defective ETC as a result of the impaired intramitochondrial metabolism is associated with a vast increase in free radical generation leading to oxidative damage that could impact development.

Cardiomyocytes are composed of bundles of myofibrils containing myofilaments. The distinct, repeating micro units of myofibrils, sarcomeres, are the fundamental contractile units of the myocytes. The mitochondria in cardiomyocytes localized to sarcomeres form intracellular energetic unit (ICEU) [26]. Catabolism favors the movement of the chemical gradient from mitochondria in the form of ATP to sarcomeres. Composed of thin and thick filaments, the thick filamentous myosin motor protein component of the cardiac sarcomere is primarily responsible for force generation. While the structural abnormalities associated with LVNC has been well described, many of the details of its mechanism have yet to be elucidated. However, studies suggest a correlation between LVNC and myocardial abnormalities with

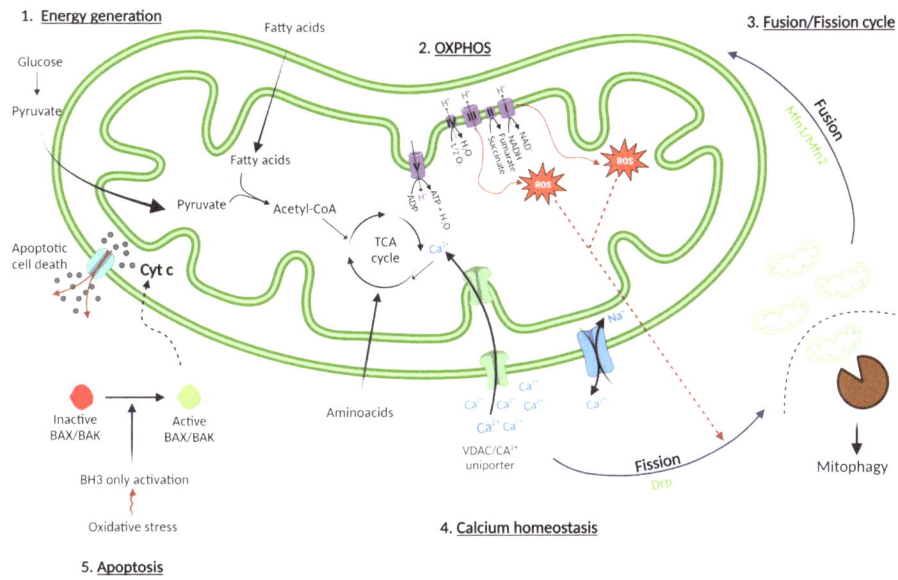

Figure 2.
A variety of roles played by Mitochondria are critical for cellular maintenance: Energy production ("powerhouse of the cell"), OXPHOS pathway, alters between fusion and fission cycle, Ca^{2+} level control and apoptosis.

energy generation, transfer and utilization as possible contributing factors to the irregular contraction and relaxation of cardiac muscles. As such, the impact of mitochondrial related gene deletion, mitochondrial function, and energy production cannot be overstated in light of the disorders arising from disruption of these processes and their impact on compaction at the early development of the LV myocardium.

3. Left ventricular noncompaction (LVNC)

Left ventricular noncompaction (LVNC), also knowns as left ventricular hyper trabeculation (LVHT) or spongy myocardium, is a rare congenital myocardial dysfunction resulting from the arrest of the compaction phase during embryogenesis. Gross histology of this heterogeneous disease condition is characterized by a spongy left ventricle (LV) myocardium, abnormal prominent trabeculations at the ventricular apex, and intra-trabeculae recesses adjacent to a well compacted LV myocardium during the final stages of cardiac development [27]. Within the ventricular cavity the double-layered ventricular myocardium consisting of epicardial and endocardial layers, there appears finger-like protrusions from the myocardium with intertrabecular recesses separating trabeculations. Pathologically these anatomical features of a noncompacted heart demonstrate a tremendously thickened endocardial layer with abnormal trabeculation and a compacted thin epicardial layer. In 1984, the first case of LVNC was described in a newborn that was also associated complications of atresia of semilunar valves and intact ventricular septum [28]. Since then, of the different phenotypes of LVNC (8 different subtypes identified to date) [29], isolated LVNCs (first reported in 1926 occurring as a result of trabeculae morphogenesis interference in the absence of any cardiac abnormalities) and congenital LVNCs are the most commonly studied. With the latter type of LVNC being associated with systemic diseases including metabolic or mitochondrial diseases, cardiomyopathies such as hypertrophic, dilated, restrictive, and arrhythmogenic, congenital heart diseases, and complex syndromes affecting vast majority of the organs and tissue [30].

While rare forms of LVNC can occur from acquired mutations, commonly LVNCs are from genetic alterations transmitted through generations [31] with around 50% of the identified LVNC patients having either autosomal dominant, autosomal recessive, or X-linked genetic inheritance patterns with multiple genes modifications [32–34] (**Figure 3**). Predominate genetic variants associated with LV noncompaction include defects in mitochondrial, sarcomeric, and cardiac genes. In addition to mitochondrial DNA mutations [35], a wide variety of mitochondrial abnormalities significantly influence LVNC including but not limited to mitochondrial dysfunction [36], metabolic myopathy altered by mitochondrial energy production [37], dysmorphic mitochondria [31, 38], mitochondrial DNA transitions (a type of DNA mutation where a purine or pyrimidine nucleotide is replaced with its complementary purine or pyrimidines, respectively) [39, 40], deficiencies in mitochondrial respiratory chain function [41], mutations in overlapping regions [42], and mitochondrial genome mutations [43]. Further supporting mitochondrial involvement, mitochondrial numbers are enriched in the cardiac muscles of individuals with LVNC, and mitochondrial DNA (mtDNA) content and copy number are also largely altered in non-compacted hearts.

4. Diagnostics and therapeutic aspects of LVNC

The occurrence of LVNC has increased in recent years with a prevalence of 0.01–0.3%, a mortality rate of 5–12%, and is predominately found in males [44]. While most LVNC patients are asymptomatic or noted to have mild symptoms of chest pain, later stages of LVNC can lead to sudden cardiac death due to compromised systolic function. Although the initial diagnosis can be at any stage in life, most individuals with LVNC go undiagnosed until the 5th decade of life. Symptoms are diverse in patients with LVNC and can include heart failure, cardiac arrhythmias, fatigue, excessive sweating, breathing difficulties, compromised growth, and abnormal weight gain, while others do not exhibit any symptoms [44–46]. Hence, early diagnosis is key for timely supportive care.

Common diagnostic tools available for LVNC include echocardiography (echo), cardiac magnetic resonance imaging (cardiac MRI or CMR), electrocardiogram (ECG), cardiac computed tomography (CT), coronary angiograms and myocardial biopsy based on the myocardial thickening [47]. In most cases the first-line diagnostic testing of any heart diseases is echo, due to its availability and being low-cost in nature. Echo criteria include (1) noncompacted/compacted ratio of the two-layered endocardium of >2, (2) left ventricular deep endomyocardial trabeculations, and (3) deep recesses filled with blood visualized on color Doppler [48, 49]. However, the detection of LVNC in its early stage of development are challenging, with only around 0.3% of the patients being referred for an echo [50, 51]. Additionally, echo diagnostics are sometimes considered to be a 'too sensitive of a method' as overdiagnosis frequently occurs, particularly in the black patient population. Therefore, serial echo diagnosis is recommended in LVNC [52].

Alternatively, CMR is a well-established, high resolution, noninvasive, albeit more expensive approach, to confirm LVNC after an initial diagnostic echo. CMR

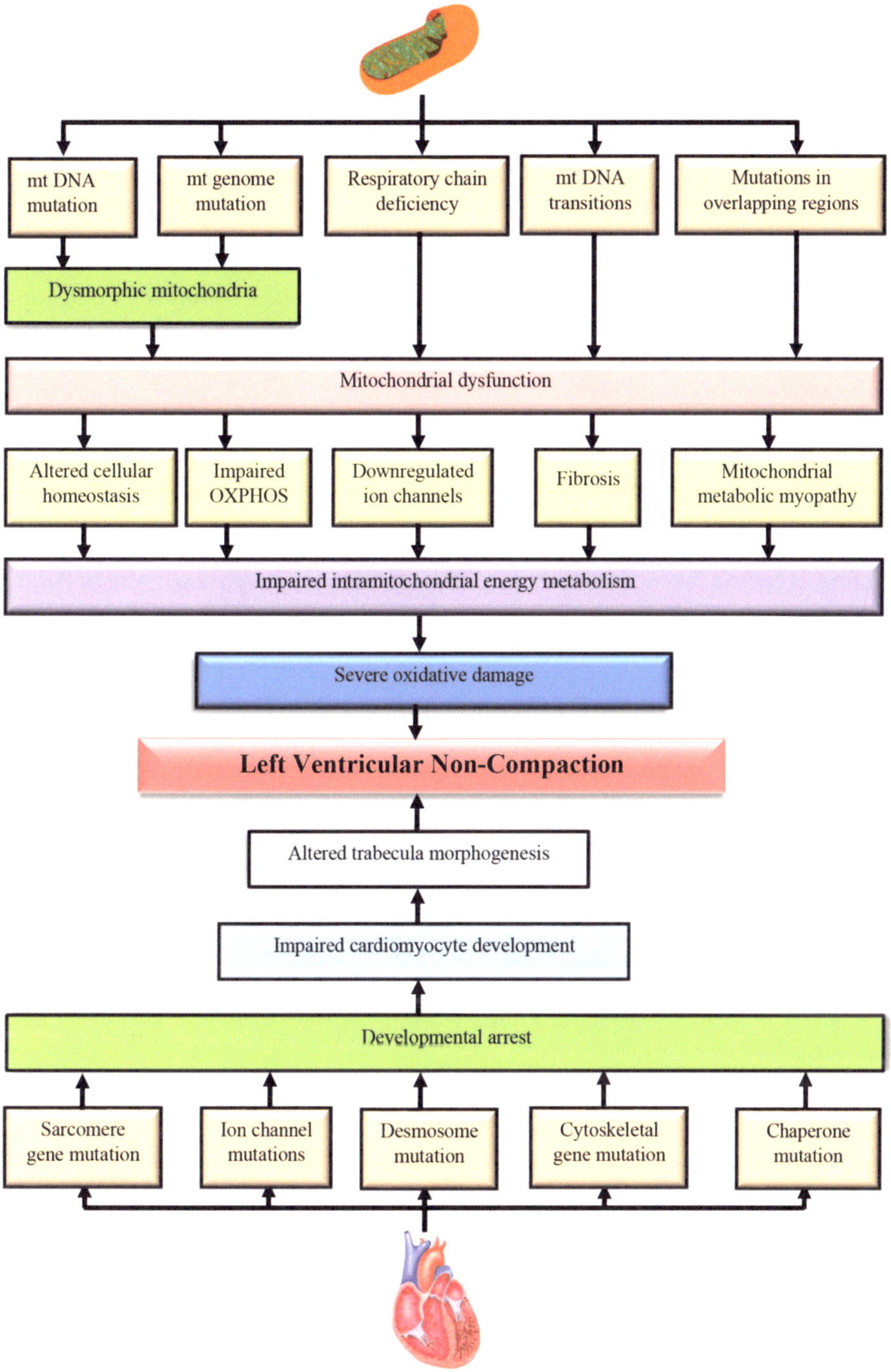

Figure 3.
Schematic overview of influencing factors in myocardial noncompaction: Differential contribution of mitochondria towards LVNC via mitochondrial dysfunction (mtDNA mutations, transitions, ETC defects, mt genome mutations) and involvement of genes associated with cardiomyopathies (sarcomeres, ion channels, cytoskeletal, chaperones, desmosomes).

offers an enhanced sensitivity, as CMR can detect myocardial trabeculations that can be enhanced with steady-state free-precession (SSFP) cine imaging [53, 54]. In CMR, the myocardial trabeculations, apex region and end-diastole ratio can be well monitored over time. Although CMR is associated with many challenges including a wide diagnostic testing timeline, high costs, and availability, it still remains the best approach as a diagnostic tool for LVNC. Unlike echo and CMR, CT imaging is less commonly used due to the ionizing radiation and lower detection ability of myocardial tissues. Nevertheless, this tool is widely used in evaluating other disease processes such as coronary arteries. Apart from the above-mentioned diagnostic tools, advances using blood for whole exome sequencing (PGxome diagnostic exome test) and copy number variation detection can be performed to study single gene defect or defects in gene sets associated with LVNC [55].

In research settings and invasive cardiac catheterization techniques, a more invasive method of histologic examination of cardiac muscle tissue biopsies is assessed. Histological analysis can identify abnormalities in the mitochondrial appearance as ragged red fibers, indicative of mitochondrial dysfunction, are suggestive of mitochondrial anomalies (Gomori Trichrome stain, **Figure 4**). A typical drawback of Gomori Trichrome Staining is the absence of these ragged red fibers in children, and therefore, it fails to detect mitochondrial disorders in neonates at early stages [56, 57]. An alternative method of early detection is the examination of cardiac tissue under electron microscopy for swollen disorganized mitochondria containing irregular cristae [57].

Importantly, around 40% of patients identified with LVNC are determined to have a familial genetic defect that impacts only cardiac function. However, while many genetic syndromes, metabolic disorders, and mitochondrial related anomalies are also associated with LVNC, in many cases the cause of LVNC is still unknown. As there is no cure to date, routine cardiac screening is an important part of the treatment of familial LVNC, with supportive therapy for LVNC patients being dependent on individual symptoms. Supportive therapy targeted to improved quality of life and overcome cardiac dysfunction includes medications to treat heart failure such as angiotensin-converting enzyme inhibitor, beta blockers, blood thinners, diuretics, and digoxin. In severe cases of LVNC, pacemaker implantation, cardioverter defibrillator, or heart transplantation is recommended. A recent case study in 2018 by

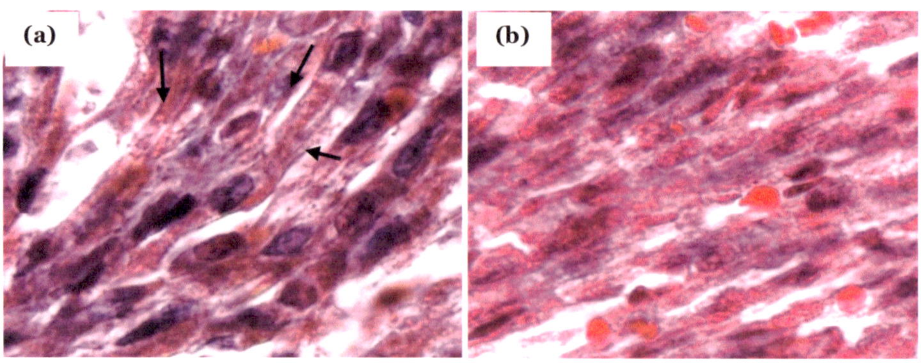

Figure 4.
Gomori Trichrome staining of cardiac tissue from an (a) hyper trabeculated heart and a (b) healthy heart: (a) arrows indicating dysmorphic mitochondria scattered as red-ragged fibers below the matrix of the membrane, (b) mitochondria appear organized and distributed across the cardiac tissue.

Kimura et al. [58], showed successful treatment of a near-fatal ventricular arrhythmia in an infant with LVNC using cardiac resynchronization therapy (CRT). These studies determined that with the implantation of a cardioverter defibrillator (preventive measure for cardiac arrest), dual chamber pacing initiation and CRT, effectively treated the mechanical dyssynchrony of the heart, with subsequent improvement in cardiac function.

Currently, there are no mechanisms to prevent LVNC or to return gain of cardiac function. While genetic testing can be done to identify gene mutations (**Table 1**) and determine the risk of passing these mutations to offspring, there are not therapeutic options to actively treat these gene mutations [74]. Future therapy that promotes personalized gene therapy could be a useful tool in treating LVNC. However, this approach could be highly challenging due to the complex genetics of LVNC.

5. Genes and related mutations associated with LVNC

A variety of gene mutations studied concerning other cardiomyopathies such as genes coding for sarcomere proteins [75], ion channels, cytoskeletal genes [76], chaperone proteins [77], and cellular signaling pathways have a significant association with LVNC [11, 78]. Specific genetic alterations include genes encoding β-myosin heavy chain (MYH7) [34, 79], α-cardiac actin (ACTC1) [80], and cardiac troponin T (TNNT2) [81], lamin A/C (LMNA) [82], ZASP (LDB3) [83], and taffazin (TAZ) [83, 84], cardiac myosin-binding protein C (MYBPC3) [85], and cardiac troponin I (TNNI3) [86] are associated with LVNC (**Table 2**).

Sarcomere gene mutations can lead to noncompaction with reduced ventricular function and hyper trabeculation [110]. Alpha-cardiac actin gene (ACTC) codes for cardiac muscle-specific alpha-actin protein, present in cardiac sarcomeres and cytoskeletal proteins, and is responsible for heart muscle contraction and generation of force to support the contraction. Novel mutations in the ACTC gene are linked to LVNC cardiomyopathies. Although, the novel protein-level amino acid sequence (A21V) mutations of ACTC1 resulting in familial LVNC are rare, it causes diverse cardiac anomalies. This resulting missense mutation in the ACTC1 gene creates structural changes to sarcomeres and their anchorage. In addition to these changes, these variants also modify the highly conserved nature of actin-like domains of the protein resulting in its destabilization with pathogenic consequences [80]. The MYH7 gene encoding for myosin heavy chain beta (MyHC-β) isoform is another primary sarcomeric protein in the adult heart. The ATPase activity of MYH7 powers the myosin power stroke within the myosin heads to convert energy that propels shortening of the sarcomeres. A heterozygous missense mutation (I467T) in MYH7 found in inherited cardiomyopathies presenting with a high penetrance and sudden death, can result in LVNC and hypertrophic cardiomyopathy (HCM) [111]. As the mutation site in MyH7 is close to the hydrophobic ATP binding pocket of the motor domain, the amino acid replacement of hydrophobic isoleucine with a non-polar threonine alters the structure subsequently effecting the ATPase activity of the motor domain [79, 80]. Cardiac Myosin binding protein C (MYBPC3) is another LVNC linked sarcomere protein. Infants with pathogenic truncating mutations in *MYBPC3* die at birth from HCM and LVNC complications. These mutations are believed to cause alterations in the primary contractile function of the heart and septal defects. However, the absolute relationship of contractile dysfunction to sarcomere protein mutations in the progression and pathophysiology of LVNC remains poorly understood [112].

Age/mean age at diagnosis	Patient gender	Complications observed	Diagnostic approach	Reference
7 years	5 males and 3 females	SVD, VA, SE, PVC, FD	Holter monitoring, intracardiac electrophysiological studies	Chin et al. [59]
47 years	24 males and 41 females	Hypokinesia, Akinesia, Dyskinesia	Echocardiography	Lofiego et al. [60]
Not reported	821 males and 627 females	LV dilatation, hypertrophy, and systolic dysfunction	Transthoracic echocardiography, MRI	Tamborini et al. [61]
33-year-old	Female	Myocardial sinusoids, high systolic ventricular pressure, external dyspnea, sinusoid anomaly	2D-echocardiography	Engberding et al. [28]
11 years	13,306 males and 12,283 females	Lower LVEF, higher LV ESV	Echocardiography	Borresen et al. [51]
47.4 years	183 males and 155 females	Lower LVEF, dyspnea, cardiomyopathy, left atrial enlargement	Transthoracic echocardiography and or MRI	Vaidya et al. [12]
90-year-old	Male	Asymptomatic until heart failure followed by progressive shortness of breath, body weakness	Color-flow Doppler echocardiography, electrocardiogram	Cevik et al. [62]
9 years	8 males and 1 female	Mostly asymptomatic, LVH	Electrocardiogram, chest X-ray, 2D-echocardiogram with Doppler interrogation	Alehan et al. [63]
53 years	71 males and 29 females	LVHT, associated neuromuscular disorders	Echocardiography	Stollberger et al. [64]
≤21 years	24 males and 18 females	Myocardial dysfunction, CVM, DCM, HCM	Echocardiography, Genetic testing (cardiomyopathy gene panel)	Miller et al. [65] (2017)
62-year-old	Female	Congestive heart failure, Bilateral crackles (mild symptoms)	Echocardiography, Color Doppler imaging	Lin et al. [66]
6-month-old	Infant (female)	Incessant ventricular fibrillation, cardiopulmonary arrest, polymorphic ventricular tachycardia, LV hypokinesis	Transthoracic echocardiography, Chest X-ray, Color Doppler imaging	Kimura et al. [58]

Age/mean age at diagnosis	Patient gender	Complications observed	Diagnostic approach	Reference
46 years	312 males and 2188 females	Cardiovascular and all-cause mortality, thromboembolic complications, ventricular arrhythmias	Echocardiography, MRI	Aung et al. [30]
41-year-old	Male	Chest pain, biatrial enlargement, right ventricular hypertrophy, global hypokinesis, lower LVEF	Electrocardiogram, MRI	Tian et al. [67]
Not reported (wide range of age groups studied)	6 males and 8 females	VSD, histiocytoid cardiomyopathy, hydrops fetalis, sudden death, heart failure	Echocardiography	Burke et al. [68]
29-year-old	Male	Dyspnea, pulmonary rales, fatigue, cardiomegaly, hepatomegaly, splenomegaly	Twelve-lead electrocardiography, twenty-four-hour Holter monitoring, speckle-tracking echocardiography, MRI, chest X-ray	Toader et al. [69]
57-year-old	Female	Heart failure, onset dyspnea	Echocardiography	Loria et al. [70]
36-year-old	Male	Shortness of breath, exercise intolerance, orthopnea, paroxysmal nocturnal dyspnea	Transesophageal echocardiogram, endomyocardial biopsy, transthoracic echocardiogram	Ayesha et al. [71]
69-year-old	Male	Atrial fibrillation, myocardial fibrosis	Electrocardiogram, post-cardiac arrest transthoracic echocardiogram	Bath et al. [72]
60-year-old	Female	Intermittent chest pain, increasing shortness of breath, decreased appetite, paroxysmal nocturnal dyspnea, orthopnea	Echocardiography, chest X-ray, CT scan	Kalavakunta et al. [73]

Table 1.
Genetic details and characteristics identified in clinical studies.

Notch signaling is a prime mediator of cardiac embryogenesis. Despite the anomalies in other signaling pathways, the dysfunction of the Notch pathway has a notable contribution to LVNC. Germline mutations in human myocardial MIB1 (mind bomb homolog 1) coding for E3 ubiquitin ligase that promotes the endocytosis of Delta and Jagged, (NOTCH ligands) are involved in LV noncompaction [113]. In these studies,

Affected genes	Gene name	Protein type	DNA variant	Cardiac manifestation	Ref no
DTNA	α-Dystrobrevin	Cytoskeletal protein	C362T, N49S	NLVNC, LVNC	[15, 83]*
LAMP2	Lysosome-associated membrane protein-2	Membrane glycoprotein	G928A transition	HCM, skeletal myopathy, DCM	[16, 87]
TAZ (G4.5)	Tafazzin	Phospholipid trans acylase	GIVS8-1C	ILVNC, DCM, BTHS	[75, 83]
HCN4	Hyperpolarization-activated cyclic nucleotide channel 4	Ion channel	G482R, Y481H	Brugada syndrome, Bradycardia, LVNC	[88]
SCN5A	Cardiac sodium channel	Ion channel	H558R	Brugada syndrome, LVNC, DCM	[89]
TMEM70	Transmembrane protein 70	Mitochondrial membrane	Y112X, 578delCA	HCM	[15]*
Nkx2–5	Nkx2-5	Transcription factor	A118S	LVNC, DCM, HF, AVB	[90]
FKBP12 (aka Fkbp1a)	Peptidyl-prolyl cis-trans isomerase	Immunophilin protein family	—	LVNC, VSD, DCM, CHD	[77, 91]
DNJAC19	Mitochondrial import inner membrane translocase subunit TIM14	DnaJ Hsp40 member C19	1G-C transversion in intron 3	DCM, DCMA	[16]*
BMP10	Bone morphogenetic protein 10	TGF-β super family proteins	V407I	LVNC, VSD, HT	[92]
LDB3	LIM-domain binding 3	Z-disk protein	G1876A, G163A	ILVNC, LVNC3, DCM, HCM	[15, 83, 93]
MYBCP3	Myosin binding protein C	Sarcomere thick filament	N948T, G490R, A833T	DCM, LVNC10	[82, 85, 94]*
MYH7	β-Myosin heavy chain 7	Sarcomere thick filament	L1793P, L387F	LVNC5, HCM, DCM	[33, 90, 94–96]*
ACTC	α-cardiac actin	Sarcomere thin filament	A21V, E101K	LVNC4	[97, 98]
TNNT2	Cardiac troponin T, type 2	Sarcomere thin filament	R141W, R131W, E96K	DCM, HCM, RCM, LVNC6, LVD	[75, 81]*
TNNI3	Cardiac troponin I	Sarcomere thin filaments	D190G, A2V	RCM, DCM	[86, 99]
TPM1	Tropomyosin-1	Actin binding protein	E40K, E54K, D159N, L113V	LVNC9, DCM, HCM	[16, 75, 99]*
LMNA	Lamin A/C	Nuclear membrane protein	R644C, R190W, V445E	LVNC	[82, 100]

Affected genes	Gene name	Protein type	DNA variant	Cardiac manifestation	Ref no
MT-ATP6	Mitochondrially encoded ATP synthase membrane subunit 6′	ATP synthase F_o subunit 6	T8528C, G8529A, C8558T, A9058G	LVNC	[101]
MT-ATP8	Mitochondrially encoded ATP synthase membrane subunit 8	ATP synthase F_o subunit 8	A8381G, C8858T	LVNC	[31, 96, 102]
MT-ND1	NADH: ubiquinone oxidoreductase core subunit 1	NADH dehydrogenase 1 enzyme	T3398C, T4216C, G15812A, A3397G	LVNC, MELAS, LHON	[40, 96]
MT-TL1	Mitochondrially encoded tRNA leucine 1	transfer RNA (UUR)	A3243G, A8344G	MELAS, MERRF	[16]
ANT2	Peroxisomal adenine nucleotide transporter-2	ADP/ATP translocase 2	G1409T polymorphism	DCM, LVNC/ LVHT	[103]
MIB1	Mindbomb homolog 1	E3 ubiquitin ligase	V943F, R530X	LVNC7, RVNC, DCM, HF	[78]
PRMD16	PR/SET Domain 16	Transcription regulator	K702X, N816S, P291L, L887P, V1101M, 1573dupC in exon 9	LVNC8, DCM	[75, 104]*
PLEC1	Plectin	Cytoskeletal protein	G4891T, G1019A	ARVC, DCM, LVNC/LVHT	[105]
MT-CYB	Cytochrome B	Component of complex III	T15693C, A15662G	LVNC, HCM	[40, 96]
ACTN2	α-Actinin 2	Cytoskeletal protein	M228T, L727R	HCM, DCM, LVNC	[106]
PRKAG2	Protein kinase AMP-activated non-catalytic subunit gamma 2	AMP-activated protein kinase (AMP-K)	H142A, T400N, N488I, E506K, R302Q	HCM, LVH	[16, 107]
PLN	Phospholamban	Integral membrane protein	R9C, L39X	DCM	[108, 109]

https://omim.org/
ILVNC, isolated left ventricular noncompaction; NLVNC, non-isolated left ventricular noncompaction; LVHT, left ventricular hyper trabeculation; RVNC, right ventricular noncompaction; AVB, Atrio ventricular block; HF, heart failure; DCM, dilated cardiomyopathy; HCM, hypertrophic cardiomyopathy; VSD, ventricular septal defect; BTHS, Barth syndrome; DCMA, dilated cardiomyopathy with ataxia syndrome; HT, hyper trabeculation; MELAS, mitochondrial encephalomyopathy; MERRF, myoclonic epilepsy with ragged-red fibers disorder; ARVC, arrhythmogenic right ventricle cardiomyopathy; CHD, congenital heart diseases; LVD, left ventricular dilation; RCM, restrictive cardiomyopathy [33].

Table 2.
Genes and associated mutations in cardiomyopathies.

MIB1 protein was noted to be vital in activating the NOTCH signaling pathway while cardiac deformity managed by two of the MIB1 autosomal dominant mutations (V943F and R530X) causes deregulation of Notch signaling resulting in LVNC. Furthermore, Luxan et al. [78] reported that myocardial inactivation of MIB1 results in the enlargement of the ventricular trabeculae and a thin compact myocardium.

Alterations in cytoskeletal genes have been linked with the LVNC development. The intermediate filament protein, lamin (lamin A/C) or LMNA, maintains the mechanical integrity of the nuclear envelope. Heterozygous LMNA gene mutations (R644C and R190W) are linked to familial and sporadic LVNC, although the mechanisms have not been elucidated to date. Furthermore, lamin A/C V445E mutations were found to be related to sudden death in LVNC patients [82]. Cardiac expressing alpha-dystrobrevin (DTNA) belongs to a dystrophin-related protein family that is significant in intracellular signal transduction. Genetic alterations in DTNA and dystrophin-associated glycoprotein complex (DAPC) located in sarcolemma provoke myocardial disorders targeting the systolic function of the heart [41]. Inactivation of DTNA leads to muscular dystrophy, skeletal myopathy, and cardiomyopathy characterized by deep trabeculations which are always observed in LVNC [76]. Congenital LVNC frequently accompanies neuromuscular disorders in patients with myotonic dystrophy type 1 (MD1), an autosomal dominant type of disorder resulting from a trinucleotide expansion (CTG nucleotide repetitions) in the dystrophia myotonica protein kinase (DMPK) gene [114].

6. Differential contribution of mitochondria towards LVNC

6.1 Mitochondrial DNA (mtDNA) mutations leading to dysmorphic mitochondria

mtDNA sequence variants are maternally inherited point mutations representing a predominate cause of inherited diseases within a tissue or organ. Studies performed on mitochondria isolated from patient's blood and *in vivo* cardiac tissues acknowledged the contribution of mtDNA mutations in the formation of cardiac noncompaction [115, 116]. In these studies, instability of cardiac-specific mtDNA is coupled to metabolic irregularities that impact cardiac functionality in response to a myriad of mitochondrial dysfunctions. Liu et al. [116] determined that hearts with noncompaction present with mitochondrial structural anomalies and have a reduced mtDNA copy number with the G4.5 gene on Xq28 that codes for acyltransferase tafazzin (TAZ); the first gene to be studied in detail in relation to the etiology of LVNC [117]. Tafazzin is a mitochondrial membrane component vital for proper functioning of the electron transport chain. This X-linked TAZ gene encodes for the mitochondrial membrane-associated phospholipid-modifying enzyme that alters cardiolipin through the addition of linoleic acid. As cardiolipin is a major player in the mitochondrial inner membrane and is requisite for the maintenance of mitochondrial shape, protein transport, and energy production within cells, it is essential for maintaining the organization of mitochondrial cristae [57]. TAZ gene mutations resulting in Bath Syndrome, perturbed mitochondrial cardiolipin metabolism and are associated with dilated cardiomyopathy. Inactivation of the TAZ gene produces dysfunctional tafazzin proteins. In this circumstance, linoleic acid is not present to alter cardiolipin. As a result, problems with normal mitochondrial shape and functions such as energy production and protein transport develop. High energy-demanding tissues including heart are more susceptible to cell death due to decreased mitochondrial energy production [118]. Furthermore, TAZ deficiency impairs cardiolipin remodeling and alters the assembly and stability of mitochondrial super complexes of complex III and IV (intermittently impacting complex V as well) in the inner mitochondrial membrane [119].

These effects occasionally result in respiratory chain activity malfunctions. Mitochondrial transcription factor A (TFAM) is a nuclear-encoded protein that regulates the transcription, packaging, and stability of the mitochondrial genome. TFAM is crucial for the development and differentiation of the mitochondrial genome [120]. It is highly likely that TFAM regulates the mtDNA copy number by binding to the mtDNA promoter region to initiate transcription. Thus, the impact of TFAM on mtDNA copy number illustrates the direct influence of TFAM in mitochondrial function. Carnitine palmitoyl transferases (CPT) are mitochondrial enzymes involved in the transportation of Acyl-CoA to the mitochondrial Matrix for β-oxidation. Located in the outer mitochondrial membrane, CPT I convert fatty acyl CoA into fatty acylcarnitine. Located in the inner mitochondrial membrane, CPT II reconverts fatty acylcarnitine into free carnitine and fatty acyl CoA for β-oxidation for energy generation. Inherited defects in CPT I, II or CPT translocases can result in failure of long-chain fatty acids transportation into the mitochondria for oxidation. This can result in a significant reduction in the ratio of free CoA to acyl CoA thus ultimately disrupting metabolic pathways and decreasing cardiac ATP production [24].

6.2 Mitochondrial dynamics and dysfunction

Adult cardiomyocytes are enriched with hypo-dynamic mitochondria that lack an interconnected reticular network. The fusion-fission cycle of cardiac mitochondria is common in cardiomyocyte mitochondrial dynamics [121]. Regulated by specialized proteins, enzymes, and adapter proteins that physically alter mitochondrial membranes, a delicate balance between mitochondrial fusion and mitochondrial fission is important in the regulation of cellular health. In adult cardiomyocytes progressive mitochondrial fission and fusion cycles occur frequently with the aid of proteins needed for the mitochondrial network remodeling. The key aspects of mitochondrial dynamics can be studied with cardiac-specific ablation of mitochondrial fission and fusion protein genes. As the cardiomyocyte mitochondria exhibit a certain degree of dynamism [122, 123], inability for the fusion or fission process could result in smaller or enlarged mitochondria, respectively. Hence, the imbalance between constant ongoing process of fusion and fission cycle are associated with increased caspases activity and subsequent cell death.

Mitochondrial dysfunction is frequently interrelated with LV noncompaction. Primary mitochondrial dysfunction arises from mutations in mitochondrial proteins involved with OXPHOS. Mitochondrial dysfunction refines mitochondrial dynamics with this phenomenon being associated with a variety of cardiac pathologies. For example, the MYH7 coding myosin protein is associated with the structure and function of cardiac sarcomere. Besides, the mutations in MYH7 linked with HCM and LVNC, makes myosin an important protein in cardiac function as defects in MYH7 expression are a common cause of cardiomyopathy [79]. Friedreich's ataxia (FRDA) is an example of a heart disease arising from mitochondrial dysfunction. FRDA is caused by the trinucleotide GAA expansion in the first intron of FXN gene (codes for mitochondrial matrix iron chaperone protein, frataxin) [123] with this triplet expansion resulting in transcription silencing and diminished frataxin expression. As a result, this mitochondrial localized protein influences iron homeostasis and respiratory control. Therefore, impaired FXN gene function in FRDA patients is associated with dysfunctional ETC complexes, specifically the complex III with high ROS levels suggesting altered mitochondrial function [124].

6.3 Mitochondrial metabolic myopathy resulting from respiratory chain complex deficiency

Mitochondrial cardiomyopathy, a distinct myocardial condition is denoted by improper cardiac muscle structure and function accompanied by genetic defects in the mitochondrial respiratory chain. Various genetic anomalies are detected in genes regulating mitochondrial activities or in genes coding for ETC complexes or in genes that code for proteins necessary in assembling and transporting.

Peroxisomal adenine nucleotide transporter-1 and 2 (ANT-1 and ANT-2) in humans are ADP/ATP carriers with two main functions; to catalyze mitochondrial-cytosol ATP/ADP exchange and regulation of the mitochondrial inner membrane mitochondrial permeability transition pore (mtPTP). The ATN-1 isoform influencing the mtPTP towards a more open state while ATN-2 is involved in the guiding the closure of the mtPTP. Within the heart, muscles, and brain ANT-1 is the predominant isoform while the second isoform ANT-2 is expressed systemically. However, ablation of ANT-1 isoform does not impair fetal development; but does result in hypertrophic cardiomyopathy in the postnatal period. In contrast, a study published in 2016 by Kokoszka et al. [125] identified the embryonic lethality of ANT-2 null mutations to be associated with a distinct cardiac developmental defect consistent with LVNC/LVHT; characterized by swollen mitochondria in cardiomyocytes and hyperproliferating cardiomyocytes. In these studies, mice with ANT-2 mutations, cardiac maturation progresses during embryonic days E9.5 and E13.5. However, by day E14.5 mice exhibit embryonic lethality. Histologic analysis of the heart revealed hyper-proliferating cardiomyocytes, decreased apoptosis, and swollen mitochondria with few cristae, and mtPTP open for transport. These findings suggest that loss of ANT-2 regulation of mtPTP closure results in cardiomyocytes maintenance in an immature state with a reduction in total number of contractile fibers and loss of organization thus paving the way for the continued immature cardiomyocyte proliferation resulting in LVNC and embryonic lethality [37].

6.4 Mitochondrial genome mutations in LVNC

In most of the reported cases, LVNC is related to the alterations in nuclear DNA encoded mitochondrial genes. Defects in the mediator of a mitochondrial fusion protein, Mitofusins 1 & 2 (MFN 1 & 2) affect the mitochondrial morphology during embryogenesis. Mediated by MFN1 and 2, mitochondrial fusion facilitates the exchange between the contents of mitochondrial membrane and matrix to help in maintaining the mitochondrial function. Mutations in any of the MFN's results in mitochondrial fragmentation that affects the symmetry of fusion and fission events [126]. As cell apoptosis is significantly influenced by the mitochondrial fusion and fission, cells lacking apoptosis related genes such as caspases 3, 7, 8, FADD, and c-FLIP are also susceptible to develop cardiac noncompaction. Caspases 3 and 7 are potential regulators of mitochondrial apoptosis. A3243G transition in tRNALeu(UUR) gene is another common mitochondrial mutation [127, 128].

The tRNALeu(UUR) gene encodes for mitochondrial transfer ribonucleic acid (tRNA) for leucine (tRNALeu) and this nucleotide alteration was studied in both HCM and LVNC [129]. Other studies show that A3243G mutation related disorders cause alterations in nearly 56 different genes, thus having a broad spectrum of impact. The A to G transition at the 3243rd position in tRNALeu (UUR) gene results in diminished glucose oxidation rate, NADH response, and mitochondrial membrane potential that ultimately affects ATP production [127, 130]. Lastly, a A8381G transition in ATPase subunit 8 genes (ATPase 8) was observed in a patient having LVNC complications [43, 102, 115]. These arising missense mutations impact within the ETC complex V that could alter the ATPase complex stability, directing to reduced ATP production [43, 131].

6.5 Mitochondrial DNA transitions in LVNC

Single mutations arising from mtDNA transitions are responsible for an abnormal diseased phenotype. mtDNA transitions mutations occur when there is a replacement of the complementary nucleotide (A replaced with G, T replaced with C and vice versa). One example is found in the mitochondrially encoded NADH: ubiquinone oxidoreductase core subunit 1 (mt-ND1) encoding gene for the NADH dehydrogenase 1 enzyme that is part of complex ETC complex I, which is active in mitochondria. Here, a single nucleotide transition (T → C) at a highly conserved nucleotide position (T3398C) is within the region of the *ND1* gene of the mt genome. This particular mtDNA transition results in the conversion of methionine to threonine at the 31st amino acid position was identified in patients suffering from cardiomyopathy [39]. A case report presented by Finsterer et al. [40] investigated the combination of A → G transition at the nucleotide position of 15,662 in novel mitochondrial cytochrome B and three of the known mutations (T3398C, T4216C, G15812A) in *ND1* gene. These above-mentioned mutations were found to be in association with left ventricular hyper trabeculation and some clinical conditions. Later studies determined that a homoplasmic A → G transition at the nucleotide position of 8381 in the ATPase8 gene, investigated by Finsterer et al. [129] resulted in an amino acid substitution of alanine to threonine. Their findings revealed the correlation of LVNC with A8381G mtDNA transition that develop later in adulthood.

6.6 Mutations in overlapping regions in LVNC

The ETC complex V, known as ATP synthase, is made up of 13 protein subunits. Two of the gene mutations in mitochondrial genome or the nuclear genes result in complex V deficiency. The mitochondrial-encoded protein subunits of complex V, ATPase 6, and ATPase 8 overlap in the mitochondrial genome and undergo polycistronic fashion of transcription. The nucleotide position 8528 is within the overlapping region that codes for ATPase 6 and ATPase 8 subunits. The phenotypic representation of point mutation affects ATPase 6 and ATPase 8 genes of complex V. This is commonly seen in identical mitochondrial mtDNA mutations in children [42]. Here, the nucleotide alteration of m. T8528C, causes a M1T in the start codon in ATPase 6 subunit (One might expect to have alterations in the protein translation initiation. However, it has not been reported so far, thus making the function of altered ATPase 6 unclear) and W55R missense mutation in ATPase 8 subunit. Additionally, 2 other overlapping mutations in G8529A and C8558T affecting both the subunits have been reported in patients exhibiting cardiomyopathies [101, 115, 132]. This kind of overlapping pathogenic mutations could cause reduced ATP synthesis by affecting mitochondrial energy production and complex I, II and III for which the mechanism is still unknown [42].

7. Conclusion

This review overlays the aspects of gene mutations relevant to mitochondrial energetics, cardiomyocyte function, and LV myocardial noncompaction. Understanding the rudimentary causes of LVNC imparts helpful information in the prognostic evaluation and early diagnosis of LV noncompaction. Further examination of mitochondrial involvement in cardiac noncompaction leading to heart failure would facilitate advances in the therapeutic treatment of this disease process.

Author details

Gowthami Mahendran[1,2] and Margaret A. Schwarz[1,2,3]*

1 Harper Cancer Research Institute, United States

2 Department of Chemistry and Biochemistry, University of Notre Dame, United States

3 Departments of Pediatrics and Anatomy, Cell Biology and Physiology, Indiana University, South Bend, Indiana, United States

*Address all correspondence to: schwarma@iu.edu

References

[1] Grant RP. The embryology of ventricular flow pathways in man. Circulation. 1962;**25**:756-779

[2] Krishnan A, Samtani R, Dhanantwari P, Lee E, Yamada S, Shiota K, et al. A detailed comparison of mouse and human cardiac development. Pediatric Research. 2014;**76**(6):500-507

[3] Dhanantwari P, Lee E, Krishnan A, Samtani R, Yamada S, Anderson S, et al. Human cardiac development in the first trimester: A high-resolution magnetic resonance imaging and episcopic fluorescence image capture atlas. Circulation. 2009;**120**(4):343-351

[4] Tan CMJ, Lewandowski AJ. The transitional heart: From early embryonic and fetal development to neonatal life. Fetal Diagnosis and Therapy. 2020;**47**(5):373-386

[5] Zhang W, Chen H, Qu X, Chang CP, Shou W. Molecular mechanism of ventricular trabeculation/compaction and the pathogenesis of the left ventricular noncompaction cardiomyopathy (LVNC). American Journal of Medical Genetics. Part C, Seminars in Medical Genetics. 2013;**163C**(3):144-156

[6] Sedmera D, Pexieder T, Hu N, Clark EB. A quantitative study of the ventricular myoarchitecture in the stage 21-29 chick embryo following decreased loading. European Journal of Morphology. 1998;**36**(2):105-119

[7] Samsa LA, Yang B, Liu J. Embryonic cardiac chamber maturation: Trabeculation, conduction, and cardiomyocyte proliferation. American Journal of Medical Genetics. Part C, Seminars in Medical Genetics. 2013;**163C**(3):157-168

[8] Keren A, Billingham ME, Popp RL. Echocardiographic recognition and implications of ventricular hypertrophic trabeculations and aberrant bands. Circulation. 1984;**70**(5):836-842

[9] Ho SY, Nihoyannopoulos P. Anatomy, echocardiography, and normal right ventricular dimensions. Heart. 2006;**92**(Suppl 1):i2-i13

[10] Kruithof BP, Kruithof-De-Julio M, Poelmann RE, Gittenberger-De-Groot AC, Gaussin V, Goumans MJ. Remodeling of the myocardium in early trabeculation and cardiac valve formation; a role for TGFbeta2. The International Journal of Developmental Biology. 2013;**57**(11-12):853-863

[11] Wengrofsky P, Armenia C, Oleszak F, Kupferstein E, Rednam C, Mitre CA, et al. Left ventricular trabeculation and noncompaction cardiomyopathy: A review. EC Clinical and Experimental Anatomy. 2019;**2**(6):267-283

[12] Vaidya VR, Lyle M, Miranda WR, Farwati M, Isath A, Patlolla SH, et al. Long-term survival of patients with left ventricular noncompaction. Journal of the American Heart Association. 2021;**10**(2):e015563

[13] Goud A, Padmanabhan S. A rare form of cardiomyopathy: Left ventricular non-compaction cardiomyopathy. Journal of Community Hospital Internal Medicine Perspectives. 2016;**6**(1):29888

[14] Stollberger C, Finsterer J, Blazek G. Left ventricular hypertrabeculation/noncompaction and association with

additional cardiac abnormalities and neuromuscular disorders. The American Journal of Cardiology. 2002;**90**(8):899-902

[15] Towbin JA. Left ventricular noncompaction: A new form of heart failure. Heart Failure Clinics. 2010;**6**(4):453-469 viii

[16] Towbin JA, Jefferies JL. Cardiomyopathies due to left ventricular noncompaction, mitochondrial and storage diseases, and inborn errors of metabolism. Circulation Research. 2017;**121**(7):838-854

[17] St-Pierre G, Steinberg C, Dubois M, Senechal M. What the cardiologist should know about mitochondrial cardiomyopathy? The Canadian Journal of Cardiology. 2019;**35**(2):221-224

[18] Greenwell AA, Gopal K, Ussher JR. Myocardial energy metabolism in non-ischemic cardiomyopathy. Frontiers in Physiology. 2020;**11**:570421

[19] Guclu A, Knaapen P, Harms HJ, Parbhudayal RY, Michels M, Lammertsma AA, et al. Disease stage-dependent changes in cardiac contractile performance and oxygen utilization underlie reduced myocardial efficiency in human inherited hypertrophic cardiomyopathy. Circulation: Cardiovascular Imaging. May 2017;**10**(5):e005604. DOI: 10.1161/CIRCIMAGING.116.005604

[20] Taanman JW. The mitochondrial genome: Structure, transcription, translation and replication. Biochimica et Biophysica Acta. 1999;**1410**(2):103-123

[21] Saada A, Bar-Meir M, Belaiche C, Miller C, Elpeleg O. Evaluation of enzymatic assays and compounds affecting ATP production in mitochondrial respiratory chain complex I deficiency. Analytical Biochemistry. 2004;**335**(1):66-72

[22] Tuppen HA, Blakely EL, Turnbull DM, Taylor RW. Mitochondrial DNA mutations and human disease. Biochimica et Biophysica Acta. 2010;**1797**(2):113-128

[23] Giorgi C, Agnoletto C, Bononi A, Bonora M, De Marchi E, Marchi S, et al. Mitochondrial calcium homeostasis as potential target for mitochondrial medicine. Mitochondrion. 2012;**12**(1):77-85

[24] Winter SC, Buist NR. Cardiomyopathy in childhood, mitochondrial dysfunction, and the role of L-carnitine. American Heart Journal. 2000;**139**(2 Pt 3):S63-S69

[25] McCormick EM, Muraresku CC, Falk MJ. Mitochondrial genomics: A complex field now coming of age. Current Genetic Medicine Reports. 2018;**6**(2):52-61

[26] Seppet EK, Eimre M, Anmann T, Seppet E, Peet N, Kaambre T, et al. Intracellular energetic units in healthy and diseased hearts. Experimental and Clinical Cardiology. 2005;**10**(3):173-183

[27] Reynen K, Bachmann K, Singer H. Spongy myocardium. Cardiology. 1997;**88**(6):601-602

[28] Engberding R, Bender F. Identification of a rare congenital anomaly of the myocardium by two-dimensional echocardiography: Persistence of isolated myocardial sinusoids. The American Journal of Cardiology. 1984;**53**(11):1733-1734

[29] Lipshultz SE, Law YM, Asante-Korang A, Austin ED, Dipchand AI, Everitt MD, et al. Cardiomyopathy in children: Classification and diagnosis: A

scientific statement from the American Heart Association. Circulation. 2019;**140**(1):e9-e68

[30] Aung N, Doimo S, Ricci F, Sanghvi MM, Pedrosa C, Woodbridge SP, et al. Prognostic significance of left ventricular noncompaction: Systematic review and meta-analysis of observational studies. Circulation: Cardiovascular Imaging. Jan 2020;**13**(1):e009712. DOI: 10.1161/CIRCIMAGING.119.009712

[31] Finsterer J, Stollberger C, Schubert B. Acquired left ventricular hypertrabeculation/noncompaction in mitochondriopathy. Cardiology. 2004;**102**(4):228-230

[32] Franz WM, Muller OJ, Katus HA. Cardiomyopathies: From genetics to the prospect of treatment. Lancet. 2001;**358**(9293):1627-1637

[33] Abbasi Y, Jabbari J, Jabbari R, Yang RQ, Risgaard B, Kober L, et al. The pathogenicity of genetic variants previously associated with left ventricular non-compaction. Molecular Genetics & Genomic Medicine. 2016;**4**(2):135-142

[34] Mazzarotto F, Hawley MH, Beltrami M, Beekman L, de Marvao A, McGurk KA, et al. Systematic large-scale assessment of the genetic architecture of left ventricular noncompaction reveals diverse etiologies. Genetics in Medicine. 2021;**23**(5):856-864

[35] Finsterer J, Harbo HF, Baets J, Van Broeckhoven C, Di Donato S, Fontaine B, et al. EFNS guidelines on the molecular diagnosis of mitochondrial disorders. European Journal of Neurology. 2009;**16**(12):1255-1264

[36] Scaglia F, Towbin JA, Craigen WJ, Belmont JW, Smith EO, Neish SR, et al. Clinical spectrum, morbidity, and mortality in 113 pediatric patients with mitochondrial disease. Pediatrics. 2004;**114**(4):925-931

[37] Kokoszka JE, Waymire KG, Flierl A, Sweeney KM, Angelin A, MacGregor GR, et al. Deficiency in the mouse mitochondrial adenine nucleotide translocator isoform 2 gene is associated with cardiac noncompaction. Biochimica et Biophysica Acta. 2016;**1857**(8):1203-1212

[38] Finsterer J, Obermann I, Milvay E. Diagnostic yield of the lactate stress test in 160 patients with suspected respiratory chain disorder. Metabolic Brain Disease. 2000;**15**(3):163-171

[39] Jaksch M, Hofmann S, Kaufhold P, Obermaier-Kusser B, Zierz S, Gerbitz KD. A novel combination of mitochondrial tRNA and ND1 gene mutations in a syndrome with MELAS, cardiomyopathy, and diabetes mellitus. Human Mutation. 1996;7(4):358-360

[40] Finsterer J, Bittner R, Bodingbauer M, Eichberger H, Stollberger C, Blazek G. Complex mitochondriopathy associated with 4 mtDNA transitions. European Neurology. 2000;**44**(1):37-41

[41] Pignatelli RH, McMahon CJ, Dreyer WJ, Denfield SW, Price J, Belmont JW, et al. Clinical characterization of left ventricular noncompaction in children: A relatively common form of cardiomyopathy. Circulation. 2003;**108**(21):2672-2678

[42] Ware SM, El-Hassan N, Kahler SG, Zhang Q, Ma YW, Miller E, et al. Infantile cardiomyopathy caused by a mutation in the overlapping region of mitochondrial ATPase 6 and 8 genes. Journal of Medical Genetics. 2009;**46**(5):308-314

[43] Perucca-Lostanlen D, Narbonne H, Hernandez JB, Staccini P, Saunieres A, Paquis-Flucklinger V, et al. Mitochondrial DNA variations in patients with maternally inherited diabetes and deafness syndrome. Biochemical and Biophysical Research Communications. 2000;**277**(3):771-775

[44] Udeoji DU, Philip KJ, Morrissey RP, Phan A, Schwarz ER. Left ventricular noncompaction cardiomyopathy: Updated review. Therapeutic Advances in Cardiovascular Disease. 2013;**7**(5):260-273

[45] Morales-Arraez D, Ventura-Cots M, Altamirano J, Abraldes JG, Cruz-Lemini M, Thursz MR, et al. Correction to: The MELD score is superior to the Maddrey discriminant function score to predict short-term mortality in alcohol-associated hepatitis: A global study. American Journal of Gastroenterology. 2022;**117**(5):818

[46] Cincinnati Children's. Available from: https://www.cincinnatichildrens.org/service/c/cardiomyopathy/types/left-ventricular-non-compaction-cardiomyopathy [Accessed: 12 August]

[47] Bennett CE, Freudenberger R. The current approach to diagnosis and management of left ventricular noncompaction cardiomyopathy: Review of the literature. Cardiology Research and Practice. 2016;**2016**:5172308

[48] Jenni R, Oechslin E, Schneider J, Attenhofer Jost C, Kaufmann PA. Echocardiographic and pathoanatomical characteristics of isolated left ventricular non-compaction: A step towards classification as a distinct cardiomyopathy. Heart. 2001;**86**(6):666-671

[49] Tian T, Liu Y, Gao L, Wang J, Sun K, Zou Y, et al. Isolated left ventricular noncompaction: Clinical profile and prognosis in 106 adult patients. Heart and Vessels. 2014;**29**(5):645-652

[50] Agarwal A, Khandheria BK, Paterick TE, Treiber SC, Bush M, Tajik AJ. Left ventricular noncompaction in patients with bicuspid aortic valve. Journal of the American Society of Echocardiography. 2013;**26**(11):1306-1313

[51] Borresen MF, Blixenkrone-Moller E, Kock TO, Sillesen AS, Vogg ROB, Pihl CA, et al. Prevalence of left ventricular noncompaction in newborns. Circulation: Cardiovascular Imaging. 2022;**15**(6):e014159

[52] Ross SB, Barratt A, Semsarian C. Time to reconsider the diagnosis of "left ventricular noncompaction" in adults? Heart, Lung & Circulation. 2022;**31**(3):301-303

[53] Gleeson TG, Mwangi I, Horgan SJ, Cradock A, Fitzpatrick P, Murray JG. Steady-state free-precession (SSFP) cine MRI in distinguishing normal and bicuspid aortic valves. Journal of Magnetic Resonance Imaging. 2008;**28**(4):873-878

[54] Paluszkiewicz J, Milting H, Kaluzna-Oleksy M, Pyda M, Janus M, Korperich H, et al. Left ventricular non-compaction cardiomyopathy-still more questions than answers. Journal of Clinical Medicine. 16 Jul 2022;**11**(14):4135. DOI: 10.3390/jcm11144135

[55] Prevention Genetics. Available from: https://www.preventiongenetics.com/testInfo?val=Left-Ventricular-Noncompaction-%28LVNC%29-Panel [Accessed August 12]

[56] Jackson MJ, Schaefer JA, Johnson MA, Morris AA, Turnbull DM, Bindoff LA. Presentation and clinical

investigation of mitochondrial respiratory chain disease. A study of 51 patients. Brain. 1995;**118**(Pt 2):339-357

[57] Meyers DE, Basha HI, Koenig MK. Mitochondrial cardiomyopathy: Pathophysiology, diagnosis, and management. Texas Heart Institute Journal. 2013;**40**(4):385-394

[58] Kimura M, Kawano K, Yaoita H, Kure S. Successful treatment of an infant with left ventricular noncompaction presenting with fatal ventricular arrhythmia treated with cardiac resynchronization therapy and an implantable cardioverter defibrillator. Case Reports in Cardiology. 2018;**2018**:1-5

[59] Chin TK, Perloff JK, Williams RG, Jue K, Mohrmann R. Isolated noncompaction of left ventricular myocardium. A study of eight cases. Circulation. 1990;**82**(2):507-513

[60] Lofiego C, Biagini E, Ferlito M, Pasquale F, Rocchi G, Perugini E, et al. Paradoxical contributions of non-compacted and compacted segments to global left ventricular dysfunction in isolated left ventricular noncompaction. The American Journal of Cardiology. 2006;**97**(5):738-741

[61] Tamborini G, Pepi M, Celeste F, Muratori M, Susini F, Maltagliati A, et al. Incidence and characteristics of left ventricular false tendons and trabeculations in the normal and pathologic heart by second harmonic echocardiography. Journal of the American Society of Echocardiography. 2004;**17**(4):367-374

[62] Cevik C, Stainback RF. Isolated left ventricular noncompaction in a 90-year-old man. Texas Heart Institute Journal. 2012;**39**(2):255-257

[63] Alehan D. Clinical features of isolated left ventricular noncompaction in children. International Journal of Cardiology. 2004;**97**(2):233-237

[64] Stollberger C, Blazek G, Winkler-Dworak M, Finsterer J. Sex differences in left ventricular noncompaction in patients with and without neuromuscular disorders. Revista Española de Cardiología. 2008;**61**(2):130-136

[65] Miller EM, Hinton RB, Czosek R, Lorts A, Parrott A, Shikany AR, et al. Genetic testing in pediatric left ventricular noncompaction. Circulation: Cardiovascular Genetics. Dec 2017;**10**(6):e001735. DOI: 10.1161/CIRCGENETICS.117.001735

[66] Lin YN, Wang YQ, Yu Y, Cao Q, Wang F, Chen SY. Left ventricular noncompaction cardiomyopathy: A case report and literature review. International Journal of Clinical and Experimental Medicine. 2014;**7**(12):5130-5133

[67] Tian J, Uddin A, Akhrass P. Left ventricular noncompaction: A rare case of nonischemic cardiomyopathy. Case Reports in Cardiology. 2019;**2019**:5637638

[68] Burke A, Mont E, Kutys R, Virmani R. Left ventricular noncompaction: A pathological study of 14 cases. Human Pathology. 2005;**36**(4):403-411

[69] Toader D, Paraschiv A, Tudorascu P, Tudorascu D, Bataiosu C, Balseanu A. Left ventricular noncompaction-a rare cause of triad: Heart failure, ventricular arrhythmias, and systemic embolic events: A case report. Journal of Medical Case Reports. 2021;**15**(1):316

[70] Loria V, Colizzi C, Vaccarella M, Franceschi F, Aspromonte N. Left ventricular noncompaction: Cause or

consequence of myocardial disease? A case report and literature review. Cardiology. 2019;**143**(3-4):100-104

[71] Ayesha B, Ahmed R, Gomceli U, Manrique C, Nicu M, Chilimuri S. A case of isolated left ventricular non-compaction cardiomyopathy in a HIV patient presenting with acute heart failure. Cardiology Research. 2019;**10**(4):236-240

[72] Bath AS, Aggarwal S, Gupta V, Kalavakunta JK. A case of left ventricular noncompaction presenting as atrial fibrillation. Cureus. 2019;**11**(3):e4309

[73] Kalavakunta JK, Tokala H, Gosavi A, Gupta V. Left ventricular noncompaction and myocardial fibrosis: A case report. International Archives of Medicine. 2010;**3**:20

[74] Shieh JT. Implications of genetic testing in noncompaction/hypertrabeculation. American Journal of Medical Genetics. Part C, Seminars in Medical Genetics. 2013;**163C**(3):206-211

[75] Klaassen S, Probst S, Oechslin E, Gerull B, Krings G, Schuler P, et al. Mutations in sarcomere protein genes in left ventricular noncompaction. Circulation. 2008;**117**(22):2893-2901

[76] Ichida F, Tsubata S, Bowles KR, Haneda N, Uese K, Miyawaki T, et al. Novel gene mutations in patients with left ventricular noncompaction or Barth syndrome. Circulation. 2001;**103**(9):1256-1263

[77] Shou W, Aghdasi B, Armstrong DL, Guo Q, Bao S, Charng MJ, et al. Cardiac defects and altered ryanodine receptor function in mice lacking FKBP12. Nature. 1998;**391**(6666):489-492

[78] Luxan G, Casanova JC, Martinez-Poveda B, Prados B, D'Amato G, MacGrogan D, et al. Mutations in the NOTCH pathway regulator MIB1 cause left ventricular noncompaction cardiomyopathy. Nature Medicine. 2013;**19**(2):193-201

[79] Hoedemaekers YM, Cohen-Overbeek TE, Frohn-Mulder IM, Dooijes D, Majoor-Krakauer DF. Prenatal ultrasound diagnosis of MYH7 non-compaction cardiomyopathy. Ultrasound in Obstetrics & Gynecology. 2013;**41**(3):336-339

[80] Frustaci A, De Luca A, Guida V, Biagini T, Mazza T, Gaudio C, et al. Novel alpha-actin gene mutation p.(Ala21Val) causing familial hypertrophic cardiomyopathy, myocardial noncompaction, and transmural crypts. Clinical-pathologic correlation. Journal of the American Heart Association. 10 Feb 2018;**7**(4):e008068. DOI: 10.1161/JAHA.117.008068

[81] Luedde M, Ehlermann P, Weichenhan D, Will R, Zeller R, Rupp S, et al. Severe familial left ventricular non-compaction cardiomyopathy due to a novel troponin T (TNNT2) mutation. Cardiovascular Research. 2010;**86**(3):452-460

[82] Liu Z, Shan H, Huang J, Li N, Hou C, Pu J. A novel lamin A/C gene missense mutation (445 V > E) in immunoglobulin-like fold associated with left ventricular non-compaction. Europace. 2016;**18**(4):617-622

[83] Xing Y, Ichida F, Matsuoka T, Isobe T, Ikemoto Y, Higaki T, et al. Genetic analysis in patients with left ventricular noncompaction and evidence for genetic heterogeneity. Molecular Genetics and Metabolism. 2006;**88**(1):71-77

[84] Ma L, Vaz FM, Gu Z, Wanders RJ, Greenberg ML. The human TAZ gene

complements mitochondrial dysfunction in the yeast taz1Delta mutant. Implications for Barth syndrome. The Journal of Biological Chemistry. 2004;**279**(43):44394-44399

[85] Van Driest SL, Vasile VC, Ommen SR, Will ML, Tajik AJ, Gersh BJ, et al. Myosin binding protein C mutations and compound heterozygosity in hypertrophic cardiomyopathy. Journal of the American College of Cardiology. 2004;**44**(9):1903-1910

[86] Kimura A, Harada H, Park JE, Nishi H, Satoh M, Takahashi M, et al. Mutations in the cardiac troponin I gene associated with hypertrophic cardiomyopathy. Nature Genetics. 1997;**16**(4):379-382

[87] Nishino I, Fu J, Tanji K, Yamada T, Shimojo S, Koori T, et al. Primary LAMP-2 deficiency causes X-linked vacuolar cardiomyopathy and myopathy (Danon disease). Nature. 2000;**406**(6798):906-910

[88] Milano A, Vermeer AM, Lodder EM, Barc J, Verkerk AO, Postma AV, et al. HCN4 mutations in multiple families with bradycardia and left ventricular noncompaction cardiomyopathy. Journal of the American College of Cardiology. 2014;**64**(8):745-756

[89] Shan L, Makita N, Xing Y, Watanabe S, Futatani T, Ye F, et al. SCN5A variants in Japanese patients with left ventricular noncompaction and arrhythmia. Molecular Genetics and Metabolism. 2008;**93**(4):468-474

[90] Gifford CA, Ranade SS, Samarakoon R, Salunga HT, de Soysa TY, Huang Y, et al. Oligogenic inheritance of a human heart disease involving a genetic modifier. Science. 2019;**364**(6443):865-870

[91] Chen H, Zhang W, Sun X, Yoshimoto M, Chen Z, Zhu W, et al. Fkbp1a controls ventricular myocardium trabeculation and compaction by regulating endocardial Notch1 activity. Development. 2013;**140**(9):1946-1957

[92] Hirono K, Saito K, Munkhsaikhan U, Xu F, Wang C, Lu L, et al. Familial left ventricular non-compaction is associated with a rare p.V407I variant in bone morphogenetic protein 10. Circulation Journal. 2019;**83**(8):1737-1746

[93] Vatta M, Mohapatra B, Jimenez S, Sanchez X, Faulkner G, Perles Z, et al. Mutations in Cypher/ZASP in patients with dilated cardiomyopathy and left ventricular non-compaction. Journal of the American College of Cardiology. 2003;**42**(11):2014-2027

[94] Schultze-Berndt A, Kuhnisch J, Herbst C, Seidel F, Al-Wakeel-Marquard N, Dartsch J, et al. Reduced systolic function and not genetic variants determine outcome in pediatric and adult left ventricular noncompaction cardiomyopathy. Frontiers in Pediatrics. 2021;**9**:722926

[95] Armel TZ, Leinwand LA. Mutations in the beta-myosin rod cause myosin storage myopathy via multiple mechanisms. Proceedings of the National Academy of Sciences of the United States of America. 2009;**106**(15):6291-6296

[96] Arbustini E, Favalli V, Narula N, Serio A, Grasso M. Left ventricular noncompaction: A distinct genetic cardiomyopathy? Journal of the American College of Cardiology. 2016;**68**(9):949-966

[97] Monserrat L, Hermida-Prieto M, Fernandez X, Rodriguez I, Dumont C, Cazon L, et al. Mutation in the alpha-cardiac actin gene associated with apical hypertrophic cardiomyopathy,

left ventricular non-compaction, and septal defects. European Heart Journal. 2007;**28**(16):1953-1961

[98] Parent JJ, Towbin JA, Jefferies JL. Left ventricular noncompaction in a family with lamin A/C gene mutation. Texas Heart Institute Journal. 2015;**42**(1):73-76

[99] Mogensen J, Kruse TA, Borglum AD. Assignment of the human cardiac troponin I gene (TNNI3) to chromosome 19q13.4 by radiation hybrid mapping. Cytogenetics and Cell Genetics. 1997;**79**(3-4):272-273

[100] Muntoni F, Bonne G, Goldfarb LG, Mercuri E, Piercy RJ, Burke M, et al. Disease severity in dominant Emery Dreifuss is increased by mutations in both emerin and desmin proteins. Brain. 2006;**129**(Pt 5):1260-1268

[101] Dautant A, Meier T, Hahn A, Tribouillard-Tanvier D, di Rago JP, Kucharczyk R. ATP synthase diseases of mitochondrial genetic origin. Frontiers in Physiology. 2018;**9**:329

[102] Finsterer J, Stollberger C, Steger C, Cozzarini W. Complete heart block associated with noncompaction, nail-patella syndrome, and mitochondrial myopathy. Journal of Electrocardiology. 2007;**40**(4):352-354

[103] Dorner A, Giessen S, Gaub R, Grosse Siestrup H, Schwimmbeck PL, Hetzer R, et al. An isoform shift in the cardiac adenine nucleotide translocase expression alters the kinetic properties of the carrier in dilated cardiomyopathy. European Journal of Heart Failure. 2006;**8**(1):81-89

[104] Arndt AK, Schafer S, Drenckhahn JD, Sabeh MK, Plovie ER, Caliebe A, et al. Fine mapping of the 1p36 deletion syndrome identifies mutation of PRDM16 as a cause of cardiomyopathy. American Journal of Human Genetics. 2013;**93**(1):67-77

[105] Bolling MC, Pas HH, de Visser M, Aronica E, Pfendner EG, van den Berg MP, et al. PLEC1 mutations underlie adult-onset dilated cardiomyopathy in epidermolysis bullosa simplex with muscular dystrophy. The Journal of Investigative Dermatology. 2010;**130**(4):1178-1181

[106] Girolami F, Iascone M, Tomberli B, Bardi S, Benelli M, Marseglia G, et al. Novel alpha-actinin 2 variant associated with familial hypertrophic cardiomyopathy and juvenile atrial arrhythmias: A massively parallel sequencing study. Circulation. Cardiovascular Genetics. 2014;**7**(6):741-750

[107] Lang T, Yu L, Tu Q, Jiang J, Chen Z, Xin Y, et al. Molecular cloning, genomic organization, and mapping of PRKAG2, a heart abundant gamma2 subunit of 5'-AMP-activated protein kinase, to human chromosome 7q36. Genomics. 2000;**70**(2):258-263

[108] Schmitt JP, Kamisago M, Asahi M, Li GH, Ahmad F, Mende U, et al. Dilated cardiomyopathy and heart failure caused by a mutation in phospholamban. Science. 2003;**299**(5611):1410-1413

[109] Haghighi K, Kolokathis F, Pater L, Lynch RA, Asahi M, Gramolini AO, et al. Human phospholamban null results in lethal dilated cardiomyopathy revealing a critical difference between mouse and human. The Journal of Clinical Investigation. 2003;**111**(6):869-876

[110] Dellefave LM, Pytel P, Mewborn S, Mora B, Guris DL, Fedson S, et al. Sarcomere mutations in cardiomyopathy with left

ventricular hypertrabeculation. Circulation. Cardiovascular Genetics. 2009;**2**(5):442-449

[111] Fiorillo C, Astrea G, Savarese M, Cassandrini D, Brisca G, Trucco F, et al. MYH7-related myopathies: Clinical, histopathological and imaging findings in a cohort of Italian patients. Orphanet Journal of Rare Diseases. 2016;**11**(1):91

[112] Hasegawa H, Komuro I. Mutations in sarcomere protein genes as a cause of heart failure. Nihon Rinsho. 2007;**65**(Suppl 4):267-272

[113] D'Amato G, Luxan G, de la Pompa JL. Notch signalling in ventricular chamber development and cardiomyopathy. The FEBS Journal. 2016;**283**(23):4223-4237

[114] Finsterer J, Stollberger C, Fazio G. Neuromuscular disorders in left ventricular hypertrabeculation/noncompaction. Current Pharmaceutical Design. 2010;**16**(26):2895-2904

[115] Tang S, Batra A, Zhang Y, Ebenroth ES, Huang T. Left ventricular noncompaction is associated with mutations in the mitochondrial genome. Mitochondrion. 2010;**10**(4):350-357

[116] Liu S, Bai Y, Huang J, Zhao H, Zhang X, Hu S, et al. Do mitochondria contribute to left ventricular non-compaction cardiomyopathy? New findings from myocardium of patients with left ventricular non-compaction cardiomyopathy. Molecular Genetics and Metabolism. 2013;**109**(1):100-106

[117] Bleyl SB, Mumford BR, Brown-Harrison MC, Pagotto LT, Carey JC, Pysher TJ, et al. Xq28-linked noncompaction of the left ventricular myocardium: Prenatal diagnosis and pathologic analysis of affected individuals. American Journal of Medical Genetics. 1997;**72**(3):257-265

[118] Saric A, Andreau K, Armand AS, Moller IM, Petit PX. Barth syndrome: From mitochondrial dysfunctions associated with aberrant production of reactive oxygen species to pluripotent stem cell studies. Frontiers in Genetics. 2015;**6**:359

[119] Karkucinska-Wieckowska A, Trubicka J, Werner B, Kokoszynska K, Pajdowska M, Pronicki M, et al. Left ventricular noncompaction (LVNC) and low mitochondrial membrane potential are specific for Barth syndrome. Journal of Inherited Metabolic Disease. 2013;**36**(6):929-937

[120] Hsieh YT, Tu HF, Yang MH, Chen YF, Lan XY, Huang CL, et al. Mitochondrial genome and its regulator TFAM modulates head and neck tumourigenesis through intracellular metabolic reprogramming and activation of oncogenic effectors. Cell Death & Disease. 2021;**12**(11):961

[121] Westermann B. Bioenergetic role of mitochondrial fusion and fission. Biochimica et Biophysica Acta. 2012;**1817**(10):1833-1838

[122] Otera H, Mihara K. Molecular mechanisms and physiologic functions of mitochondrial dynamics. Journal of Biochemistry. 2011;**149**(3):241-251

[123] Dorn GW 2nd. Mitochondrial dynamism and heart disease: Changing shape and shaping change. EMBO Molecular Medicine. 2015;**7**(7):865-877

[124] Rotig A, de Lonlay P, Chretien D, Foury F, Koenig M, Sidi D, et al. Aconitase and mitochondrial iron-sulphur protein deficiency in Friedreich ataxia. Nature Genetics. 1997;**17**(2):215-217

[125] Kokoszka JE, Waymire KG, Levy SE, Sligh JE, Cai J, Jones DP, et al. The ADP/

ATP translocator is not essential for the mitochondrial permeability transition pore. Nature. 2004;**427**(6973):461-465

[126] Chen H, Detmer SA, Ewald AJ, Griffin EE, Fraser SE, Chan DC. Mitofusins Mfn1 and Mfn2 coordinately regulate mitochondrial fusion and are essential for embryonic development. The Journal of Cell Biology. 2003;**160**(2):189-200

[127] Finsterer J. Genetic, pathogenetic, and phenotypic implications of the mitochondrial A3243G tRNALeu(UUR) mutation. Acta Neurologica Scandinavica. 2007;**116**(1):1-14

[128] Shanske S, Pancrudo J, Kaufmann P, Engelstad K, Jhung S, Lu J, et al. Varying loads of the mitochondrial DNA A3243G mutation in different tissues: Implications for diagnosis. American Journal of Medical Genetics. Part A. 2004;**130A**(2):134-137

[129] Finsterer J, Stollberger C, Wegmann R, Janssen LA. Acquired left ventricular hypertrabeculation/noncompaction in myotonic dystrophy type 1. International Journal of Cardiology. 2009;**137**(3):310-313

[130] de Andrade PB, Rubi B, Frigerio F, van den Ouweland JM, Maassen JA, Maechler P. Diabetes-associated mitochondrial DNA mutation A3243G impairs cellular metabolic pathways necessary for beta cell function. Diabetologia. 2006;**49**(8):1816-1826

[131] Mkaouar-Rebai E, Kammoun F, Chamkha I, Kammoun N, Hsairi I, Triki C, et al. A de novo mutation in the adenosine triphosphatase (ATPase) 8 gene in a patient with mitochondrial disorder. Journal of Child Neurology. 2010;**25**(6):770-775

[132] Jonckheere AI, Hogeveen M, Nijtmans LG, van den Brand MA, Janssen AJ, Diepstra JH, et al. A novel mitochondrial ATP8 gene mutation in a patient with apical hypertrophic cardiomyopathy and neuropathy. Journal of Medical Genetics. 2008;**45**(3):129-133

Chapter 10

Perspective Chapter: Cardiovascular Post-Acute COVID-19 Syndrome – Definition, Clinical Scenarios, Diagnosis, and Management

Claudio Stefano Centorbi, Enrica Garau, Leonardo Borsi, Valerio Brambilla, Lorenzo Brambilla and Davide Lazzeroni

Abstract

Post-acute COVID-19 syndrome (PACS) describes the clinical condition of some SARS-CoV-2-infected patients in which a wide range of signs and symptoms that persist for several months after the acute phase of the disease. Cardiovascular symptoms including chest pain, dyspnea, elevated blood pressure, palpitations, inappropriate tachycardia, fatigue, and exercise intolerance are common in this condition. Some infected patients develop cardiovascular diseases such as myocarditis, pericarditis, new or worsening myocardial ischemia due to obstructive coronary artery disease, microvascular dysfunction, stress cardiomyopathy, thromboembolism, cardiovascular sequelae of pulmonary disease, arrhythmias, while others have cardiovascular symptoms without objective evidence of cardiovascular abnormalities. In the present chapter, definition, spectrum of manifestations, clinical scenarios, diagnosis, management, and therapy of cardiovascular PACS will be discussed.

Keywords: SARS-CoV2, COVID-19, post-acute COVID-19 syndrome, long-COVID-19, cardiovascular disease, myocardial injury, cardiopulmonary exercise testing, postural orthostatic tachycardia syndrome, post-COVID-19 rehabilitation

1. Introduction

1.1 Post-acute COVID-19 syndrome introduction

Severe acute respiratory syndrome coronavirus 2 (SARS-CoV-2), the pathogen responsible for coronavirus disease 2019 (COVID-19), has caused morbidity and mortality at an unprecedented level worldwide [1]. Scientific interest is progressively shifting from the acute phase toward the subacute and long-term consequences of COVID-19, which can affect many organ systems [2]. As replication-competent

SARS-CoV-2 has not been isolated after 3 weeks, literature defined post-acute COVID-19 syndrome (PACS) as "persistent symptoms and/or delayed or long-term complications of SARS-CoV-2 infection beyond 4 weeks from the onset of symptoms" [3], which can be further divided into two categories:

- Subacute or ongoing symptomatic COVID-19, which includes symptoms and abnormalities present from 4 to 12 weeks beyond acute COVID-19;

- Chronic or post-COVID-19 syndrome, which includes symptoms and abnormalities persisting or present beyond 12 weeks of the onset of acute COVID-19 and not attributable to alternative diagnoses [4–6].

  A large constellation of symptoms has been associated with PACS, of which the most common include fatigue (53.1%), dyspnea (43.4%), joint pain (27.3%), and chest pain (21.7%) [3]. Moreover, more than half of patients experiencing three or more symptoms [7]. Long COVID was the first term used to describe the range of signs and symptoms that can appear suddenly and last for months to years after SARS-CoV-2 infection [8]. The patient community as a whole coined this phrase in the spring of 2020 [9], and others such as post-COVID-19 condition, post-acute sequelae of SARS-CoV-2 infection, and post-COVID syndrome soon followed. Patients-researchers with long COVID, later known as the Patient-Led Research Collaborative, wrote the first article on prolonged symptoms of COVID-19, and long COVID continues to be the term of choice for patients [10]. As a result, the diagnostic criteria and outcomes employed vary greatly. The WHO, the UK National Institute for Health and Care Excellence, and the US Centres for Disease Control and Prevention are just a few organizations that have developed their own terminologies and definitions [11, 12]. It is noteworthy that long COVID is still frequently used by researchers as a fairly general word covering persistent signs and symptoms that remain or emerge after acute SARS-CoV-2 infection for any amount of time, while other names have much more specific definitions [13]. This highlights how, although long COVID is not always caused by viral persistence, it is difficult to determine with precision when acute COVID-19 ends [13]. Moreover, data about the length of long-term viral persistence are limited, a further item leading to lack of concordance between researchers. **Table 1** summarized different terms used to describe post-COVID-19 sequelae.

  Since there is a lack of universally accepted diagnostic criteria, the exact epidemiology of PACS is still not known, and the prevalence rates are extremely different between COVID-19 severity, different world area, different pandemic waves or viral variants as well as between different samples. For these reasons, differences in prevalence data of PACS may range from 30 to 90% of patients [3]. **Figure 1** shows different post-COVID-19 nomenclatures and typical post-acute COVID-19 symptoms arranged within the shape of SARS-CoV2.

1.2 Post-acute COVID-19 syndrome and cardiovascular disease introduction

The first case of SARS-CoV-2 was discovered on December 31, 2019, in Wuhan, China. In March 2020, the COVID-19 pandemic's epicenter began to shift to Latin America, Europe, and the United States. Cardiac symptoms, such as chest pain, fatigue, shortness of breath, and palpitations, might last for months in some SARS-CoV-2 patients [14]. Myocardial injury and involvement have been seen in both

Nomenclature	Definition
Long COVID	Can be broadly defined as «signs, symptoms, and sequelae that continue or develop after acute COVID-19 or SARS-CoV-2 infection for any period of time»
Post-acute-COVID-19 syndrome	Persistent symptoms and/or delayed or long-term complications of SARS-CoV-2 infection beyond 4 weeks from the onset of symptoms.
	The term is further divided into two categories: 1. subacute or ongoing symptomatic COVID-19, which includes symptoms and abnormalities present from 4–12 weeks beyond acute COVID-19: 2. chronic or post-COVID-19 syndrome, which includes symptoms and abnormalities persisting or present beyond 12 weeks of the onset of acute COVID-19 and not attributable to alternative diagnoses.
Post-COVID-19 condition	Post-COVID-19 condition occurs in individuals with a history of probable or confirmed SARS-CoV-2 infection, usually 3 months from the onset of COVID-19 with symptoms that last for at least 2 months and cannot be explained by an alternative diagnosis; symptoms might be new onset after initial recovery from an acute COVID-19 episode or persist from the initial illness; symptoms might also fluctuate or relapse over time; a separate definition might be applicable for children
Persistent symptoms or COVID-19 consequences	Persistent signs and symptoms that continue or develop after acute COVID-19 for any period of time
COVID-19 long haulers	Common term used to refer to subjects with post-COVID-19 conditions or long COVID-19.
Ongoing symptomatic COVID-19	Signs and symptoms of COVID-19 from 4 weeks up to 12 weeks
Post-acute sequelae of SARS CoV-2 infection	Persistent or new symptoms after COVID-19 infection; the definition will be revised in an iterative manner based on existing data, medical literature, and feedback from patient representatives, patients, and the scientific community; updated definitions might be used to implement a strategy to modify deeper phenotyping
Post-COVID conditions	An umbrella term for the wide range of physical and mental health consequences experienced by some patients that are present four or more weeks after SARS-CoV-2 infection, including by patients who had initial mild or asymptomatic acute infection.

Table 1.
Post-COVID-19 nomenclature.

symptomatic and asymptomatic individuals [14]. This evidence has been seen in both laboratory and imaging studies, and patients hospitalized for COVID-19 have been shown to have a variety of cardiac testing abnormalities (such as electrocardiographic abnormalities and elevated cardiac biomarkers), as well as a variety of cardiovascular complications (such as myocardial damage, thrombosis, and arrhythmia) [15–18]. The literature is starting to define the specific types of Cardiovascular disease (CVD), such as myocardial injury, arrhythmias, heart failure (HF), vascular dysfunction, and thromboembolic disease, that appear to be a consequence of severe infection. Comorbid CVD has been linked to a more severe course and increased mortality of COVID-19, according to numerous studies [19–22]. A meta-analysis by Figliozzi et al. revealed that having a history of CVD tripled the odds of developing a severe course of COVID-19, which was defined as death, severe COVID-19 infection, hospitalization in an intensive care unit (ICU), use of mechanical ventilation, or disease progression [23]. Congestive HF was discovered as a potential outcome of a COVID-19 as

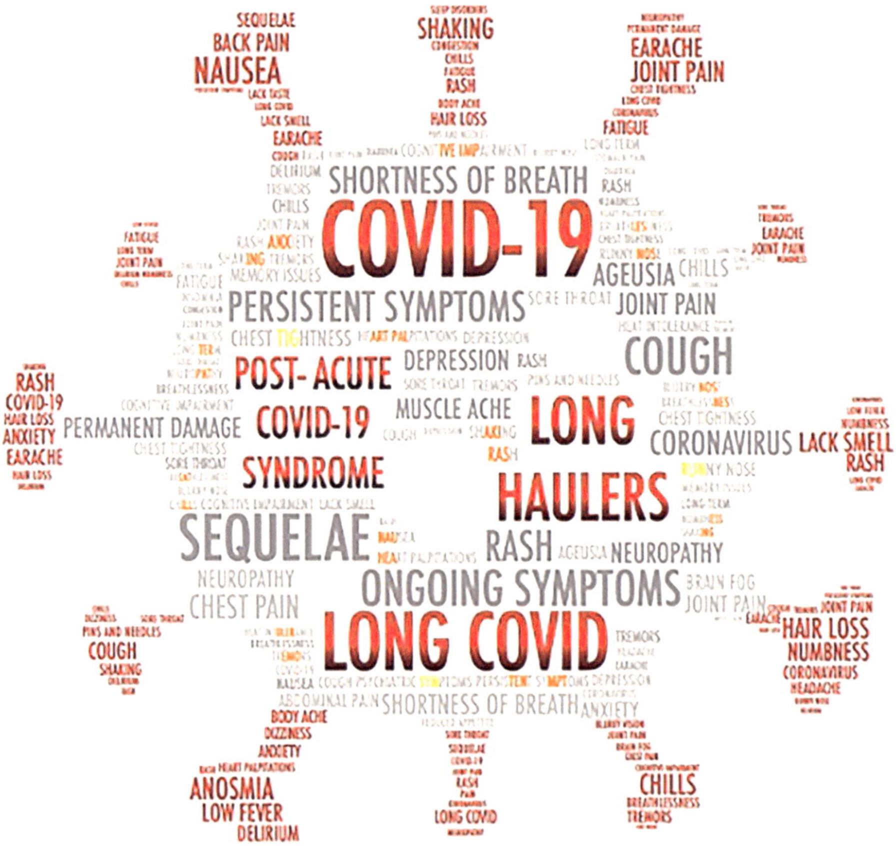

Figure 1.
Different post-COVID-19 nomenclatures and typical post-acute COVID-19 symptoms arranged within the shape of SARS.

well as a risk factor for a more severe course and greater mortality [24]. Moreover, in comparison with CVD, CV risk factors are linked to a higher probability of a more severe course and a higher mortality. Different studies reported how diabetes mellitus, chronic kidney disease, and hypertension are linked to COVID-19 and PACS [25–28]. However, prognostic factors of COVID-19 severity still represent a scientific challenge, since even subjects with the same genotype and infected by the same virus may show marked difference in disease severity [29].

2. Cardiovascular PACS: pathophysiology and spectrum of diseases

PACS describe constellation of new, returning, or persistent symptoms experienced by patients 4 or more weeks after SARS-CoV-2 infection [30]. Patients with this condition can experience potentially wide-ranging symptoms of every organ system with varying impacts on quality of life. COVID-19 caused severe acute respiratory syndrome coronavirus 2 (SARS-CoV-2) but, in addition to systemic and respiratory complications, may manifest acute cardiovascular syndrome and myocardial involvement (**Figure 2**).

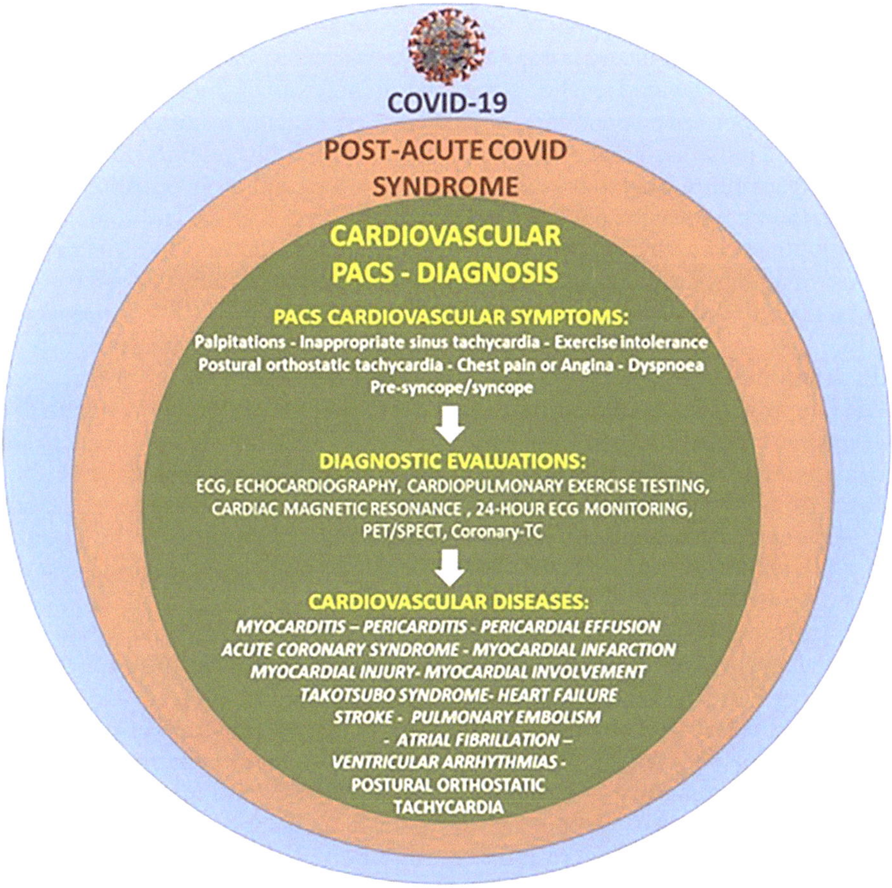

Figure 2.
From COVID-19 to PACS cardiovascular symptoms and cardiovascular disease.

During the acute phase, several mechanisms have been proposed to directly or indirectly justify myocardial injury:

- direct cytotoxic injury [31]
- dysregulation of renin–angiotensin–aldosterone system or autonomic function [32]
- endothelitis and thrombo-inflammation [33]
- dysregulated immune response with cytokine release [34]

SARS-CoV-2 binds on transmembrane angiotensin-converting enzyme 2 (ACE2) to enter in the host cells including type 2 pneumocytes, macrophages, endothelial cells, pericytes, and cardiac myocytes, leading to inflammation and multiorgan failure. The infection of endothelial cells or pericytes could lead to microvascular and macrovascular dysfunction with intravascular thrombosis. The immune over-reactivity contributes to potentially destabilize atherosclerotic plaques and explain the possible development of the acute coronary syndrome. The progression of systemic inflammation and immune cell overactivation, leading to a "cytokine storm" (abnormal elevated level of cytokines) in infection of the respiratory tract and particularly of type 2 pneumocytes, leads to severe acute respiratory syndrome. It has been demonstrated that activated T cells and macrophages may infiltrate infected myocardium, thereby resulting in the development of myocarditis. Similarly, the viral invasion could cause directly myocyte damage and contribute to the development of arrhythmias and left ventricular dysfunction [14]. The pattern of myocardial injury following SARS-CoV-2 infection was initially derived from autopsy. In early autopsy series of 80 consecutive SARS-CoV-2 PCR-positive cases, only four patients (5%) had definition of cardiac injury [35]. In a subsequent autopsy study, a definite diagnosis of myocarditis was demonstrated in 7, 2, to 14% of cases, while interstitial macrophage infiltration was found in 86% of patients, pericarditis and right ventricular injury in 19%, respectively [36, 37]. However, subsequent studies demonstrated that only 1.4% met the well-established histological criteria [38] for myocarditis, suggesting that true myocarditis was relatively rare [39–41]. Lindner et al. [42] demonstrated the presence of SARS-CoV-2 viral particles in the hearts and in particular in interstitial cells including pericytes and macrophages and not within cardiomyocytes.

Cardiac troponin is frequently elevated in COVID-19 patients [43] and indicates myocardial injury. As a consequence of the above-mentioned mechanisms, myocardial injury during COVID-19 includes myocarditis and pericarditis [44], acute coronary syndrome secondary to obstructive coronary artery disease (myocardial infarction type 1) [45] or to oxygen augmented demand (myocardial infarction type 2) [45–49], multisystem inflammatory syndrome in children (MIS-C) and in adults (MIS-A) [50–52], takotsubo/stress cardiomyopathy [53, 54], acute or pulmonale resulting from macro-pulmonary or micro-pulmonary emboli [45, 55], exacerbation of chronic conditions like preexisting heart failure or acute viral infection unmasking subclinical heart disease [56–60]. Since more of these etiologies may coexist, identifying a specific underlying cause during acute phase sometimes may be really challenging.

After the acute phase, PACS may occur in patients who have experienced varying degrees of COVID-19-related disease, from asymptomatic infection to critical illness. Chest pain, dyspnea, and palpitations are some of the key symptoms that draw attention to the cardiovascular system. These symptoms may underlie a COVID-19-related cardiovascular disease that developed or exacerbated during or after infection. For this reason, it is therefore necessary to distinguish cardiovascular complications that can occur during the early post-acute or in chronic phase of COVID-19 (post-acute COVID-19 syndrome with cardiovascular disease, PACS-CVD) from cardiovascular symptoms that extend beyond acute infection, but which are not correlated with a cardiovascular disease (post-acute COVID-19 syndrome with cardiovascular symptoms, PACS-CVS) [61].

Mechanisms for the development of cardiovascular disease after COVID-19 infection are still poorly understood, and several hypotheses have been suggested:

- chronic inflammatory response evoked by persistent viral reservoirs in the heart following the acute infection with consequent tissue damage and chronic myocardial fibrosis that leads to impaired ventricular compliance, perfusion, stiffness, contractility and potential arrhythmias [62].

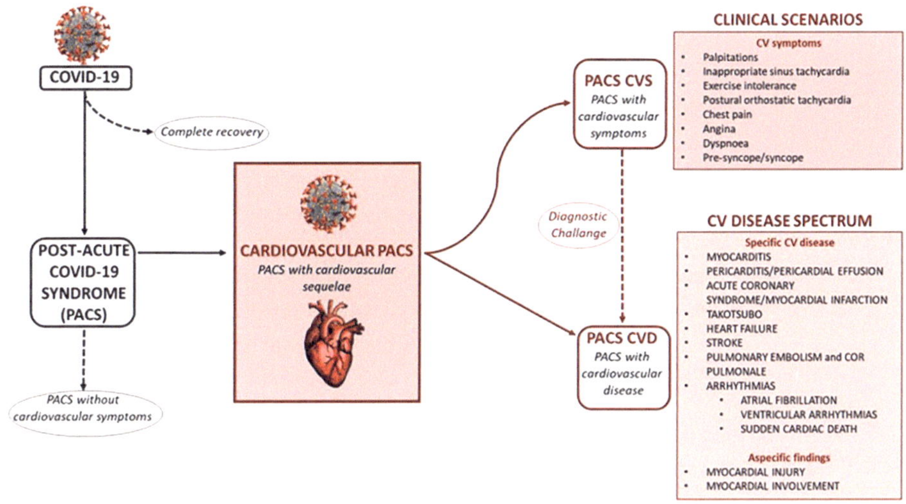

Figure 3.
PACS cardiovascular symptoms and PACS cardiovascular disease.

- autoimmune response to cardiac antigens through molecular mimicry [63]. In fact, Wang et al. identify a wide range of autoantibodies against humoral and tissue antigens in patients with severe COVID-19 [64–66]; in other studies, autoantibodies against cholinergic and adrenergic receptors were found [67, 68]. Moreover, cytokine profile analysis and proteomic studies revealed increased expression of prothrombotic factors beyond acute infection [69, 70], thereby justifying increased rate of thrombo-embolic events and/or pulmonary hypertension.

Figure 3 shows differences between PACS with cardiovascular symptoms and cardiovascular disease as well as different clinical scenarios and disease spectrum of cardiovascular PACS.

2.1 PACS-cardiovascular disease

CVD refers cardiovascular conditions that manifest 4 weeks after SARS-CoV-2 infection and includes all forms of myocardial involvement that can be development during acute phase of infection:

- Myocarditis

- Pericarditis

- New or worsening myocardial ischemia due to obstructive coronary artery disease, augmented demand, or microvascular dysfunction (acute coronary syndrome and myocardial infarction)

- Stress cardiomyopathy (Takotsubo syndrome)

- Thromboembolism and cardiovascular involvement of pulmonary disease (e.g. pulmonary hypertension with right ventricular failure)

- Multisystem inflammatory syndrome in adults (MIS-A) and children (MIS-C).
- Arrhythmias (e.g. atrial fibrillation (AF), premature ventricular beats, and ventricular tachycardias).

Discerning whether PACS-CVD began in acute infection, during illness resolution, or as a new condition post-recovery may be challenging.

- **Myocarditis:** it is defined by the presence of cardiac symptoms such as chest pain, dyspnea, palpitations, and syncope associated with:
    - Laboratory: elevated cardiac troponin;
    - Electrocardiogram (ECG): abnormal electrocardiographic findings (diffuse T-wave inversion and ST segment elevation);
    - Echocardiography: left ventricular wall motion abnormalities in noncoronary distribution;
    - cardiac magnetic resonance (CMR) patterns: non-ischemic late gadolinium enhancement pattern (usually sub-epicardial) with prolonged native T1 and T2 relaxation times;
    - Histopathologic findings on biopsy or postmortem evaluation: inflammatory myocardial infiltrates associated with myocyte degeneration and necrosis;
    - Absence of critical epicardial coronary artery disease (defined using noninvasive coronary imaging and or coronary angiography).

Prevalence and incidence of myocarditis in COVID-19 infection are highly variable [71]. Autopsy results among COVID-19 patients showed mixed data. In a study by Halushka et al, classic myocarditis was identified in 7.2%, non-myocarditis inflammatory infiltrate in 12.6%, single-cell ischemia in 13.7%, and acute myocardial infarction in 4.7% [72]. Regarding echocardiographic data in patients hospitalized for COVID-19 suggest that myocardial dysfunction may be present in up to 40% [73, 74]. On the other hand, cardiac magnetic resonance (CMR), the most sensitive imaging modality for identifying myocardial (and pericardial) involvement, has been used in several studies to evaluate symptomatic and asymptomatic individuals with COVID-19, in both hospital and ambulatory settings. In a study of 100 patients (33% hospitalized), non-ischemic LGE was found in 20% and prolonged native T1 and T2 relaxation times in 73% and 60%, respectively [75]. Similar findings have been observed in other CMR studies, with variable degrees of LGE and mapping abnormalities [76–81]. When performed in athletes as screening protocol, various abnormalities have been noted with 0.6–3% of subjects meeting modified Lake Louise criteria for clinical myocarditis [82–84]. Variability in observed findings with CMR likely reflects differences in the populations studied, in timing of CMR relative to infection onset as well as in the specific imaging protocols that could affect interpretations of imaging data. Several mechanisms have been proposed by which SARS-CoV-2 may contribute to myocarditis such as direct virus invasion, host inflammatory or immune responses, and microvascular angiopathy. Moreover, emerging data seem to indicate other mechanisms such as a maladaptive host immune response with excessive activation of innate immune pathways, a surge of pro-inflammatory cytokines, a deregulated thrombo-inflammation, a thrombotic microangiopathy, an endothelial dysfunction, and a mechanism of molecular mimicry [85–88]. Other hypotheses may include augmented demand ischemia, stress cardiomyopathy, and hypoxia-induced myocardial injury [89]. While the acute inflammation and myocardial injury have been well attended, the long-term effects of myocarditis are completely unknown. Most infected patients experience mild form of myocarditis with self-limiting symptoms and without persistence of LGE; other patients, in the chronic phase, experience various degrees of systolic dysfunction (with symptoms related to heart failure) and/or cardiac arrhythmias (e.g. atrial fibrillation, supraventricular, and/or ventricular tachyarrhythmias) because of extensive myocardial fibrosis [90, 91].

- **Pericarditis:** it represents another cardiac manifestation of COVID-19 and is defined by the presence of two or more of the following features [92]:

    - pericardial chest pain;
    - pericardial friction rub;
    - PR depression and or diffuse concave upward ST elevation on ECG;
    - new or worsening pericardial effusion during infection.

  In some cases, it may be associated with myocardial involvement (myo-pericarditis). The pathogenesis of acute and chronic pericarditis and myo-pericarditis in COVID-19 patients is not still understood. Direct virus-mediated cytotoxicity and dysregulation of the immune system are the key in the pathogenesis of SARS-CoV-2 infection leading to an overproduction of pro-inflammatory cytokines resulting a cytokine storm, an immune-mediated inflammation that affects myocardium and pericardium and an ACE 2 receptor downregulation in acute and long COVID-19 play a fundamental role in pericardial involvement [93, 94]. Data on pericardial disease are relatively scarce. A systematic review including studies on adult patients undergoing any type of cardiac assessment after COVID-19 recovery reported a prevalence of pericardial enhancement in 63/758 patients (8%) and of pericardial effusion in 99/758 patients (13%) [95]. Only few studies reported a formal clinical diagnosis of myo-pericarditis (2%) and pericarditis (0.5%) [96]. Based on studies, pericarditis appears to be common in the acute infection but rare in the post-acute period of COVID-19, while small pericardial effusions may be relatively common in the post-acute phase of COVID-19 [97]. In hospitalized patients with COVID-19, diffuse acute ST changes consistent with pericarditis were present in 12% of subjects [98]. In competitive athletes screened after COVID-19, pericarditis was present in 0.3% of cases [99]. In the post-acute period of COVID-19, a pericardial effusion was identified in a proportion of patients ranging from 5 to 20% [100, 101].

- **Myocardial ischemia:** Virus damage of endothelial cells or pericytes leads to microvascular and macrovascular dysfunction [102], thereby potentially destabilizes atherosclerotic plaques. Moreover, hypercoagulability state linked to inflammation also predisposes to intravascular thrombosis. All these mechanisms may explain acute coronary events that occur during the acute phase of infection such as acute coronary syndrome with myocardial infarction type 1 secondary to atherosclerotic plaque instability or intravascular thrombosis. Arrhythmias or systemic hypoxia also contribute to augmented oxygen demand and may cause myocardial injury with myocardial infarction type 2 (without obstructive coronary disease). During acute phase, myocardial injury, assessed by troponin elevation, complicate a share of hospitalized patients with COVID-19, particularly patients who require intensive care. In post-infection phase, patients could experience signs and symptoms of inducible ischemia due to the instability of an unknown or known critical epicardial coronary artery disease, or due to the presence of coronary microvascular dysfunction in the absence of obstructive coronary artery disease [61]. About 20–30% of patients hospitalized with COVID-19 show elevations in troponin levels, often because of myocardial infarction type 2 that is the most common manifestation of myocardial injury during infection [103, 104]. The real risk of ACS and of myocardial injury in the setting of post-COVID-19 infection is unknown.

- **Stress-induced cardiomyopathy (Takotsubo syndrome):** it represents a clinical syndrome characterized by a transient reversible wall motion abnormality of the left ventricle in the absence of significant obstructive coronary artery disease [105]. Takotsubo syndrome is typically associated with intense emotional or physical stress and is most commonly in women (>90%). The pathophysiology of Takotsubo syndrome is not well understood. It seems that intense sympathetic overstimulation by catecholamines (catecholamine-mediated myocardial stunning) results in myocardial stunning as a direct effect of catecholamines on cardiomyocytes, hyperdynamic contractility, epicardial spasm, and microvascular dysfunction [106]; moreover, autonomic dysfunction may persist long after the acute phase of Takotsubo [107]. Some reports have demonstrated that Takotsubo cardiomyopathy represents a complication of COVID-19 [108, 109]. It is noteworthy that all patients with COVID-19, in addition to typical predisposing/triggering factors for Takotsubo syndrome (e.g. hyperadrenergic tone or microvascular/endothelial dysfunction), experience a strong emotional stress linked to the fear of the potentially lethal consequences of the infection (emotional stress) [110, 111]. Emblematic and curious is the case of a patient with a previous history of anxiety, who, during a hospitalization for COVID-19, develops a Takotsubo syndrome immediately after the communication of the death of her husband, also hospitalized for COVID-19 [112]. Interesting studies have showed that patients with COVID-19 can have high level of cortisol, higher than patients undergoing major surgery [113]. The high levels of cortisol and catecholamines can have a "toxic" effect on cardiomyocytes in COVID-19 patients and could play a role in the development of Takotsubo syndrome [114]. Although tending to have a benign prognosis, during the acute phase Takotsubo syndrome may be complicated with severe ventricular systolic dysfunction, severe mitral insufficiency resulting in signs and symptoms of heart failure/cardiogenic shock, obstruction of the outflow tract of the left ventricle, intracavitary thrombosis, and atrial and ventricular arrhythmias. It is also known that recovery of ventricular function can be variable over time and that, in the long-term, myocardial fibrosis can be observed despite complete recovery of the systolic function of the left ventricle [115]. In post-COVID-19 phase, patients may experience persistence of signs and symptoms of heart failure with or without complete recovery of systolic function and the onset or persistence of arrhythmias often linked to the presence of myocardial fibrosis.

- **Thromboembolism and cardiovascular sequelae of pulmonary disease:** The most severe form of COVID-19-associated with interstitial pneumonia is the acute respiratory distress syndrome (ARDS) [116]. Precapillary pulmonary hypertension is a frequent finding attributed to hypoxic pulmonary vasoconstriction, microvascular thrombosis, and sometimes pulmonary vascular remodeling [117]. The reflex vascular regulation of the pulmonary circulation in the presence of poorly oxygenated areas can significantly reduce the blood flow directed to atelectatic areas to improve the ventilation/perfusion ratio increasing right ventricular afterload [118]. On the other hand, COVID-19 infection exposes to a greater risk of venous thromboembolisms. About 20% of patients with COVID-19 shows coagulation abnormalities, which might cause venous and pulmonary thromboembolism [119], from segmental and subsegmental pulmonary embolisms (often pauci-symptomatic) to bilateral pulmonary embolisms with further deterioration of gas exchanges [120–122], thereby leading to acute right heart failure [123]. Cardiac involvement may involve varying degrees of right ventricular systolic dysfunction up to cardiogenic shock with hemodynamic instability. The real impact of pulmonary embolism during severe manifestations from COVID-19 is likely to be underestimated, since generally only patients in whom there is a clinical suspicion undergoes pulmonary CT angiography. However, a study revealed that 40% of COVID-19 patients with elevated D-dimer and who underwent a thoracic CT angiography had pulmonary embolism, often segmental [124]. A recent metanalysis showed that 20% of patients hospitalized for COVID-19 infection develop pulmonary embolism as a complication during hospitalization. However, it clearly emerged that only a minimal part of the patients had undergone pulmonary CT angiography indicating that the result is probably underestimated [125]. In chronic stages of infection, patients could complain of dyspnea and signs and symptoms of heart failure secondary to chronic pulmonary hypertension with right ventricular dysfunction.

- **MIS-A and MIS-C:** Systemic inflammation is one of the pathophysiological keys of COVID-19 infection. This inflammatory state often persists during the convalescent phase. This post-infection hyperinflammatory phase can lead a multisystem inflammatory syndrome that was seen for the first time in April 2020 [126–128] in pediatric population and was called multisystem inflammatory syndrome (MIS-C). Successively, a similar multisystem hyperinflammatory state was observed in adults and was called multisystem inflammatory syndrome in adults (MIS-A) [129]. The exact pathophysiology of MIS-A and MIS-C remains unclear. Possible pathophysiological the mechanisms for both syndromes include the formation of autoantibodies, antibody recognition of persistent viral antigens on infected cells and, particularly for MIS-C, hyperinflammatory response due to viral super antigens, abnormal immune response to the SARS-COV 2 virus with some similarities to Kawasaki disease, macrophage activation syndrome, or cytokine storm. The diagnostic criteria of both syndromes are similar: a previous SARS COV2 infection and hyperinflammatory state associated with dysfunction of at least two between cardiovascular, pulmonary, gastrointestinal, cutaneous, nervous, hematological, and renal systems [130, 131]. The exact incidence of MIS-A and MIS-C is largely unknown.

- **Arrhythmias:** Arrhythmias are frequently reported in COVID-19 patients. Atrial fibrillation (AF) being the most common form. The pathophysiology of COVID-19-related AF is not well understood. Proposed mechanisms include reduction in angiotensin-converting enzyme 2 (ACE2) receptor availability, cytokine storm, direct viral endothelial damage, electrolytes, and acid base abnormalities in the acute phase of severe illness and increased adrenergic drive [132]. Based on literature data, among COVID-19 patients, AF was detected in 19–21% of all cases [133–135] and in patients with severe pneumonia, ARDS) and sepsis, the incidence of during hospitalization is usually higher [136, 137]. The real incidence of atrial fibrillation in post-COVID-19 period is unknown. Increased post-infectious adrenergic tone, any persistent cardiac involvement during infection (e.g. myocarditis and chronic pulmonary heart) or the presence of predisposing illness (e.g. arterial hypertension, ischemic heart disease, mitral regurgitation, and hypertensive heart) represent the most important predisposing factors. Management of AF should be set up according to current guidelines [138, 139]. Ventricular arrhythmias are less frequent during infection and may be caused by myocardial injury secondary to myocarditis or ischemic myocardial damage, by the presence of electrolyte or acid base imbalances or by the concomitant use of QTc-interfering drugs, especially in intensive care. In post-COVID-19 period, ventricular arrhythmias, at rest or during exercise, should represent "red flags" of cardiac involvement, even in asymptomatic patients.

2.2 PACS cardiovascular symptoms

CVS include a series of heterogeneous cardiovascular symptoms without objective evidence of cardiovascular disease using standard diagnostic tests. Exercise intolerance and tachycardia are the most common reported symptoms together to postural orthostatic tachycardia syndrome (POTS) post-exertional malaise and chronic fatigue syndrome. Chest pain and dyspnea with or without exercise intolerance including memory impairment and attention deficit with poor executive function (frequently described as brain fog) and sleep disturbance are other symptoms reported. There are not established timeline for diagnosing PACS-CVS but it should be considered when cardiovascular symptoms persist beyond a time frame typical for acute infection severity and expected recovery based on age and status of underlying health and without the evidence of cardiovascular impairment because of COVID-19 infection. Ten to 30% of patients seem to experience prolonged symptoms following SARS-CoV-2 infection related to cardiovascular system [140]. In a study one-third of patients with COVID-19 noted at least one symptom and nearly 15% experienced 3 or more symptoms lasting 12 weeks or longer [141]. Different mechanisms have been proposed for PACS-CVS: inflammation [142] immune activation [142, 143] viral persistence [144] triggering of latent viruses [145] endothelial dysfunction [146, 147] impaired exercise metabolism [148] and cardiac deconditioning following viral infection [149, 150].

2.3 Post-COVID-19 Tachycardia, exercise intolerance with post-exertional malaise and chronic fatigue syndrome

Inappropriate sinus tachycardia and exercise intolerance are often associated after COVID-19 infection. It is usually an inappropriate compensatory response that reflects dysautonomia, hyperadrenergic, and inflammatory post-infection state and the presence of metabolism alterations and immune dysfunction [151–153]. Deconditioning represents a final common pathway starting from these two conditions. There are reduced circulating volume and cardiac atrophy with a shift in the LV pressure-volume curve because of hypovolemia and reduced stroke volume with compensatory tachycardia [149–151]. Once symptoms develop, a downward spiral characterized by short periods of bedrest that produce exercise intolerance, post-exertional malaise, and tachycardia leads to further inactivity and worsening of cardiovascular deconditioning with even more debilitating symptoms and chronic fatigue [35]. Patients with COVID-19 reported at home chronic fatigue and dyspnea by 30% and 15%, respectively, at 6 months [152].

Post-COVID-19 Postural Orthostatic Tachycardia Syndrome: Inappropriate tachycardia represents one of the most common cardiovascular sequelae of PACS as well as the most common cause of exercise intolerance in individuals without exertional desaturation. Symptoms often include both cardiac symptoms (palpitations, light-headedness, chest discomfort, dyspnea, or pre-syncope) and non-cardiac symptoms (brain fog, headache, nausea, tremulousness, blurred vision, and exercise intolerance or fatigue) [153]. The presence of inappropriate tachycardia may result in significant limitations on functional capacity as well as in daily living activities such as doing housework or bathing [154]. In the absence of orthostatic hypotension, postural orthostatic tachycardia syndrome (POTS) is defined by an increase in heart rate of >30 beats per minute in those aged >19 years or >40 beats per minute in those aged 120 beats per minute during the 10-minute active stand test. Orthostatic hypotension is defined by a drop in systolic blood pressure of at least 20 mm Hg or diastolic blood pressure of at least 10 mm Hg within 3 min of standing [154]. Figure shows symptoms, diagnostic criteria, mechanisms, and therapy of post-COVID-19 POTS as well as a tachogram and autonomic function data of a case of post COVID-19 male with symptomatic POTS due to hyper-adrenergic response to orthostatic position (**Figure 4**).

Under normal conditions, the assumption of upright posture affects an instantaneous shift of ≈500 mL of blood from the thorax to the lower abdomen and legs, a secondary shift of plasma volume (10–25%) out of the vasculature and into the interstitial tissue, which decreases venous return to the heart (preload), and further affects a decline in cardiac filling and BP [154]. In response of preload reduction, in order to maintain blood pressure homeostasis, the baroreceptors trigger a compensatory decrease in parasympathetic tone as well as an increase in sympathetic activation, that result in an increase in HR and systemic vasoconstriction [154]. The net hemodynamic effect of transition to upright posture is a 10- to 20-bpm increase in HR, a negligible change in systolic BP, and a ≈5-mmHg increase in diastolic BP [149]. Orthostatic dysregulation occurs when this gravitational regulatory mechanism does not respond properly. Patients can present with orthostatic hypotension (seen in autonomic nervous system failure) or with orthostatic tachycardia [154]. Patients with POTS typically maintain (or even increase) their BP on standing. The cardinal hemodynamic feature in POTS is that HR increases excessively and is associated with multiple symptoms on standing that improve with recumbence [154]. Of note,

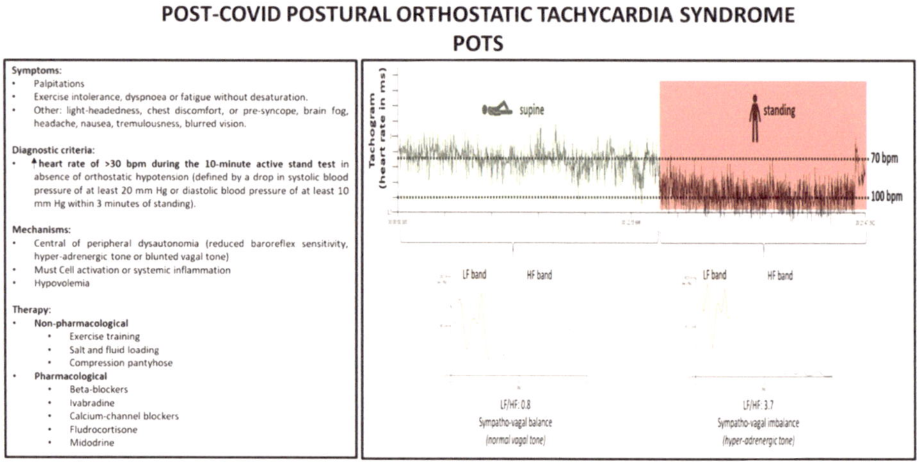

Figure 4.
Evaluation, diagnostic criteria, mechanisms, and therapy of post-COVID POTS.

tachycardia should last for more than 30 to induce symptoms. It is also important that the patient stands quietly for the full 10 min, as an increase in heart rate may take time. Initial evaluation requires supine blood pressure, saturation, and heart rate measurements, followed by periodic re-assessment in standing position as well as during a 6-minute walking test. Exercise testing should also recommend in patients with exercise intolerance, especially in those with chest pain or discomfort; cardio-pulmonary exercise testing (CPET) could be useful in order to evaluate patients with exercise intolerance and dyspnea, since it allows to differentiate between cardiac, pulmonary, or peripheral causes. Ambulatory rhythm monitoring should also be considered to exclude arrhythmia and define the pattern of heart rate elevation [61]. Whereas the latter can likely be done with a 24- to 48-hour Holter monitor, longer-duration monitoring (e.g. extended Holter monitor and event monitor) should be considered in those with episodic palpitations, depending on their reported frequency [61]. Mobile health devices capable of heart rate and ECG monitoring can also help in evaluation and surveillance monitoring during recovery [61]. **Figure 5** shows proposed diagnostic workup for post-COVID-19 POTS.

The benefits of exercise training following bedrest deconditioning and that resulting from POTS [155–158] are well described. To achieve these effects, however, specific types of exercise training are recommended. For patients unable to tolerate upright exercise, recumbent or semi-recumbent exercise (e.g. rowing, swimming, or cycling) is recommended initially, with transition to upright exercise over time as orthostatic intolerance resolves [159, 160]. Exercise duration should be short initially and increased gradually as functional capacity increases, with submaximal level of intensity. In fact, since autonomic dysfunction represents the main cause of POTS, physical exercise represents the most powerful therapy able to positive modulate autonomic function, thereby improving functional capacity, even in the presence of cardiovascular disease [161]. Other non-pharmacological interventions should be also considered such as: salt and fluid loading (5–10 g or 1–2 teaspoons of table salt per day as well as 2–3 liters of water or an electrolyte-balanced fluid per day), support stockings, avoid factors that contribute to dehydration (alcohol and/or caffeine, excessive heat exposure [162]. Although no pharmacological therapies are currently approved

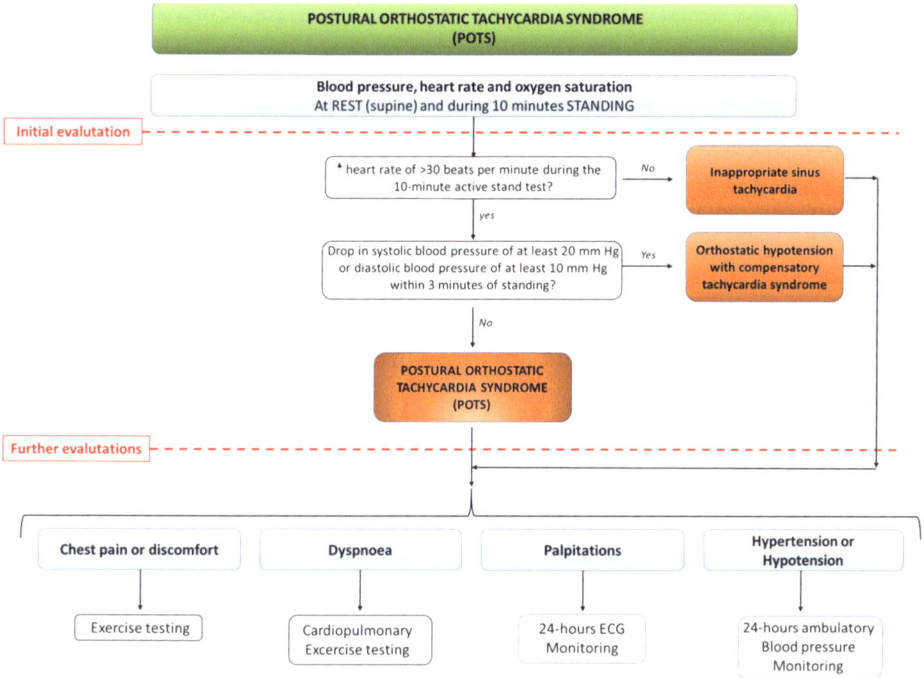

Figure 5.
Diagnostic work-up for post-COVID POTS.

for POTS treatment in PAC, low-dose beta-blocker (e.g. bisoprolol, metoprolol, nebivolol, and propranolol) or a non-dihydropyridine calcium-channel blocker (e.g. diltiazem and verapamil) may be used empirically in order to slow heart rate. On the other hand, nonselective beta-blockers (e.g. propranolol) may help to control symptoms in POTS patients [163, 164], especially in those with coexisting anxiety or migraine. Moreover, ivabradine has also been used in those with severe fatigue exacerbated by beta-blockers and calcium-channel blockers. A trial of 22 patients with POTS an improvement in heart rate and quality of life was observed following treatment with ivabradine for 1 month [165]. Fludrocortisone (up to 0.2 mg taken at night) may also be used in conjunction with salt loading to increase blood volume and help with orthostatic intolerance (AHA). Finally, midodrine (2.5–10 mg) may help with orthostatic intolerance, with the first dose taken in the morning before getting out of bed and the last dose taken no later than 4 pm [162].

2.4 Post-COVID-19 angina or chest pain

Chest pain represents one of the symptoms most frequently encountered in patients with previous Sars-Cov-2 infection. Ischemic chest pain (angina) can be related to coronary involvement by thrombotic or vasospasm mechanism or microvascular disease, instead non-ischemic chest pain can be found in the case of pericarditis or myocarditis. Sometimes, non-cardiac chest pain can be experienced by originating from the lungs or pulmonary circulation, aorta or mediastinum for lymphadenitis. A careful anamnesis on the characteristics of the symptom allows to address the diagnostic workup (see figure work-up). Troponin values together with the ECG and echocardiogram must be used to exclude the hypothesis of ischemic or non-ischemic myocardial injury. Stress test, better if cardiopulmonary exercise testing, allows to highlight inducible ischemia as well as to differentiate between cardiac, peripheral, or ventilatory causes of chest pain. Echocardiography or myocardial scintigraphy (SPECT) with pharmacological or physical stress in association with anatomical study of coronary artery with angio-TC or invasive coronary angiography allow the diagnosis of obstructive or microcirculatory coronary disease in specific cases. Particularly if microvascular dysfunction is suspected, Positron Emission Tomography (PET) for myocardial perfusion assessment may be particularly useful [166, 167]. Finally, invasive coronary vasomotor test helps in coronary vasospasm evaluation, but it must be performed in specialized centers [166, 167]. In the case of non-cardiac chest pain, anatomical study (chest X-ray, chest CT, and possible pulmonary angio-TC) associated with a functional study (arterial O2 saturation, resting spirometry, and cardiopulmonary exercise testing) together with the determination of the D-dimer can help to identify any thrombo-embolic or pulmonary parenchymal disease resulting from COVID-19 infection. Additional targeted diagnostics examination such as chest angio-TC or PET study must be reserved for patients with specific diagnostic suspicions such as aortic or mediastinal disease.

2.5 Post-COVID-19 dyspnea

Since lung disease represents the major manifestation of SARS-COV2, a careful cardio-respiratory physical examination represents the first assessment to investigate causes of post-COVID-19 dyspnea, followed by arterial oxygen saturation (both at rest and during the 6-minute Walking Test). Subsequently, an anatomical study of the respiratory system with chest X-ray associated with a functional study with Spirometry at rest will be necessary. Chest computed tomography or computed tomography pulmonary angiogram should be reserved for patients with highly suspicious and/or suggestive findings of significant pulmonary, parenchymal, and/or vascular involvement (history of moderate or severe COVID-19-related disease, elevated D-dimer levels during the acute phase, risk factors for venous thromboembolism). When pulmonary causes were excluded, the diagnostic process must include the study of the cardiovascular system (see figure work-up). ECG allows to exclude cardiac rhythm abnormalities (e.g., tachyarrhythmias such as atrial fibrillation), new conduction abnormalities that may underlie left or right ventricular dysfunction, or to observe anomalies indicative of myocardial necrosis-ischemia. Echocardiography allows the analysis of the left ventricle and can highlight a systolic dysfunction with global or segmental kinetics anomalies suggestive for myocardial injury, giving the clinical suspicion of myocarditis or ischemic event. Right ventricular dilatation and systolic dysfunction associated with pulmonary hypertension and dilated pulmonary circulation may be suggestive of pulmonary thromboembolism and/or moderate or severe pulmonary parenchymal disease. Pericardial effusion may be a suggestive finding for a pericardial event. Laboratory tests with blood gas analysis may help and must include the determination of the hemoglobin values, of BNP (in the suspicion of heart failure), of the troponin values (to highlight any chronic myocardial damage), of D-dimer (in the suspect of a thrombo-embolic event or of the oxygen saturation and partial pressure values and of the acid-base balance). The most informative test for patients with post-COVID-19 dyspnea is still the cardiopulmonary exercise Testing (CPET) [168]. CPET allows to assess the presence of myocardial ischemia (reduced values of VO2/WR slope, reduced oxygen pulse, and ST abnormalities), of ventilatory dysfunction (high VE/VCO2 slope values, trend anomalies, and PET-O2 and PET-CO2 values), of muscle-metabolic inefficiency (altered anaerobic threshold and reduced oxygen uptake extraction slope values) or aortic stiffness [169]. Moreover, post-COVID-19 unexplained dyspnea without cardiopulmonary abnormalities is common with PACS and may relate to deconditioning with poor cardiovascular fitness. In a study, 59% of patients with COVID-19 had persistent dyspnea at 3 months [170]. On Cardiopulmonary exercise testing (CPET), patients with post-COVID-19 dyspnea had lower peak VO2, lower VO2 at anaerobic threshold, and data suggestive of muscular inefficiency such as lower oxygen uptake extraction slope (**Figure 6**).

Finally, third-level assessments can be reserved for those patients with a picture that is not yet perfectly clear but is suspected of specific pathologies. If inducible ischemia is highlighted, pharmacological or exercise eco stress or myocardial scintigraphy, coronary computed tomographic angiography (CCTA) or invasive coronary angiography can be performed. Instead, if myocarditis is suspected, it will be necessary to perform a contrast-enhanced cardiovascular magnetic resonance imaging to

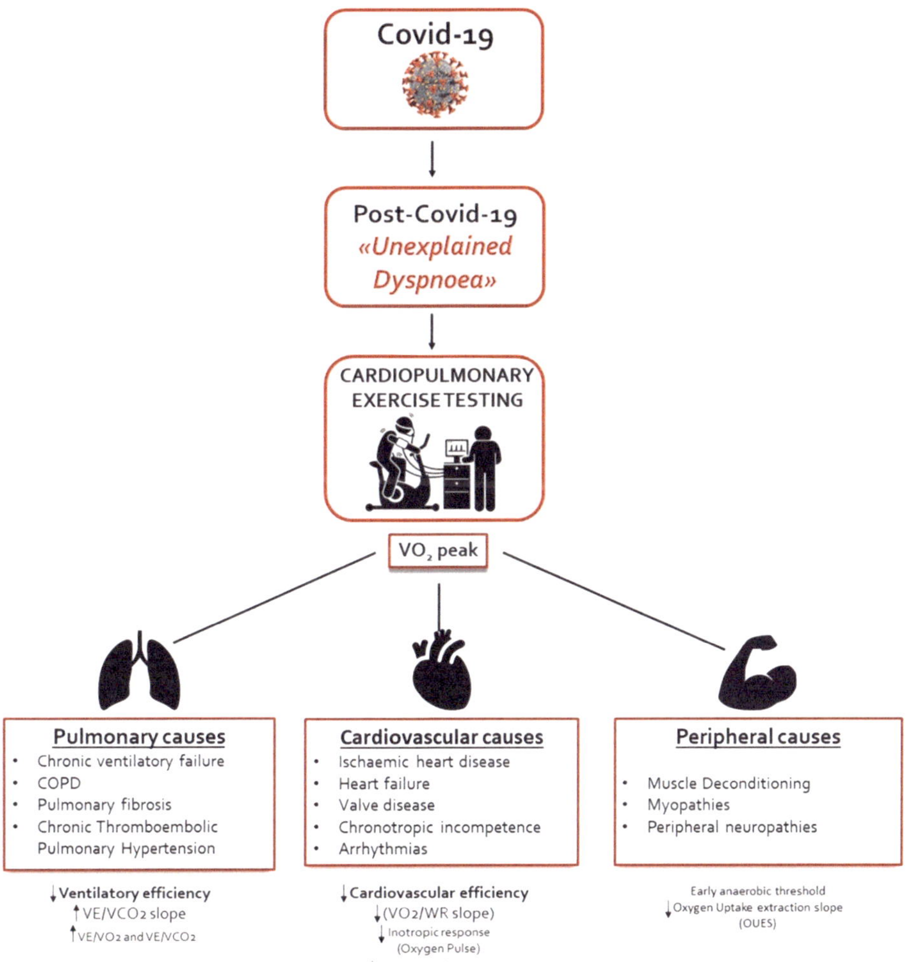

Figure 6.
Cardiopulmonary exercise testing evaluation in post-COVID patients.

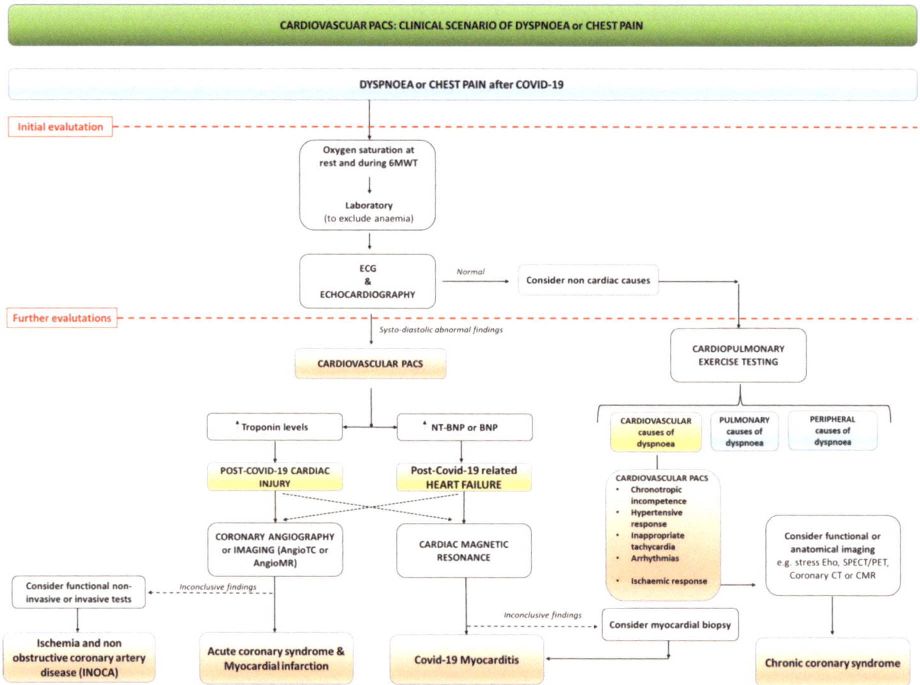

Figure 7.
Diagnostic work-up for post COVID-19 dyspnea and chest pain.

assess the possible presence of myocardial damage with myocardial fibrosis. Cardiac biopsy should be evaluated only in special cases. **Figure** 7 shows proposed diagnostic workup for post-COVID-19 dyspnea and chest pain.

2.6 Post-COVID-19 fatigue

Fatigue is a typical feature of coronavirus disease 2019 (COVID-19) in both the acute and chronic phases. In a meta-analysis, the prevalence of fatigue was 23% in acute COVID-19 infection [171]. Persistence for weeks or months beyond the acute phase of infection is common [172]. Up to 46% of patients report fatigue lasting weeks to months post-COVID-19 infection [173]. The degree of fatigue can be subjective, or it can be objectively quantified as a reduction in muscle strength on physical examination [173]. Fatigue is reported both in its "physical" (loss of energy and feeling of heaviness) and "mental" (a feeling of brain fog). Fatigue is often perceived as more intense and persistent in the presence of reduced physical or cognitive activity [174], and complete anamnestic evaluation is crucial to clarify the nature of the symptoms, mechanisms of onset, and impact in patient's quality of life. Cardio-respiratory physical examination with laboratory tests with the values of hemoglobin, glycemia, C-reactive protein, troponin, D-dimer and BNP, and arterial oxygen saturation are of crucial importance. ECG and echocardiography represent the first-level tests for cardiovascular assessment. Chest X-ray and spirometry, on the other hand, represent the first step in analyzing the respiratory system. Cardiopulmonary exercise test (CPET) allows to quantify exercise limitation through the direct measurement of oxygen consumption values (VO_2), thereby allowing to discriminate between a cardiac or ventilatory or peripheral cause such as dys-autonomic deconditioning or muscle inefficiency. Finally, a correct evaluation of the neuro-phycological and cognitive functions is also important, to exclude possible other causes of fatigue such as anxious, depressive syndrome, or post-traumatic stress disorder. Further examinations will be considered based on the findings observed during the diagnostic process.

3. PACS therapy

Since, nowadays, no specific therapy for cardiovascular diseases associated with COVID-19 or PACS (e.g., myocarditis, acute coronary syndrome, pericarditis, Takotsubo syndrome, atrial or ventricular arrhythmias, and heart failure) are available, the standard of care reported by international cardiac guidelines represents the recommended therapeutic strategy for each specific vascular sequela of the PACS. Although current evidence for of long COVID treatment is lacking, many clinical trials on therapy for CV sequelae treatment of long COVID and are currently underway. Moreover, both SARS-Cov2 acute infection specific therapy and vaccinations are opening up promising scenarios in the prevention and treatment of COVID-19 sequelae. In fact, more than 700 studies related to COVID-19 and more than 100 on long term are ongoing (see International Clinical Trials Registry Platform (ICTRP) (who.int) and see Search of: COVID-19—List Results—ClinicalTrials.gov), thereby suggesting the hope for a "new era" in the treatment of this, in many respects, unknown pathology. Studies include a wide range of therapy such as: rehabilitation programs (for the treatment of fatigue, dyspnea, inappropriate tachycardia, POTS, and cognitive decline), immunomodulatory therapies (e.g. steroids, laranilubmab, tocilizumab, atorvastatin, and colchicine), anti-thrombotic (e.g. aspirin), or anti-coagulation (e.g. apixaban). Although a large amount of evidence confirms a lack of benefit of aspirin in reducing mortality among hospitalized [175] and non-hospitalized outpatients [176], promising results were produced in support of anticoagulation [177]. The multiplatform adaptive randomized controlled clinical trial [178] reported an improved survival in moderately ill patients treated with therapeutic dose of heparin, but not in critical illness. In contrast, other studies [179–181] reported no difference in primary outcome measures among patients receiving therapeutic vs. prophylactic dose anticoagulation. Therefore, further research is therefore needed to better understand the long-term benefits of anticoagulation in patients. Although anti-inflammatory drugs such as dexamethasone [182] and tocilizumab [183] or antivirals such as remdesivir [184] represent the most used and effective therapeutic armamentarium in patients with severe COVID-19, whether they are able to prevent cardiovascular sequelae or to reduce the impact of long-COVID-19 after the acute phase is still unclear. In conclusion, nowadays, the most effective way of preventing serious complications from SARS-CoV-2 infection is represented by SARS-Co2 vaccination [185–191]. Early data [192] have recently suggested the possibility that of long COVID symptoms could be alleviated through vaccination. More specifically, of 900 people with long COVID, only 18.7% of patients reported a deterioration on clinical status, while 56.7% of vaccinated showed an overall improvement in clinical sequelae.

Finally, since the acute phase of COVID-19 is complicated by several multisystem sequelae in a vast majority of subjects, rather than a single drug, subjects with PACS need a multidisciplinary approach aimed at managing each single PACS sequela. This multidisciplinary approach, including clinical, cardiological, pneumological, neurological psychological, and physiotherapeutic evaluation, is generally provided

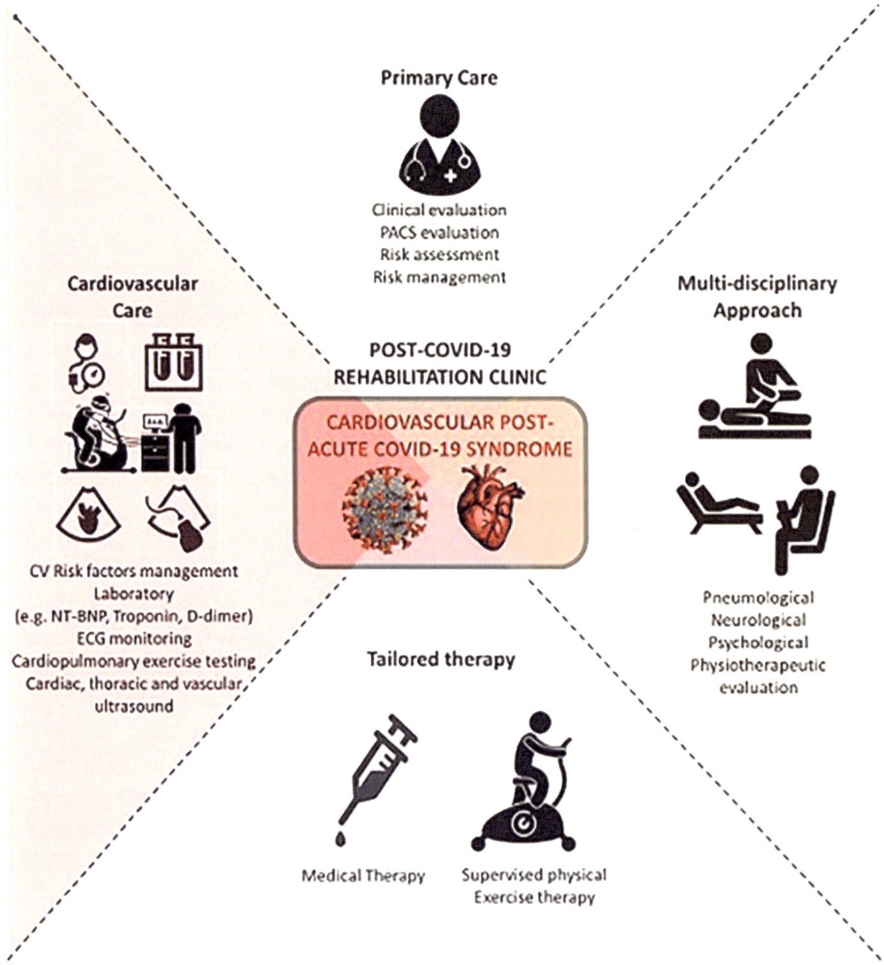

Figure 8.
PACS evaluation and therapy.

by the rehabilitation program of chronic diseases (e.g. cardiac or pulmonary rehabilitation) [193]. For these reasons, on top of the aforementioned therapies, a specific post-COVID-19 rehabilitation approach represents new hope in fighting against the sequelae of PACS (**Figure 8**). In fact, results from early post-COVID-19 rehabilitation registry and trials showed an improvement in dyspnea, anxiety, muscle strength, walking capacity, sit-to-stand performance, and quality of life; on the other hand, results on pulmonary function are still inconsistent [194].

4. Future directions and conclusions

Since many aspects of the PACS remain unclear, further studies will be needed to shed light on the following aspects. First, establish the prevalence SARS-CoV-2-induced CV injury and CV sequelae of PACS. Second, define univocal and universal diagnostic criteria for long-COVID-19, based not only on clinical symptoms but also on specific biomarkers.

Third, identify novel therapeutic solutions or novel use of old drugs to prevent and treat or COVID-19 long-term CV injury. Finally, he long-term prognostic impact of cardiovascular sequelae of SARS-CoV-2 infection in both healthy subjects as well as in patients with preexisting cardiac diseases (e.g. ischemic heart disease, heart failure) is evaluated in order to clarify whether SARS-Cov2 infection or its sequelae beyond the acute phase of COVID-19 may represent a novel risk factor for future cardiovascular disease. In fact, data from the national healthcare databases from the US Department of Veterans Affairs including a large cohort of 153,760 individuals with COVID-19 compared to two sets of control cohorts (5,637,647 contemporary controls and 5,859,411 historical controls) showed that, beyond the first 30 days after infection, individuals with COVID-19 are at increased risk of incident cardiovascular disease spanning several categories, including cerebrovascular disorders, dysrhythmias, ischemic and non-ischemic heart disease, pericarditis, myocarditis, heart failure, and thromboembolic disease [194, 195]. Moreover, these risks and burdens were evident even among individuals who were not hospitalized during the acute phase of the infection and increased in a graded fashion according to the care setting during the acute phase (non-hospitalized, hospitalized, and admitted to intensive care), thereby providing novel evidence of post-COVID-19 cardiovascular prognostic impact. In particular, if these data will be confirmed, the presence of a SARS-Cov2 infection as well as a history of PACS should be considered in the future as a novel parameter in cardiovascular risk estimation beyond traditional cardiovascular risk factors.

Conflict of interest

The authors declare no conflict of interest.

Figures and tables, part of the manuscript, were drawn by the authors and therefore are to be considered an original contribution.

Author details

Claudio Stefano Centorbi[1*], Enrica Garau[1], Leonardo Borsi[2], Valerio Brambilla[2], Lorenzo Brambilla[3] and Davide Lazzeroni[2]

1 Brotzu Hospital, Paediatric Cardiology and Congenital Heart Disease Unit, Cagliari, Italy

2 Fondazione Don Carlo Gnocchi, Parma, Italy

3 IRCCS Fondazione Don Carlo Gnocchi, Milan, Italy

*Address all correspondence to: doc.centorbi@gmail.com

References

[1] Dong E, Du H, Gardner L. An interactive web-based dashboard to track COVID-19 in real time. The Lancet Infectious Diseases. 2020;**20**:533-534

[2] Gupta A et al. Extrapulmonary manifestations of COVID-19. Nature Medicine. 2020;**26**:1017-1032

[3] Van Kampen JJA et al. Duration and key determinants of infectious virus shedding in hospitalized patients with coronavirus disease-2019 (COVID-19). Nature Communications. 2021;**12**:267

[4] Datta SD, Talwar A, Lee JT. A proposed framework and timeline of the spectrum of disease due to SARS-CoV-2 infection:illness beyond acute infection and public health implications. Journal of the American Medical Association. 2020;**324**:2251-2252

[5] Greenhalgh T, Knight M, A'Court C, Buxton M, Husain L. Management of post-acute COVID-19 in primary care. British Medical Journal. 2020;**370**:m3026

[6] Shah W, Hillman T, Playford ED, Hishmeh L. Managing the long term effects of COVID-19: Summary of NICE, SIGN, and RCGP rapid guideline. British Medical Journal. 2021;**372**:n136

[7] Nalbandian A, Sehgal K, Gupta A, et al. Post-acute COVID-19 syndrome. Nature Medicine. 2021;**27**:601-615. DOI: 10.1038/s41591-021-01283-z

[8] Callard F, Perego E. How and why patients made long Covid. Social Science Medicine. 2021;**268**:113426

[9] Munblit D, Nicholson TR, Needham DM, et al. Studying the post-COVID-19 condition: Research challenges, strategies, and importance of Core Outcome Set development. BMC Medicine. 2022;**20**:50

[10] Davis HE, Assaf GS, McCorkell L, et al. Characterizing long COVID in an international cohort: 7 months of symptoms and their impact. EClinicalMedicine. 2021;**38**:101019

[11] UK National Institute for Health and Care Excellence. COVID-19 rapid guideline: Managing the long-term effects of COVID-19. March 1, 2022. https://www.nice.org.uk/guidance/ng188/resources/covid19-rapid-guideline-managing-the-longterm-effects-of-covid19-pdf-51035515742 (Accessed February 14, 2022).

[12] US Centers for Disease Control and Prevention. Evaluating and caring for patients with post-COVID conditions: Interim guidance. June 14, 2021. https://www.cdc.gov/coronavirus/2019-ncov/hcp/clinical-care/post-covid-index.html (Accessed February 14, 2022).

[13] Munblit D, O, Hara ME, Akrami A, Perego E, Olliaro P, Needham DM. Long COVID: Aiming for a consensus. Lancet Respiratin Med;**10**:632-634. DOI: 10.1016/S2213-2600(22)00135-7

[14] The Task Force for the management of COVID-19 of the European Society of Cardiology. European Society of Cardiology guidance for the diagnosis and management of cardiovascular disease during the COVID-19 pandemic: Part 1—epidemiology, pathophysiology, and diagnosis. European Heart Journal. 2022;**43**:1033-1058

[15] Carfì A, Bernabei R, Landi F, et al. Persistent symptoms in patients after acute COVID-19. Journal of the American Medical Association. 2020;**324**:603-605

[16] Logue JK, Franko NM, McCulloch DJ, et al. Sequelae in adults at 6 months after COVID-19 infection. JAMA Network Open. 2021;**4**:e210830

[17] Sandoval Y, Januzzi JL Jr, Jaffe AS. Cardiac troponin for assessment of myocardial injury in COVID-19: JACC review topic of the week. Journal of the American College of Cardiology. 2020;**76**:1244-1258

[18] Giustino G, Croft LB, Stefanini GG, et al. Charac- terization of myocardial injury in patients with COVID- 19. Journal of the American College of Cardiology. 2020;**76**:2043-2055

[19] Puntmann VO, Carerj ML, Wieters I, et al. Outcomes of cardiovascular magnetic resonance imaging in pa- tients recently recovered from coronavirus disease 2019 (COVID-19). JAMA Cardiology. 2020;**5**:1265-1273

[20] Del Sole F, Farcomeni A, Loffredo L, et al. Features of severe COVID-19: A sys- tematic review and meta-analysis. European Journal of Clinical Investigation. 2020;**50**:e13378

[21] Zhou F, Yu T, Du R, et al. Clinical course and risk factors for mortality of adult inpatients with COVID-19 in Wuhan, China: A retrospective cohort study. Lancet. 2020;**395**:1054-1062

[22] Inciardi RM, Adamo M, Lupi L, et al. Characteristics and outcomes of patients hospitalized for COVID-19 and cardiac disease in Northern Italy. European Heart Journal. 2020;**41**:1821-1829

[23] Figliozzi S, Masci PG, Ahmadi N, et al. Predictors of adverse prognosis in COVID-19: A systematic review and meta-analysis. European Journal of Clinical Investigation. 2020;**50**:e13362

[24] Tomasoni D, Inciardi RM, Lombardi CM, et al. Impact of heart failure on the clinical course and outcomes of patients hospitalized for COVID-19. Results of the Cardio-COVID-Italy multicentre study. European Journal of Heart Failure. 2020;**22**:2238-2247

[25] Barron E, Bakhai C, Kar P, et al. Associations of type 1 and type 2 diabetes with COVID-19-related mortality in England: A whole-population study. The Lancet Diabetes and Endocrinology. 2020;**8**:813-822

[26] Ssentongo P, Ssentongo AE, Heilbrunn ES, Ba DM, Chinchilli VM. Association of cardiovascular disease and 10 other pre-existing comorbidities with COVID-19 mortality: A systematic review and meta-analysis. PLoS One. 2020;**15**:e0238215

[27] Grasselli G, Zangrillo A, Zanella A, et al. COVID-19 Lombardy ICU Network. Baseline characteristics and outcomes of 1591 patients infected with SARS- CoV-2 admitted to ICUs of the Lombardy Region, Italy. JAMA. 2020;**323**:1574-1581

[28] Wu C, Chen X, Cai Y, et al. Risk factors associated with acute respiratory distress syndrome and death in patients with coronavirus disease 2019 pneumonia in Wuhan, China. JAMA Internal Medicine. 2020;**180**:934-943

[29] Lazzeroni D, Concari P, Moderato L. Simultaneous COVID-19 in monozygotic twins. Annals of Internal Medicine. 2021;**174**:717-719

[30] Centers for Disease Control and Prevention. PostCOVID conditions. Accessed January 5, 2022. https://www.cdc.gov/coronavirus/2019-ncov/long-term-effects/index.htm

[31] Dong E, Du H, Gardner L. An interactive web-based dashboard to

track COVID-19 in real time. The Lancet Infectious Diseases. 2020;**20**:533-534

[32] Perego E, Callard F, Stras L, Melville-Johannesson B, Pope R, Alwan N. Why we need to keep using the patient made term "Long Covid". 2020. https://blogs.bmj.com/bmj/2020/10/01/why-we-need-to-keep-using-the-patient-made-term-longcovid/

[33] National Institute for Health and Care Excellence. COVID-19 rapid guideline: Managing the long-term effects of COVID-19. NICE guideline [NG188]. 2020. https://www.nice.org.uk/guidance/ng188

[34] Nalbandian A, Sehgal K, Gupta A, Madhavan MV, McGroder C, Stevens JS, et al. Post-acute COVID-19 syndrome. Nature Medicine. 2021;**27**:601-615

[35] Edler C, Schroder AS, Aepfelbacher M, Fitzek A, Heinemann A, Heinrich F, et al. Dying with SARS-CoV-2 infection—an autopsy study of the first consecutive 80 cases in Hamburg, Germany. International Journal of Legal Medicine. 2020;**134**:1275-1284

[36] Basso C, Leone O, Rizzo S, De Gaspari M, van der Wal AC, Aubry MC, et al. Pathological features of COVID-19-associated myocardial injury: A multicentre cardiovascular pathology study. European Heart Journal. 2020;**41**:3827-3835

[37] Halushka MK, Vander Heide RS. Myocarditis is rare in COVID-19 autopsies: Cardiovascular findings across 277 postmortem examinations. Cardiovascular Pathology. 2021;**50**:107300

[38] Aretz HT. Myocarditis: The Dallas criteria. Human Pathology. 1987;**18**:619-624

[39] Fox SE, Vander Heide RS. COVID-19: The heart of the matter—pathological changes and a proposed mechanism. Journal of Cardiovascular Pharmacology and Therapeutics. 2021;**26**:217-224

[40] Hooper JE, Padera RF, Dolhnikoff M, da Silva LFF, Duarte-Neto AN, Kapp ME, et al. A postmortem portrait of the coronavirus disease 2019 (COVID-19) pandemic: A large multi-institutional autopsy survey study. Archives of Pathology & Laboratory Medicine. 2021;**145**:529-535

[41] Kawakami R, Sakamoto A, Kawai K, Gianatti A, Pellegrini D, Nasr A, et al. Pathological evidence for SARS-CoV-2 as a cause of myocarditis: JACC review topic of the week. Journal of the American College of Cardiology. 2021;**77**:314-325

[42] Lindner D, Fitzek A, Bräuninger H, Aleshcheva G, Edler C, Meissner K, et al. Association of cardiac infection with SARS-CoV-2 in confirmed COVID-19 autopsy cases. JAMA Cardiology. 2020;**5**:1281-1285

[43] Giustino G, Croft LB, Stefanini GG, Bragato R, Silbiger JJ, Vicenzi M, et al. Characterization of myocardial injury in patients with COVID-19. Journal of the American College of Cardiology. 2020;**76**:2043-2055

[44] Singer ME, Taub IB, Kaelber DC. Risk of myocarditis from COVID-19 infection in people under age 20: A population-based analysis. medRxiv. Published online July 27, 2021. 10.1101/2021.07.23. 21260998

[45] Thygesen K, Alpert JS, Jaffe AS, et al. Fourth universal definition of myocardial infarction (2018). Journal of the American College of Cardiology. 2018;**72**:2231-2264

[46] Halushka MK, Vander Heide RS. Myocarditis is rare in COVID-19 autopsies: Cardiovascular findings

across 277 postmortem examinations. Cardiovascular Pathology. 2021;**50**:107300

[47] Cornelissen A, Kutyna M, Cheng Q, Sato Y, Kawakami R, Sakamoto A, et al. Effects of simulated COVID-19 cytokine storm on stent thrombogenicity. Cardiovascular Revascular Medicine. Feb 2022;**35**:129-138. DOI: 10.1016/j.carrev.2021.03.023. Epub: 2021 Apr 8. PMID: 33863660; PMCID: PMC8026249

[48] Huang C, Wang Y, Li X, et al. Clinical features of patients infected with 2019 novel coronavirus in Wuhan, China. Lancet. 2020;**395**:497-506

[49] Lala A, Johnson KW, Januzzi JL, et al. Prevalence and impact of myocardial injury in patients hospitalized with COVID-19 infection. Journal of the American College of Cardiology. 2020;**76**:533-546

[50] Wang D, Hu B, Hu C, et al. Clinical characteristics of 138 hospitalized patients with 2019 novel coronavirusinfected pneumonia in Wuhan, China. JAMA. 2020;**323**:1061-1069

[51] Webster G, Patel AB, Carr MR, et al. Cardiovascular magnetic resonance imaging in children after recovery from symptomatic COVID-19 or MIS-C: A prospective study. Journal of Cardiovascular Magnetic Resonance. 2021;**23**:86

[52] Theocharis P, Wong J, Pushparajah K, et al. Multimodality cardiac evaluation in children and young adults with multisystem inflammation associated with COVID-19. European Heart Journal Cardiovascular Imaging. 2021;**22**:896-903

[53] Nune A, Iyengar KP, Goddard C, et al. Multisystem inflammatory syndrome in an adult following the SARS-CoV-2 vaccine (MIS-V). BML Case Reports. 2021;**14**(7):e243888

[54] Meyer P, Degrauwe S, Van Delden C, et al. Typical takotsubo syndrome triggered by SARS-CoV-2 infection. European Heart Journal. 2020;**41**:1860

[55] Nguyen D, Nguyen T, De Bels D, et al. A case of Takotsubo cardiomyopathy with COVID 19. European Heart Journal Cardiovascular Imaging. 2020;**21**:1052

[56] Alvarez-Garcia J, Jaladanki S, Rivas-Lasarte M, et al. New heart failure diagnoses among patients hospitalized for COVID-19. Journal of the American College of Cardiology. 2021;**77**:2260-2262

[57] Goyal P, Reshetnyak E, Khan S, et al. Clinical characteristics and outcomes of adults with a history of heart failure hospitalized for COVID-19. Circulation. 2021;**14**:e008354

[58] Kirkegaard C, Falcó-Roget A, Sánchez-Montalvá A, Valls Á, Clofent D, Campos-Varela I, et al. Incidence and risk factors for early readmission after hospitalization for SARS-CoV-2 infection: Results from a retrospective cohort study. Infection. Apr 2022;**50**(2):371-380. DOI: 10.1007/s15010-021-01662-1. Epub: 2021 Jul 30. PMID: 34331263; PMCID: PMC8323963

[59] Yoo J, Grewal P, Hotelling J, et al. Admission NTproBNP and outcomes in patients without history of heart failure hospitalized with COVID-19. ESC Heart Failure. 2021;**8**:4278-4287

[60] Al-Aly Z, Xie Y, Bowe B. High-dimensional characterization of post-acute sequelae of COVID-19. Nature. 2021;**594**:259-264

[61] Writing Committee, Gluckman TJ, Bhave NM, Allen LA, Chung EH, Spatz ES, et al. 2022 ACC Expert Consensus Decision Pathway on Cardiovascular Sequelae of COVID-19 in

Adults: Myocarditis and Other Myocardial Involvement, Post-Acute Sequelae of SARS-CoV-2 Infection, and Return to Play: A Report of the American College of Cardiology Solution Set Oversight Committee. Journal of American College Cardiology. 2022;**79**:1717-1756. DOI: 10.1016/j.jacc.2022.02.003

[62] Pollack A, Kontorovich AR, Fuster V, Dec GW. Viral myocarditis—diagnosis, treatment options, and current controversies. Nature Reviews. Cardiology. 2015;**12**:670-680

[63] Blagova O, Varionchik N, Zaidenov V, Savina P, Sarkisova N. Anti-heart antibodies levels and their correlation with clinical symptoms and outcomes in patients with confirmed or suspected diagnosis COVID-19. European Journal of Immunology. 2021;**51**:893-902

[64] Wang EY, Mao T, Klein J, Dai Y, Huck JD, Jaycox JR, et al. Diverse functional autoantibodies in patients with COVID-19. Nature. 2021;**595**:283-288

[65] Franke C, Ferse C, Kreye J, Reincke SM, Sanchez-Sendin E, Rocco A, et al. High frequency of cerebrospinal fluid autoantibodies in COVID-19 patients with neurological symptoms. Brain Behavior Immunity. 2021;**93**:415-419. Long COVID/ post-acute sequelae of COVID-19 17 Downloaded from https://academic.oup.com/eurheartj/advance-article/doi/10.1093/eurheartj/ehac031/6529562 by guest on 22 February 2022

[66] Richter AG, Shields AM, Karim A, Birch D, Faustini SE, Steadman L, et al. Establishing the prevalence of common tissue-specific autoantibodies following severe acute respiratory syndrome coronavirus 2 infection. Clinical and Experimental Immunology. 2021;**205**:99-105

[67] Konstantinov K, Von Mikecz A, Buchwald D, Jones J, Gerace L, Tan E. Autoantibodies to nuclear envelope antigens in chronic fatigue syndrome. Journal of Clinical Investigation. 1996;**98**:1888-1896

[68] Loebel M, Grabowski P, Heidecke H, Bauer S, Hanitsch LG, Wittke K, et al. Antibodies to β adrenergic and muscarinic cholinergic receptors in patients with Chronic Fatigue Syndrome. Brain, Behavior, and Immunity. 2016;**52**:32-39

[69] Talla A, Vasaikar SV, Lemos MP, Moodie Z, Pebworth M-PL, Henderson KE, et al. Longitudinal immune dynamics of mild COVID-19 define signatures of recovery and persistence. bioRxiv 2021. DOI: 10.1101/2021.05.26.442666

[70] Von Meijenfeldt FA, Havervall S, Adelmeijer J, Lundström A, Magnusson M, Mackman N, et al. Sustained prothrombotic changes in COVID-19 patients 4 months after hospital discharge. Blood Advances. 2021;**5**:756-759

[71] Mele D, Flamigni F, Rapezzi C, Ferrari R. Myocarditis in COVID-19 patients: Current problems. International Emergency Medicine. 2021;**16**:1123-1129. DOI: 10.1007/s11739-021-02635-w

[72] Halushka MK, Vander Heide RS. Myocarditis is rare in COVID-19 autopsies: Cardiovascular findings across 277 postmortem examinations. Cardiovascular Pathology. 2021;**50**:107300

[73] Szekely Y, Lichter Y, Taieb P, et al. Spectrum of cardiac manifestations in COVID-19: A systematic echocardiographic study. Circulation. 2020;**142**:342-353

[74] Sun W, Zhang Y, Wu C, et al. Incremental prognostic value of

biventricular longitudinal strain and high-sensitivity troponin I in COVID-19 patients. Echocardiography. 2021;**38**:1272-1281

[75] Puntmann VO, Carerj ML, Wieters I, et al. Outcomes of cardiovascular magnetic resonance imaging in patients recently recovered from coronavirus disease 2019 (COVID-19). JAMA Cardiology. 2020;**5**:1265-1273

[76] Esposito A, Palmisano A, Natale L, Ligabue G, Peretto G, Lovato L, et al. Cardiac magnetic resonance characterization of myocarditis-like acute cardiac syndrome in COVID-19. JACC Cardiovascular Imaging. 2020;**13**:2462-2465. DOI: 10.1016/j.jcmg.2020.06.003

[77] Huang L, Zhao P, Tang D, et al. Cardiac involvement in patients recovered from COVID-2019 identified using magnetic resonance imaging. JACC. Cardiovascular Imaging. 2020;**13**:2330-2339

[78] Knight DS, Kotecha T, Razvi Y, et al. COVID-19: Myocardial injury in survivors. Circulation. 2020;**142**:1120-1122

[79] Kotecha T, Knight DS, Razvi Y, et al. Patterns of myocardial injury in recovered troponin-positive COVID-19 patients assessed by cardiovascular magnetic resonance. European Heart Journal. 2021;**42**:1866-1878

[80] Joy G, Artico J, Kurdi H, et al. Prospective casecontrol study of cardiovascular abnormalities 6 months following mild COVID-19 in healthcare workers. JACC. Cardiovascular Imaging. 2021;**14**:2155-2166

[81] Galea N, Marchitelli L, Pambianchi G, et al. T2- mapping increase is the prevalent imaging biomarker of myocardial involvement in active COVID-19: A Cardiovascular Magnetic Resonance study. Journal of Cardiovascular Magnetic Resonance. 2021;**23**:68

[82] Daniels CJ, Rajpal S, Greenshields JT, et al. Prevalence of clinical and subclinical myocarditis in competitive athletes with recent SARS-CoV-2 infection: Results from the Big Ten COVID-19 Cardiac Registry. JAMA Cardiology. 2021;**6**:1078-1087

[83] Martinez MW, Tucker AM, Bloom OJ, et al. Prevalence of inflammatory heart disease among professional athletes with prior COVID-19 infection who received systematic return-to-play cardiac screening. JAMA Cardiology. 2021;**6**:745-752

[84] Moulson N, Petek BJ, Drezner JA, et al. SARS-CoV2 cardiac involvement in young competitive athletes. Circulation. 2021;**144**:256-266

[85] Chau VQ, Giustino G, Mahmood K, et al. Cardiogenic shock and hyperinflammatory syndrome in young males with COVID-19. Circulation. Heart Failure. 2020;**13**:e007485

[86] Skendros P, Mitsios A, Chrysanthopoulou A, et al. Complement and tissue factor-enriched neutrophil extracellular traps are key drivers in COVID-19 immunothrombosis. The Journal of Clinical Investigation. 2020;**130**:6151-6157

[87] Fox SE, Falgout L, Vander Heide RS. COVID-19 myocarditis: Quantitative analysis of the inflammatory infiltrate and a proposed mechanism. Cardiovascular Pathology. 2021;**54**:107361

[88] Bajaj R, Sinclair HC, Patel K, et al. Delayed-onset myocarditis following

COVID-19. The Lancet Respiratory Medicine. 2021;**9**:e32-e34

[89] Hendren NS, Drazner MH, Bozkurt B, et al. Description and proposed management of the acute COVID-19 cardiovascular syndrome. Circulation. 2020;**141**:1903-1914

[90] Ammirati E et al. Prevalence, characteristics, and outcomes of COVID-19-associated acute myocarditis. Circulation. 2022;**145**:1123-1139. DOI: 10.1161/CIRCULATIONAHA.121.056817

[91] Palmisano A, Gambardella M, Angelo T, Vignale D, Ascione R, Gatti M, et al. Advanced cardiac imaging in the spectrum of COVID-19 related cardiovascular involvement. Clinical Imaging. 2022;**90**:78-89. DOI: 10.1016/j.clinimag.2022.07.009

[92] Adler Y, Charron P, Imazio M, et al. 2015 ESC Guidelines for the diagnosis and management of pericardial diseases: The Task Force for the Diagnosis and Management of Pericardial Diseases of the European Society of Cardiology (ESC) Endorsed by: The European Association for Cardio-Thoracic Surgery (EACTS). European Heart Journal. 2015;**36**:2921-2964

[93] Chen G, Wu D, Guo W, et al. Clinical and immunological features of severe and moderate coronavirus disease 2019. The Journal of Clinical Investigation. 2020;**130**:2620-2629

[94] Crook H, Raza S, Nowell J, Young M, Edison P. Long covid-mechanisms, risk factors, and management. BMJ. 2021;**374**:n1648

[95] Ramadan MS, Bertolino L, Zampino R, Durante-Mangoni E, Iossa D, Ursi MP, et al. Cardiac sequelae after coronavirus disease 2019 recovery: A systematic review. Clinical Microbiology Infection. 2021;**27**:1250-1261

[96] Hall J, Myall K, Lam JL, Mason T, Mukherjee B, West A, et al. Identifying patients at risk of post-discharge complications related to COVID-19 infection. Thorax. 2021;**76**:408-411

[97] Carubbi F, Alunno A, Leone S, Di Gregorio N, Mancini B, Viscido A, et al. Pericarditis after SARS-CoV-2 infection: Another pebble in the mosaic of long COVID? Viruses. 2021;**13**:1997. DOI: 10.3390/v13101997

[98] Angeli F, Spanevello A, De Ponti R, Visca D, Marazzato J, Palmiotto G, et al. Electrocardiographic features of patients with COVID-19 pneumonia. European Journal of Medicine. 2020;**78**:101-106

[99] Martinez MW, Tucker AM, Bloom OJ, Green G, DiFiori JP, Solomon G, et al. Prevalence of Inflammatory Heart Disease Among Professional Athletes With Prior COVID-19 infection who received systematic return-to-play cardiac screening. JAMA Cardiology. 2021;**6**:745

[100] Puntmann VO, Carerj ML, Wieters I, Fahim M, Arendt C, Hoffmann J, et al. Outcomes of Cardiovascular Magnetic Resonance Imaging in Patients Recently Recovered From Coronavirus Disease 2019 (COVID-19). JAMA Cardiology. 2020;**5**:1265

[101] Kotecha T, Knight DS, Razvi Y, Kumar K, Vimalesvaran K, Thornton G, et al. Patterns of myocardial injury in recovered troponin-positive COVID-19 patients assessed by cardiovascular magnetic resonance. European Heart Journal. 2021;**42**:1866

[102] Prasad M, Leon M, Lerman LO, Lerman A. Viral endothelial dysfunction: A unifying mechanism for COVID-19.

Mayo Clinic Proceedings. 2021;**96**:3099-3108. DOI: 10.1016/j.mayocp.2021.06.027

[103] Majure DT, Gruberg L, Saba SG, Kvasnovsky C, Hirsch JS, Jauhar R. Usefulness of elevated troponin to predict death in patients with COVID-19 and myocardial injury. The American Journal of Cardiology. 2021;**138**:100-106. DOI: 10.1016/ j.amjcard.2020.09.060

[104] Lippi G, Lavie CJ, Sanchis-Gomar F. Cardiac troponin I in patients with coronavirus disease 2019 (COVID-19): Evidence from a meta-analysis. Progress in Cardiovascular Diseases. 2020;**63**(3):390-391. DOI: 10.1016/j.pcad.2020.03.001

[105] Templin C et al. Clinical features and outcomes of takotsubo (stress) cardiomyopathy. New England Journal of Medicine. 2021;**373**:929-938

[106] Lyon AR, Citro R, Schneider B, Morel O, Ghadri JR, Templin C, et al. Pathophysiology of Takotsubo Syndrome: JACC State-of-the-Art Review. Journal of the American College of Cardiology. 2021;**77**(7):902-921. DOI: 10.1016/j.jacc.2020.10.060. PMID: 33602474

[107] Lazzeroni D, Bini M, Castiglioni P, Moderato L. Autonomic function in Takotsubo syndrome long after the acute phase. International Journal of Cardiology. 2017;**231**:222-224. DOI: 10.1016/j.ijcard.2017.01.002

[108] Nguyen D, Nguyen T, de Bels D, Castro RJ. A case of Takotsubo cardiomyopathy with COVID 19. European Heart Journal of Cardiovascular Imaging. 1 Sep 2020;**21**(9):1052. DOI: 10.1093/ehjci/jeaa152. PMID: 32395765; PMCID: PMC7239208

[109] Sala S, Peretto G, Gramegna M, Palmisano A, Villatore A, Vignale D, et al. Acute myocarditis presenting as a reverse Tako-Tsubo syndrome in a patient with SARS-CoV-2 respiratory infection. European Heart Journal. 2020;**41**:1861-1862. DOI: 10.1093/eurheartj/ehaa286

[110] Lazzeroni D, Bini M, Castiglioni P, Moderato L, Ciracì C, Camaiora U, et al. Anxiety disorders and stressful events in Takotsubo syndrome. Cardiology Journal. 2018;**25**(4):495-500. DOI: 10.5603/CJ.a2017.0136

[111] Moderato L, Lazzeroni D, Oppo A, Dell, Orco F, Moderato P, Presti G. Acute stress response profiles in health workers facing SARS-CoV-2. Frontiers in Psychology. 2021;**12**:660156. DOI: 10.3389/fpsyg.2021.660156

[112] Moderato L, Monello A, Lazzeroni D, Binno S, Giacalone R, Ferraro S, et al. Takotsubo syndrome during SARS-CoV-2 pneumonia: A possible cardiovascular complication. G Ital Cardiology (Rome). 2020;**21**(6):417-420. DOI: 10.1714/3359.33323

[113] Tan T, Khoo B, Mills EG, Phylactou M, Patel B, Eng PC, et al. Association between high serum total cortisol concentrations and mortality from COVID-19. The Lancet Diabetes and Endocrinology. 2020;**8**:659-660

[114] Shah RM, Shah M, Shah S, Li A, Jauhar S. Takotsubo syndrome and COVID-19: Associations and implications. Current Problem Cardiology. 2021;**46**(3):100763. DOI: 10.1016/j.cpcardiol.2020.100763

[115] Citro R, Prota C, Silverio A, Bossone E. Takotsubo: concetti emergenti in tema di diagnosi, prognosi e terapia [Takotsubo syndrome: Emerging concepts about diagnosis, prognosis and therapy]. G Ital Cardiology (Rome). 2019;**20**(9):512-522. DOI: 10.1714/3207.31840

[116] Grasselli G, Zangrillo A, Zanella A, et al. Baseline characteristics and outcomes of 1591 patients infected with SARSCoV-2 admitted to ICUs of the Lombardy Region, Italy. JAMA. 2020;**323**:1574-1581

[117] Ryan D, Frohlich S, McLoughlin P. Pulmonary vascular dysfunction in ARDS. Annals of Intensive Care. 2014;**4**:28

[118] Morrell NW, Nijran KS, Biggs T, Seed WA. Magnitude and time course of acute hypoxic pulmonary vasoconstriction in man. Respiration Physiology. 1995;**100**:271-281

[119] Wichmann D, Sperhake JP, Lütgehetmann M, Steurer S, Edler C, Heinemann A, et al. Autopsy findings and venous thromboembolism in patients with COVID-19: A Prospective Cohort Study. Annals of Internal Medicine. 18 Aug 2020;**173**(4):268-277. DOI: 10.7326/M20-2003. Epub: 2020 May 6. PMID: 32374815; PMCID: PMC7240772

[120] Bompard F, Monnier H, Saab I, Tordjman M, Abdoul H, Fournier L, et al. Pulmonary embolism in patients with Covid-19 pneumonia. The European Respiratory Journal. 30 Jul 2020;**56**(1):2001365. DOI: 10.1183/13993003.01365-2020. PMID: 32398297; PMCID: PMC7236820

[121] Poissy J, Goutay J, Caplan M, Parmentier E, Duburcq T, Lassalle F, et al. Lille ICU haemostasis COVID-19 Group. pulmonary embolism in patients with COVID-19: Awareness of an increased prevalence. Circulation. 14 Jul 2020;**142**(2):184-186. DOI: 10.1161/CIRCULATIONAHA.120.047430. Epub: 2020 Apr 24. PMID: 32330083

[122] Creel-Bulos C, Hockstein M, Amin N, et al. Acute cor pulmonale in critically ill patients with Covid-19. The New England Journal of Medicine. 2020;**382**:e70

[123] Szekely Y, Lichter Y, Taieb P, Banai A, Hochstadt A, Merdler I, et al. Spectrum of cardiac manifestations in COVID-19: A systematic echocardiographic study. Circulation. 28 Jul 2020;**142**(4):342-353. DOI: 10.1161/CIRCULATIONAHA.120.047971. Epub: 2020 May 29. PMID: 32469253; PMCID: PMC7382541

[124] Chen J, Wang X, Zhang S, et al. Findings of acute pulmonary embolism in COVID-19 patients. The SFAR website. https://sfar.org/download/the-lancet-infectious-diseases-findings-of-acute-pulmonary-embolism-in-covid-19-patients.

[125] Zuin M, Bilato C, Quadretti L, Vatrano M, Navaro M, Rigatelli G, et al. Tasso di embolia polmonare acuta nei pazienti ospedalizzati per COVID-19 in Italia. Metanalisi aggregata [Incidence of acute pulmonary embolism in hospitalized COVID-19 Italian patients. A pooled meta-analysis]. G Ital Cardiology (Rome). 2022;**23**(4):233-243. DOI: 10.1714/3766.37530

[126] Riphagen S, Gomez X, Gonzalez-Martinez C, Wilkinson N, Theocharis P. Hyperinflammatory shock in children during COVID-19 pandemic. Lancet. 2020;**395**:1607-1608. DOI: 10.1016/S0140-6736(20)31094-1

[127] Jiang L, Tang K, Levin M, et al. COVID-19 and multisystem inflammatory syndrome in children and adolescents. Lancet Infective Diseases. 2020;**20**:e276-e288. DOI: 10.1016/S1473-3099(20)30651

[128] Gupta S, Malhotra N, Gupta N, Agrawal S, Ish P. The curious case of

coronavirus disease 2019 (COVID-19) in children. The Journal of Pediatrics. 2020;**222**:258-259. DOI: 10.1016/j.jpeds.2020.04.062

[129] Morris SB, Schwartz NG, Patel P, et al. Godfred-Cato S. case series of multisystem inflammatory syndrome in adults associated with SARS-CoV-2 infection - United Kingdom and United States, march-august 2020. MMWR. Morbidity and Mortality Weekly Report. 2020;**69**:1450-1456. DOI: 10.15585/mmwr.mm6940e1

[130] Centers for Disease Control and Prevention (CDC). Multisystem inflammatory syndrome in adults (MIS-A) case definition information for healthcare providers. Available at https://www.cdc.gov/mis/mis-a/hcp.html [Accessed 15th August 2021]

[131] CDC Health Alert Network. Mulitsystem Inflammatory Syndrome in Children (MIS-C) Associated with Coronavirus Disease 2019. 2019 (COVID-19). Available online: https://emergency.cdc.gov/han/2020/han00432.asp [Accessed 23 May 2020]

[132] Kochi AN, Tagliari AP, Forleo GB, Fassini GM, Tondo C. Cardiac and arrhythmic complications in patients with COVID-19. Journal of Cardiovascular Electrophysiology. 2020;**31**(5):1003-1008

[133] Inciardi RM, Adamo M, Lupi L, Cani DS, Di Pasquale M, Tomasoni D, et al. Characteristics and outcomes of patients hospitalized for COVID-19 and cardiac disease in Northern Italy. European Heart Journal. 2020;**41**(19):1821-1829

[134] Gopinathannair R, Merchant FM, Lakkireddy DR, Etheridge SP, Feigofsky S, Han JK, et al. COVID-19 and cardiac arrhythmias: A global perspective on arrhythmia characteristics and management strategies. Journal of Intervention Card Electrophysiology. Nov 2020;**59**(2):329-336. DOI: 10.1007/s10840-020-00789-9. Epub: 2020 Jun 3. PMID: 32494896; PMCID: PMC7268965

[135] Ambrus DB, Benjamin EJ, Bajwa EK, Hibbert KA, Walkey AJ. Risk factors and outcomes associated with new-onset atrial fibrillation during acute respiratory distress syndrome. Journal of Critical Care. 2015;**30**(5):994-997

[136] Klein Klouwenberg PM, Frencken JF, Kuipers S, Ong DS, Peelen LM, van Vught LA, et al. Incidence, predictors, and outcomes of new-onset atrial fibrillation in critically ill patients with sepsis. A Cohort Study. American Journal of Respiratory Critical Care Medicine. 2017;**195**(2):205-211

[137] Walkey AJ, Hammill BG, Curtis LH, Benjamin EJ. Long-term outcomes following development of new-onset atrial fibrillation during sepsis. Chest. 2014;**146**(5):1187-1195

[138] Visseren FLJ, Mach F, Smulders YM, Carballo D, Koskinas KC, Bäck M, et al. 2021 ESC Guidelines on cardiovascular disease prevention in clinical practice. European Heart Journal. 2021;**42**(34):3227-3337. DOI: 10.1093/eurheartj/ehab484

[139] January CT, Wann LS, Calkins H, Chen LY, Cigarroa JE, Cleveland JC, et al. 2019 AHA/ACC/HRS Focused Update of the 2014 AHA/ACC/HRS Guideline for the Management of Patients With Atrial Fibrillation: A Report of the American College of Cardiology/American Heart Association Task Force on Clinical Practice Guidelines and the Heart Rhythm Society in Collaboration With the Society of Thoracic Surgeons. Circulation. 2019;**140**(2):e125-e151. DOI: 10.1161/CIR.0000000000000665

[140] Logue JK, Franko NM, McCulloch DJ, et al. Sequelae in adults at 6 months after COVID-19 infection. JAMA Network Open. 2021;**4**:e210830

[141] Whitaker M, Elliott J, Chadeau-Hyam M, et al. Persistent symptoms following SARS-CoV-2 infection in a random community sample of 508,707 people. medRxiv. 2021;**18**(9):e1003777. DOI: 10.1101/2021.06.28.21259452

[142] Peluso MJ, Lu S, Tang AF, Durstenfeld MS, Ho HE, Goldberg SA, et al. Markers of immune activation and inflammation in individuals with post-acute sequelae of SARS-CoV-2 infection. The Journal of Infectious Diseases. 1 Dec 2021;**224**(11):1839-1848. DOI: 10.1093/infdis/jiab490. PMID: 34677601; PMCID: PMC8643408

[143] Wang EY, Mao T, Klein J, et al. Diverse functional autoantibodies in patients with COVID-19. Nature. 2021;**595**:283-288

[144] Visvabharathy L, Hanson BA, Orban ZS, Lim PH, Palacio NM, Jimenez M, et al. T cell responses to SARS-CoV-2 in people with and without neurologic symptoms of long COVID. medRxiv [Preprint]. 21 Oct 2022:**2021**.08.08.21261763. DOI: 10.1101/2021.08.08.21261763. PMID: 34401886; PMCID: PMC8366804

[145] Gold JE, Okyay RA, Licht WE, et al. Investigation of long COVID prevalence and its relationship to EpsteinBarr virus reactivation. Pathogens. 2021;**10**(6):763

[146] Evans PC, Rainger GE, Mason JC, et al. Endothelial dysfunction in COVID-19: A position paper of the ESC Working Group for Atherosclerosis and Vascular Biology, and the ESC Council of Basic Cardiovascular Science. Cardiovascular Research. 2020;**116**:2177-2184

[147] Charfeddine S, Ibn H, Amor H, Jdidi J, et al. Long COVID 19 syndrome: Is it related to microcirculation and endothelial dysfunction? Insights from TUN-EndCOV Study. Frontier in Cardiovascular Medicine. 2021;**8**:745758

[148] Baratto C, Caravita S, Faini A, et al. Impact of COVID-19 on exercise pathophysiology: A combined cardiopulmonary and echocardiographic exercise study. Journal of Applied Physiology. 2021;**130**:1470-1478

[149] Clavario P, De Marzo V, Lotti R, Barbara C, Porcile A, Russo C, et al. Cardiopulmonary exercise testing in COVID-19 patients at 3 months follow-up. International Journal of Cardiology. 1 Oct 2021;**340**:113-118. DOI: 10.1016/j.ijcard.2021.07.033. Epub: 2021 Jul 24. PMID: 34311011; PMCID: PMC8302817

[150] Rinaldo RF, Mondoni M, Parazzini EM, et al. Deconditioning as main mechanism of impaired exercise response in COVID-19 survivors. The European Respiratory Journal. 2021;**58**(2):2100870

[151] Raj SR, Arnold AC, Barboi A, et al. Long-COVID postural tachycardia syndrome: An American Autonomic Society statement. Clinical Autonomic Research. 2021;**31**:365-368

[152] Benarroch EE. “Dysautonomia”: A plea for precision. Clinical Autonomic Research. 2021;**31**:27-29

[153] Ahmed A, Pothineni N, Charate R, et al. Inappropriate Sinus Tachycardia: Etiology, pathophysiology, and management. Journal of the American College of Cardiology. 2022;**79**(24):2450-2462. DOI: 10.1016/j.jacc.2022.04.019

[154] Raj SR. Postural tachycardia syndrome (POTS). Circulation.

2013;**127**(23):2336-2342. DOI: 10.1161/CIRCULATIONAHA.112.144501

[155] Saltin B, Blomqvist G, Mitchell JH, et al. Response to exercise after bed rest and after training. Circulation. 1968;**38**:VII1-VII78

[156] Hastings JL, Krainski F, Snell PG, et al. Effect of rowing ergometry and oral volume loading on cardiovascular structure and function during bed rest. Journal of Applied Physiology. 2012;**112**:1735-1743

[157] Fu Q, Vangundy TB, Galbreath MM, et al. Cardiac origins of the postural orthostatic tachycardia syndrome. Journal of the American College of Cardiology. 2010;**55**:2858-2868

[158] Shibata S, Fu Q, Bivens TB, et al. Short-term exercise training improves the cardiovascular response to exercise in the postural orthostatic tachycardia syndrome. The Journal of Physiology. 2012;**590**:3495-3505

[159] Lindsay RK, Wilson JJ, Trott M. et al, What are the recommendations for returning athletes who have experienced long term COVID-19 symptoms? Annals of Medicine. 2021;**53**:1935-1944

[160] Fu Q, Levine BD. Exercise and non-pharmacological treatment of POTS. Autonomic Neuroscience. 2018;**215**:20-27

[161] Lazzeroni D, Castiglioni P, Bini M, Faini A, Camaiora U, Ugolotti PT, et al. Improvement in aerobic capacity during cardiac rehabilitation in coronary artery disease patients: Is there a role for autonomic adaptations? European Journal of Preventive Cardiology. 2017 Mar;**24**(4):357-364. DOI: 10.1177/2047487316681341

[162] Bryarly M, Phillips LT, Fu Q, et al. Postural orthostatic tachycardia syndrome: JACC focus seminar. Journal of the American College of Cardiology. 2019;**73**:1207-1228

[163] Arnold AC, Okamoto LE, Diedrich A. et al, Lowdose propranolol and exercise capacity in postural tachycardia syndrome: A randomized study. Neurology. 2013;**80**:1927-1933

[164] Raj SR, Black BK, Biaggioni I, et al. Propranolol decreases tachycardia and improves symptoms in the postural tachycardia syndrome: Less is more. Circulation. 2009;**120**:725-734

[165] Taub PR, Zadourian A, Lo HC, et al. Randomized trial of ivabradine in patients with hyperadrenergic postural orthostatic tachycardia syndrome. Journal of the American College of Cardiology. 2021;**77**:861-871

[166] Espejo C, Mejia-Renteria H, Travieso A, et al. Myocardial ischaemia of non-obstructive origin as a cause of new onset anginal chest pain in the long COVID syndrome. European Heart Journal. 2021;**42**

[167] Gulati M, Levy PD, Mukherjee D, et al. 2021 AHA/ ACC/ASE/CHEST/SAEM/SCCT/SCMR Guideline for the evaluation and diagnosis of chest pain: A report of the American College of Cardiology/American Heart Association Joint Committee on Clinical Practice Guidelines. Journal of the American College of Cardiology. 2021;**78**:e187-e285

[168] Mancini DM, Brunjes DL, Lala A, Trivieri MG, Contreras JP, Natelson BH. Use of cardiopulmonary stress testing for patients with unexplained dyspnea post-coronavirus disease. JACC Heart Failure. 2021;**9**:927-937. DOI: 10.1016/j.jchf.2021.10.002

[169] Lazzeroni D, Moderato L, Breviario F, De Finis A, Catellani G,

Marazzi PL, et al. Relationship between aortic stiffness and cardiorespiratory fitness in primary and secondary cardiovascular prevention patients. European Journal of Preventive Cardiology. 2022;**28**(18):e45-e48. DOI: 10.1093/eurjpc/zwaa090

[170] Aparisi A, Ybarra-Falcon C, Garcia-Gomez M, et al. Exercise ventilatory inefficiency in post-COVID-19 syndrome: Insights from a prospective evaluation. Journal of Clinical Medicine. 2021;**10**(12):2591

[171] Borges do Nascimento IJ, von Groote TC, O'Mathuna DP, et al. Clinical, laboratory and radiological characteristics and outcomes of novel coronavirus (SARS- CoV-2) infection in humans: A systematic review and series of meta-analyses. PLoS One. 2020;**15**:e0239235

[172] Katz BZ, Collin SM, Murphy G, et al. The international Collaborative on Fatigue Following Infection (COFFI). Fatigue. 2018;**6**:106-121

[173] Sandler CX, Wyller VBB, Moss-Morris R, Buchwald D, Crawley E, Hautvast J, et al. Long COVID and post-infective fatigue syndrome: A review. Open Forum Infective Diseases. 2021;**8**:ofab440

[174] Bennett BK, Goldstein D, Chen M, et al. Characterization of fatigue states in medicine and psychiatry by structured interview. Psychosomatic Medicine. 2014;**76**:379-388

[175] RECOVERY Collaborative Group. Aspirin in patients admitted to hospital with COVID-19 (RECOVERY): A randomised, controlled, open-label, platform trial. Lancet. 2022;**399**:143-151

[176] Connors JM, Brooks MM, Sciurba FC, Krishnan JA, Bledsoe JR, Kindzelski A, et al. Effect of antithrombotic therapy on clinical outcomes in outpatients with clinically stable symptomatic COVID-19: The ACTIV-4B randomized clinical trial. JAMA. 2021;**326**:1703-1712

[177] REMAP-CAP Investigators; ACTIV-4a Investigators; ATTACC Investigators, Goligher EC, Bradbury CA, McVerry BJ, et al. Therapeutic anticoagulation with heparin in critically ill patients with Covid-19. The New England Journal of Medicine. 2021;**385**:777-789

[178] Lawler PR, Goligher EC, Berger JS, Neal MD, McVerry BJ, Nicolau JC, et al. Therapeutic anticoagulation with heparin in noncritically Ill patients with Covid-19. The New England Journal of Medicine. 2021;**385**:790-802

[179] Lopes RD, Furtado RH, Macedo AVS, Bronhara B, Damiani LP, Barbosa LM, et al. Therapeutic versus prophylactic anticoagulation for patients admitted to hospital with COVID-19 and elevated D-dimer concentration (ACTION): An open-label, multicentre, randomised, controlled trial. Lancet. 2021;**397**:2253-2263

[180] Sadeghipour P, Talasaz A, Rashidi F, Sharif-Kashani B, Beigmohammadi M, Farrokhpour M, et al. Effect of inter-mediate-dose vs standard-dose prophylactic anticoagulation on thrombotic events, extracorporeal membrane oxygenation treatment, or mortality among patients with COVID-19 admitted to the intensive care unit: The INSPIRATION randomized clinical trial. JAMA. 2021;**325**:1620-1630

[181] Sholzberg M, Tang GH, Rahhal H, AlHamzah M, Kreuziger LB, Ní Áinle F, et al. Heparin for moderately Ill patients with Covid-19. medRxiv [Preprint]. 12 Jul 2021:**2021**.07.08.21259351. DOI: 10.1101/2021.07.08.21259351. Update

in: BMJ. 2021 Oct 14;375:n2400. PMID: 34268513; PMCID: PMC8282099

[182] Collaborative Group RECOVERY, Horby P, Lim WS, Emberson JR, Mafham M, Bell JL, et al. Dexamethasone in hospitalized patients with Covid-19. The New England Journal of Medicine. 2021;**384**:693-704

[183] Stone JH, Frigault MJ, Serling-Boyd NJ, Fernandes AD, Harvey L, Foulkes AS, et al. Efficacy of tocilizumab in patients hospitalized with Covid-19. The New England Journal of Medicine. 2020;**383**:2333-2344

[184] Beigel JH, Tomashek KM, Dodd LE, Mehta AK, Zingman BS, Kalil AC, et al. Remdesivir for the treatment of Covid-19—final report. The New England Journal of Medicine. 2020;**383**:1813-1826

[185] McDonald I, Murray SM, Reynolds CJ, Altmann DM, Boyton RJ. Comparative systematic review and meta-analysis of reactogenicity, immunogenicity and efficacy of vaccines against SARS-CoV-2. NPJ Vaccines. 2021;**6**:74

[186] Polack FP, Thomas SJ, Kitchin N, Absalon J, Gurtman A, Lockhart S, et al. Safety and efficacy of the BNT162b2 mRNA Covid-19 vaccine. The New England Journal of Medicine. 2020;**383**:2603-2615

[187] Haas EJ, Angulo FJ, McLaughlin JM, Anis E, Singer SR, Khan F, et al. Impact an effectiveness of mRNA BNT162b2 vaccine against SARS-CoV-2 infections and COVID-19 cases, hospitalisations, and deaths following a nationwide vaccination campaign in Israel: An observational study using national surveillance data. Lancet. 2021;**397**:1819-1829

[188] Sadoff J, Gray G, Vandebosch A, Cárdenas V, Shukarev G, Grinsztejn B, et al. Safety and efficacy of single-dose Ad26.COV2.S vaccine against Covid-19. The New England Journal of Medicine. 2021;**384**:2187-2201

[189] Logunov DY, Dolzhikova IV, Shcheblyakov DV, Tukhvatulin AI, Zubkova OV, Dzharullaeva AS, et al. Safety and efficacy of an rAd26 and rAd5 vector-based heterologous prime-boost COVID-19 vaccine: An interim analysis of a randomised controlled phase 3 trial in Russia. Lancet. 2021;**397**:671-681

[190] Tanriover MD, Doğanay HL, Akova M, Güner HR, Azap A, Akhan S, et al. Efficacy and safety of an inactivated whole-virion SARS-CoV-2 vaccine (CoronaVac): Interim results of a double-blind, randomised, placebo-controlled, phase 3 trial in Turkey. Lancet. 2021;**398**:213-222

[191] Shinde V, Bhikha S, Hoosain Z, Archary M, Bhorat Q, Fairlie L, et al. Efficacy of NVX-CoV2373 Covid-19 vaccine against the B.1.351 variant. The New England Journal of Medicine. 2021;**384**:1899-1909

[192] Strain WD, Sherwood O, Banerjee A, Vvd T, Hishmeh L, Rossman J. The impact of COVID vaccination on symptoms of long COVID. An international survey of people with lived experience of long COVID. SSRN 2021. doi:10.2139/ssrn. 3868856.

[193] Arienti C, Campagnini S, Brambilla L, Fanciullacci C, Lazzarini SG, Mannini A, et al. The methodology of a "living" COVID-19 registry development in a clinical context. Journal of Clinical Epidemiology. 2022;**142**:209-217. DOI: 10.1016/j.jclinepi.2021.11.022

[194] Fugazzaro S, Contri A, Esseroukh O, Kaleci S, Croci S, Massari M,

et al. Rehabilitation interventions for post-acute COVID-19 syndrome: A systematic review. International Journal of Environmental Research Public Health. 2022;**19**(9):5185. DOI: 10.3390/ijerph19095185

[195] Xie Y, Xu E, Bowe B, et al. Long-term cardiovascular outcomes of COVID-19. Nature Medicine. 2022;**28**:583-590. DOI: 10.1038/s41591-022-01689-3